Aktuelle Probleme
aus dem Gebiet der Cancerologie III

Aktuelle Probleme aus dem Gebiet der Cancerologie III

Drittes Heidelberger Symposion

Herausgegeben von

H. Lettré und G. Wagner

Mit 90 Abbildungen

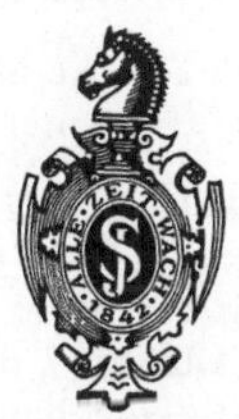

Springer-Verlag Berlin Heidelberg New York 1971

ISBN-13: 978-3-540-05359-0 e-ISBN-13: 978-3-642-65159-5
DOI: 10.1007/978-3-642-65159-5

Satz-, Druck- und Bindearbeiten: Universitätsdruckerei Mainz GmbH

Vorwort

Der hier vorgelegte dritte Band der Publikationsreihe „Aktuelle Probleme aus dem Gebiet der Cancerologie" faßt die Vorträge zusammen, die auf dem aus Anlaß des 80. Geburtstags von Prof. Dr. K. H. BAUER vom Deutschen Krebsforschungszentrum veranstalteten 3. Heidelberger Krebssymposion vom 23.–25. September 1970 gehalten wurden. Bewußt wurde dabei davon Abstand genommen, andererorts bereits erschienene oder in Druck gegebene Vorträge nochmals in extenso wiederzugeben; von diesen Beiträgen wird hier nur jeweils eine kurze Zusammenfassung gebracht.

Neben einigen eingeladenen Gastrednern, die dem Symposion gewisse programmatische Akzente setzten, kommen in den Tagungsbeiträgen vorwiegend die Wissenschaftler des Deutschen Krebsforschungszentrums zu Wort. Somit gibt der Tagungsbericht zugleich einen Einblick in die derzeitigen Arbeitsgebiete und Projekte der 7 Institute des Heidelberger Zentrums.

Wir danken dem Verein zur Förderung der Krebsforschung in Deutschland e. V. für die finanzielle Unterstützung und dem Springer-Verlag für sein Entgegenkommen bei der Drucklegung und die vorzügliche Ausstattung auch dieses Bandes.

Heidelberg, im April 1971 H. LETTRÉ G. WAGNER

Inhaltsverzeichnis

A.

1. Wissenschaftliche Sitzung am Mittwoch, den 23. 9. 1970

(Vorsitz: D. SCHMÄHL)

(Vorsitz: Kl. MUNK)

B.

2. Wissenschaftliche Sitzung am Donnerstag, den 24. 9. 1970

(Vorsitz: E. HECKER)

(Vorsitz: Kl. GOERTTLER)

C.

3. Wissenschaftliche Sitzung am Donnerstag, den 24. 9. 1970

(Vorsitz: H. LETTRÉ)

D.

Round-table-Diskussion über „Konzeptionshemmer und Krebsentstehung"

(Vorsitz: Kl. GOERTTLER)

E.

4. Wissenschaftliche Sitzung am Freitag, den 25. 9. 1970

(Vorsitz: K. E. Scheer)

(Vorsitz: G. Wagner)

Liste der Referenten, Co-Autoren und Sitzungsleiter

BACH, H., Dr. med.
Institut für experimentelle Pathologie
am Deutschen Krebsforschungszentrum
Heidelberg

BARTSCH, H., Dr. rer. nat.
Biochemisches Institut
am Deutschen Krebsforschungszentrum
Heidelberg

BEHEIM, P., Dr. rer. nat.
Institut für experimentelle
Krebsforschung
am Deutschen Krebsforschungszentrum
Heidelberg

DALLENBACH, F., M. D., Priv. Doz. Dr. med.
Institut für experimentelle Pathologie
am Deutschen Krebsforschungszentrum
Heidelberg

DÖNGES, K. H., Dr. rer. nat.
Institut für experimentelle
Krebsforschung
am Deutschen Krebsforschungszentrum
Heidelberg

FISCHER, H., Dr. med.
Institut für Virusforschung
am Deutschen Krebsforschungszentrum
Heidelberg

FUSENIG, N. E., Dr. med.
Biochemisches Institut
am Deutschen Krebsforschungszentrum
Heidelberg

GEORGI, P., Priv. Doz. Dr. med.
Institut für Nuklearmedizin
am Deutschen Krebsforschungszentrum
Heidelberg

GOERTTLER, Kl., Prof. Dr. med.
Institut für experimentelle Pathologie
am Deutschen Krebsforschungszentrum
Heidelberg

GRANZOW, Ch., Dr. med.
Institut für experimentelle
Krebsforschung
am Deutschen Krebsforschungszentrum
Heidelberg

GRUNDMANN, E., Prof. Dr. med.
Institut für experimentelle Toxikologie
der Farbenfabriken Bayer A. G.
Wuppertal-Elberfeld

HAAG, D., Dipl.-Phys.
Institut für vergleichende und
experimentelle Pathologie
am Pathologischen Institut
der Universität
Heidelberg

HAHN, E. C., Ph. D.
Institut für Virusforschung
am Deutschen Krebsforschungszentrum
Heidelberg

HECKER, E., Prof. Dr. rer. nat.
Biochemisches Institut
am Deutschen Krebsforschungszentrum
Heidelberg

HILLEMANNS, H. G., Prof. Dr. med.
Universitäts-Frauenklinik
Freiburg i. Br.

HUNT, W. A., Ph. D.
Wissenschaftliches Zentrum der
IBM Deutschland
Heidelberg

IMMICH, H., Prof. Dr. med.
Institut für Dokumentation,
Information und Statistik
am Deutschen Krebsforschungszentrum
Heidelberg

IVERSEN, O. H., Prof. Dr. med.
Institutt for General og Eksperimentell
Patologi, Rikshospitalet
Oslo, Norwegen

KARATSCHAI, M., Dr. med.
Institut für experimentelle Pathologie
am Deutschen Krebsforschungszentrum
Heidelberg

KINZEL, V., Dr. med.
Institut für experimentelle Pathologie
am Deutschen Krebsforschungszentrum
Heidelberg

KÖHLER, C., Dipl. Volksw.
Institut für Dokumentation,
Information und Statistik
am Deutschen Krebsforschungszentrum
Heidelberg

KRAUTKRÄMER, H., Dr. phil.
Süddeutscher Rundfunk
Sendestelle Heidelberg-Mannheim
Heidelberg

KREIBICH, G., Dr. rer. nat.
Biochemisches Institut
am Deutschen Krebsforschungszentrum
Heidelberg

KRÜGER, F. W., Dr. rer. nat.
Institut für experimentelle Toxikologie
und Chemotherapie
am Deutschen Krebsforschungszentrum
Heidelberg

LETTRÉ, H., Prof. Dr. phil.
Institut für experimentelle
Krebsforschung
am Deutschen Krebsforschungszentrum
Heidelberg

LORENZ, W. J., Priv. Doz. Dr. rer. nat.
Institut für Nuklearmedizin
am Deutschen Krebsforschungszentrum
Heidelberg

LUDWIG, G., Dr. phil.
Institut für Virusforschung am
Deutschen Krebsforschungszentrum
Heidelberg

LUIG, H., Dipl.-Phys.
Institut für Nuklearmedizin
am Deutschen Krebsforschungszentrum
Heidelberg

MEDER, H. G., Dr. rer. nat.
Wissenschaftliches Zentrum
der IBM Deutschland
Heidelberg

MUNK, Kl., Prof. Dr. ed.
Institut für Virusforschung
am Deutschen Krebsforschungszentrum
Heidelberg

NIU, M. C., Prof. Ph. D.
Department of Biology
Temple University
Philadelphia, U. S. A.

OPFERKUCH, J., Dipl.-Chem.
Biochemisches Institut
am Deutschen Krebsforschungszentrum
Heidelberg

OSSWALD, H., Prof. Dr. med.
Institut für experimentelle Toxikologie
und Chemotherapie
am Deutschen Krebsforschungszentrum
Heidelberg

PAWELETZ, N., Priv. Doz. Dr. rer. nat.
Institut für experimentelle
Krebsforschung
am Deutschen Krebsforschungszentrum
Heidelberg

PISTOR, P., Dipl.-Phys.
Wissenschaftliches Zentrum
der IBM Deutschland
Heidelberg

PONTÉN, J., Prof., Ph. D.
The Wallenberg Laboratory
University of Uppsala
Uppsala, Schweden

RYTÖMAA, T., Dr. med.
II. Department of Pathology,
University of Helsinki
Helsinki, Finnland

SANDOR, L., Dr. med.
Institut für Dokumentation,
Information und Statistik
am Deutschen Krebsforschungszentrum
Heidelberg

SAUER, G., Priv. Doz. Dr. phil.
Institut für Virusforschung
am Deutschen Krebsforschungszentrum
Heidelberg

SCHEER, K. E., Prof. Dr. med.
Institut für Nuklearmedizin
am Deutschen Krebsforschungszentrum
Heidelberg

SCHENK, P., Priv. Doz. Dr. med.
Universitäts-Strahlenklinik
(Czerny-Krankenhaus)
Heidelberg

SCHERF, H. R., Dr. rer. nat.
Institut für experimentelle Toxikologie
und Chemotherapie
am Deutschen Krebsforschungszentrum
Heidelberg

SCHMÄHL, D., Prof. Dr. med.
Institut für experimentelle Toxikologie
und Chemotherapie
am Deutschen Krebsforschungszentrum
Heidelberg

SCHMIDLIN, P., Dr. rer. nat.
Institut für Nuklearmedizin
am Deutschen Krebsforschungszentrum
Heidelberg

SCHMIDT, R., Apotheker
Biochemisches Institut
am Deutschen Krebsforschungszentrum
Heidelberg

SINN, H., Dr. rer. nat.
Institut für Nuklearmedizin
am Deutschen Krebsforschungszentrum
Heidelberg

STAEMMLER, H. J., Prof. Dr. med.
Frauenklinik der
Städtischen Krankenanstalten
Ludwigshafen

SÜSS, R., Dr. rer. nat.
Institut für experimentelle Pathologie
am Deutschen Krebsforschungszentrum
Heidelberg

TASCA, C., Dr. med.
Institut für experimentelle Pathologie
am Deutschen Krebsforschungszentrum
Heidelberg

TAUXE, W. N., M. D.
Section of Clinical Pathology,
Mayo Clinic and Mayo Foundation
Rochester/Minn., U. S. A.

TRAUT, M., Dr. rer. nat.
Biochemisches Institut
am Deutschen Krebsforschungszentrum
Heidelberg

VOLM, M., Dr. rer. nat.
Institut für experimentelle Pathologie
am Deutschen Krebsforschungszentrum
Heidelberg

WAGNER, G., Prof. Dr. med.
Institut für Dokumentation,
Information und Statistik
am Deutschen Krebsforschungszentrum
Heidelberg

WALCH, G., Dr. rer. nat.
Wissenschaftliches Zentrum der
IBM Deutschland
Heidelberg

WANZEK, L., Dr. med.
Frauenarzt
Schwetzingen

WAYSS, K., Dr. rer. nat.
Institut für experimentelle Pathologie
am Deutschen Krebsforschungszentrum
Heidelberg

WEISBURGER, J. H., M. D.
National Cancer Institute,
National Institutes of Health
Bethesda/Md., U. S. A.

WERNER, D., Priv. Doz. Dr. rer. nat.
Institut für experimentelle
Krebsforschung
am Deutschen Krebsforschungszentrum
Heidelberg

Wesch, H., Dipl.-Phys.
Institut für Nuklearmedizin
am Deutschen Krebsforschungszentrum
Heidelberg

Westermark, B., Ph. D.
The Wallenberg Laboratory
University of Uppsala
Uppsala, Schweden

Wiessler, M., Dr. rer. nat.
Institut für experimentelle Toxikologie
und Chemotherapie
am Deutschen Krebsforschungszentrum
Heidelberg

Wolff-Terroine, M., Ph. D.
Service de Documentation Scientifique
de l'Institut Gustave-Roussy
Villejuif, Frankreich

Zimmerer, J., Dr. rer. nat.
Institut für Nuklearmedizin
am Deutschen Krebsforschungszentrum
Heidelberg

A.

1. Wissenschaftliche Sitzung am Mittwoch, den 23. 9. 1970

Vorsitz: D. Schmähl und Kl. Munk

Chemical Carcinogens, Cancer Research, and the Prevention of Cancer

By

J. H. Weisburger and Elizabeth K. Weisburger

It is an honor indeed to represent the National Cancer Institute of the U. S. Public Health Service in this significant symposium organized by the German Cancer Research Center on the occasion of the 80th birthday of Prof. Dr. K. H. Bauer.

As a young medical student Prof. Bauer lived at the time when the problem of experimental induction of cancer was born. Fischer noted reversible hyperplasia in animals treated with scarlet red [*25*]. Shortly thereafter Yamagiwa and Ichikawa succeeded in inducing cancer in rabbits and published their findings in German [*94*]. These were no doubt most exciting findings at that time. In many ways, one envies Prof. Bauer for having seen and lived with these pioneers. However, Prof. Bauer has himself become heavily involved as a pioneer in his own right. His interests extend along a broad front of cancer studies, from surgery to experimental chemotherapy and cancer causation. As an author, Prof. Bauer has contributed importantly to the original literature. Yet he is also well known as a seasoned interpreter of the existing facts in his monumental work „Das Krebsproblem" [*4*].

My purpose today is to review briefly the present status of some select aspects of research in the area of chemical carcinogenesis and causation of cancer.

Some Evidence that Environmental Factors Play a Role in the Genesis of Human Cancers

There is now existing in world literature a wealth of information on cancer incidence in various populations in the world, collected under the aegis of UICC and WHO in *Europe*, our own National Cancer Institute and the Sloan-Kettering Institute in the *United States*, Prof. Segi *et al.* at Tohoku University in *Japan*, and under the impetus of Prof. J. Higginson at the International Agency for Research on Cancer (Lyon) in *Africa*. Some of the underlying statistics are highly reliable; other reports are

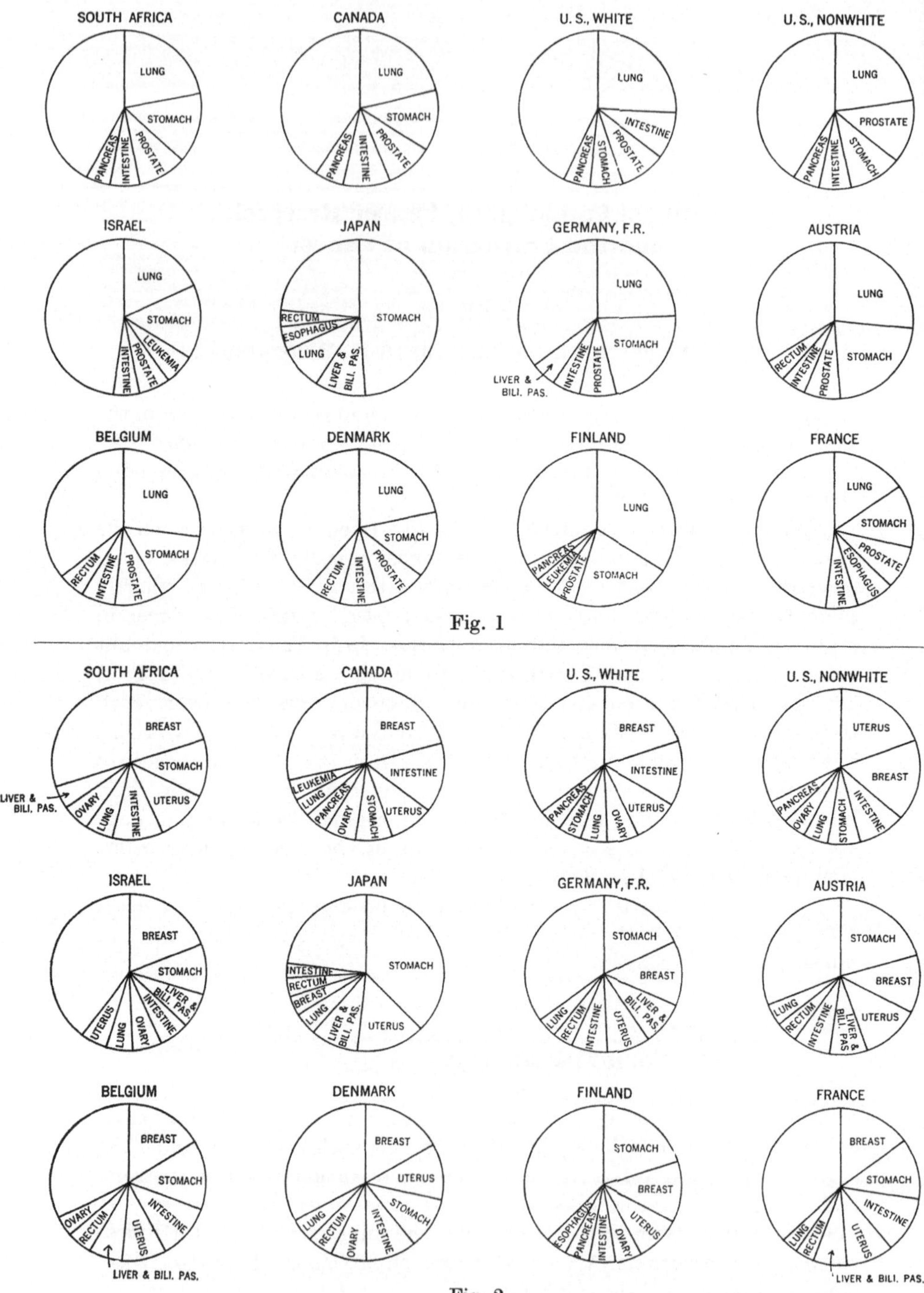

Fig. 1

Fig. 2

Figs. 1 and 2. Ratio of deaths from different neoplasms among males (Fig. 1) and females (Fig. 2) countries, 1964/65 (from [72])

based on developing efforts in this area and require further refinement. However, from the combined demographic effort, it is quite apparent and obvious that cancer incidence in various parts of the world is different. For example, in the Federal Republic of Germany cancer in the stomach and in the liver in men and in women is sufficiently high to warrant a special graph in the report of SEGI *et al.* [*72*] (Figs. 1 and 2). On the other hand, in the United States primary liver cancer is much less of a problem, and is not even included in the graph. Cancer of the stomach is likewise appreciably lower and has been decreasing over the last 30 years. In contrast, in Japan gastric cancer in males accounts for almost half of all cases of cancer seen, whereas cancer of the colon, rectum, prostate or breast is relatively unimportant. It is well known that in the United States and other western countries the reverse is true. Such differences are also apparent at other target organs such as for example shown in detail in Figs. 3–5, taken from the most recent publication of SEGI *et al.* Even within the overall statistical evaluation there are pronounced regional differences. For example, South Africa assumes an intermediate rate with respect to liver cancer (Fig. 5). However, among certain of the Bantu tribes in that country hepatocellular carcinoma is not only the most prevalent type but is often fatal to the males at most remarkably young age, with an average between 25 and 30 years. Within the city of Hamburg MAASS *et al.* [*50*] recently reported a highly localized distribution of certain types of cancer. At the second Heidelberger Symposion MACDONALD and WOLF [*51*] dealt with differences in cancer incidence in 3 regions in Texas. There are no doubt other highly localized factors which contribute to the occurrence of certain types of neoplasms.

In part, such findings could be interpreted in terms of genetics. By this one means that the overall responsiveness of the total living system to a given carcinogenic challenge would depend in part on heritable characteristics. There are numerous instances in animal tests where qualitative and quantitative incidence and also the target organs were a function of genetic factors. Also in man, for example, the incidence of prostatic cancer appeared to be more common in individuals with blood group A [*5*].

However, genetically motivated responses do not seem to exert the most striking, overriding control over the eventual development of cancer. Thus, studies on migrants or various ethnic groups, pioneered in the United States by HAENSZEL, WYNDER *et al.* [*34, 76, 92, 93*] have demonstrated that Japanese migrants, first to Hawaii and then the U. S. mainland, acquire in successive generations the cancer incidence typical of the host country, and do not retain that of the parent region of origin. Similar findings were made with select migrants from Europe, in particular Poland and Scandinavia. Even in cases of internal migration within

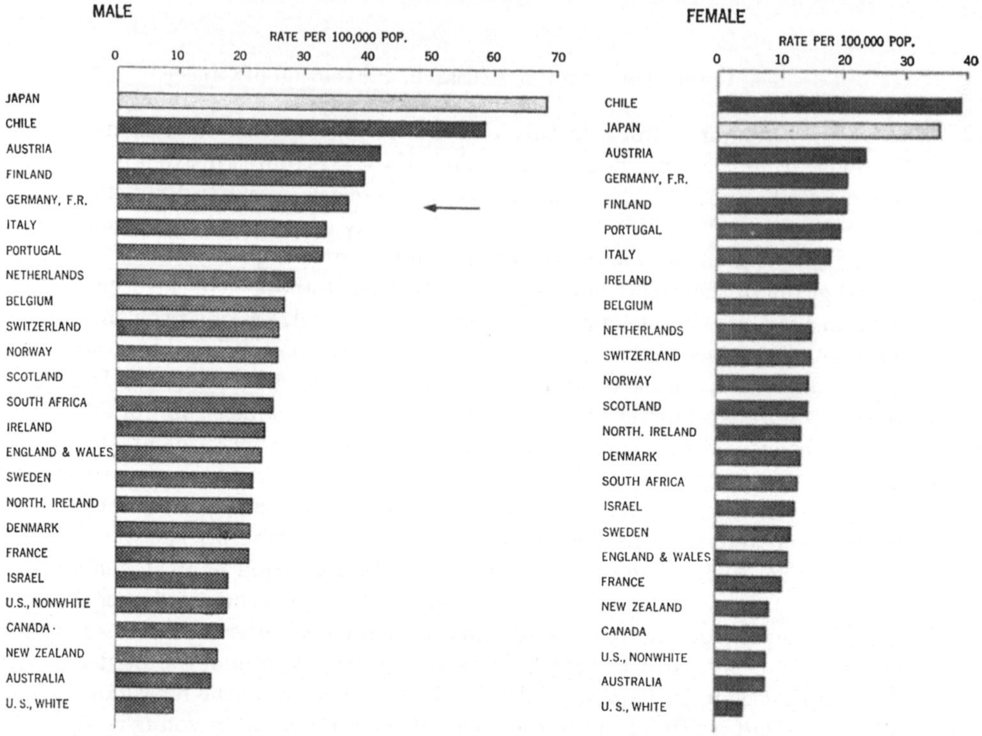

MALE

RATE PER 100,000 POP.

0 10 20 30 40 50 60 70

JAPAN
CHILE
AUSTRIA
FINLAND
GERMANY, F.R.
ITALY
PORTUGAL
NETHERLANDS
BELGIUM
SWITZERLAND
NORWAY
SCOTLAND
SOUTH AFRICA
IRELAND
ENGLAND & WALES
SWEDEN
NORTH. IRELAND
DENMARK
FRANCE
ISRAEL
U.S., NONWHITE
CANADA
NEW ZEALAND
AUSTRALIA
U. S., WHITE

FEMALE

RATE PER 100,000 POP.

0 10 20 30 40

CHILE
JAPAN
AUSTRIA
GERMANY, F.R.
FINLAND
PORTUGAL
ITALY
IRELAND
BELGIUM
NETHERLANDS
SWITZERLAND
NORWAY
SCOTLAND
NORTH. IRELAND
DENMARK
SOUTH AFRICA
ISRAEL
SWEDEN
ENGLAND & WALES
FRANCE
NEW ZEALAND
CANADA
U.S., NONWHITE
AUSTRALIA
U. S., WHITE

Fig. 3. Age-adjusted death rates for malignant neoplasms of the stomach, 1964/65 (from [*72*])

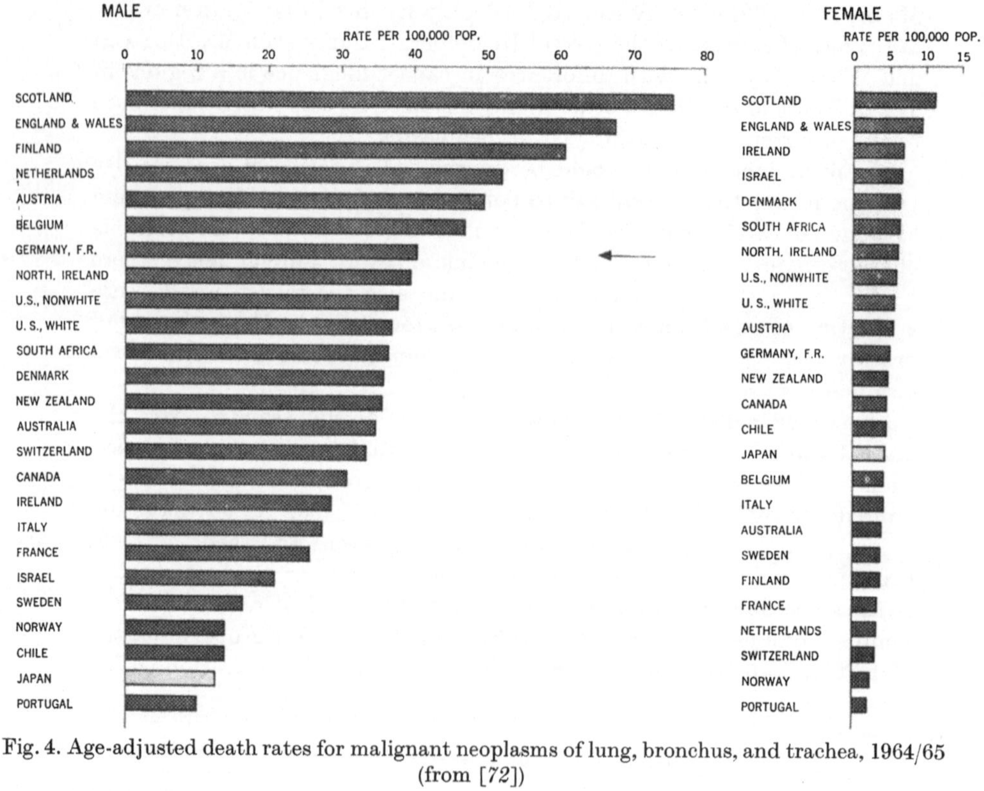

MALE

RATE PER 100,000 POP.

0 10 20 30 40 50 60 70 80

SCOTLAND
ENGLAND & WALES
FINLAND
NETHERLANDS
AUSTRIA
BELGIUM
GERMANY, F.R.
NORTH. IRELAND
U.S., NONWHITE
U. S., WHITE
SOUTH AFRICA
DENMARK
NEW ZEALAND
AUSTRALIA
SWITZERLAND
CANADA
IRELAND
ITALY
FRANCE
ISRAEL
SWEDEN
NORWAY
CHILE
JAPAN
PORTUGAL

FEMALE

RATE PER 100,000 POP.

0 5 10 15

SCOTLAND
ENGLAND & WALES
IRELAND
ISRAEL
DENMARK
SOUTH AFRICA
NORTH. IRELAND
U.S., NONWHITE
U. S., WHITE
AUSTRIA
GERMANY, F.R.
NEW ZEALAND
CANADA
CHILE
JAPAN
BELGIUM
ITALY
AUSTRALIA
SWEDEN
FINLAND
FRANCE
NETHERLANDS
SWITZERLAND
NORWAY
PORTUGAL

Fig. 4. Age-adjusted death rates for malignant neoplasms of lung, bronchus, and trachea, 1964/65 (from [*72*])

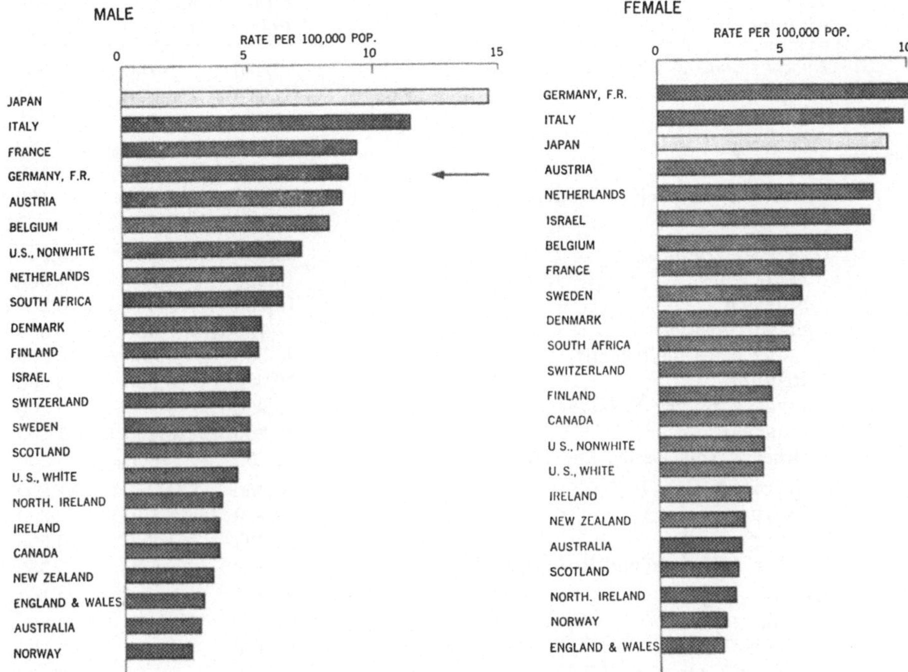

Fig. 5. Age-adjusted death rates for malignant neoplasms of liver and biliary passages, 1964/65 (from [*72*])

a country CORREA *et al.* [*12*] observed development of gastric cancer in the population of Cali, Columbia typical of certain regional incidence patterns. Depending on the age at migration, the influence of the total environment in the parent country made itself felt, suggesting that carcinogenic influences are impressed early in life.

Thus, it can be concluded from these demographic considerations that for many types of cancer in man the problem of detecting and analysing exogenous factors as causative elements will remain an important endeavor for the practical goal of eventual prevention. That success can be achieved by this means is not unrealistic, considering the case histories with some occupational cancers. BOYLAND [*7*] and BURDETTE [*10*] at a recent symposium in Boston also viewed cancer in man chiefly as the end result of environmental chemical challenges.

In the United States a recent estimate by the Statistical Research Section of the American Cancer Society shows that fatalities due to cancer amounted to almost 17% of deaths due to all causes in the United States. In 1970 approximately 330,000 individuals, 180,000 males and 150,000 females, will die of cancer (Table). The death rate is about 60%

Table. *Estimated Cancer Deaths by Sex and Site in the United States of America in 1970*)*

SITE All Sites	Total 330,000	Males 180,000	Females 150,000
Buccal Cavity & Pharynx	6,950	5,100	1,850
Lip	125	100	25
Tongue	1,625	1,200	425
Salivary Glands	650	400	250
Floor of Mouth	500	400	100
Other & Unspecified Mouth	1,100	700	400
Pharynx	2,950	2,300	650
Digestive Organs	98,000	52,500	45,500
Esophagus	6,100	4,600	1,500
Stomach	15,600	9,300	6,300
Small Intestine	750	400	350
Large Intestine (Colon)	35,300	16,400	18,900
Rectum	10,500	5,900	4,600
Liver & Biliary Passages	9,900	4,700	5,200
Pancreas	18,200	10,400	7,800
Other & Unspecified Digestive	1,650	800	850
Respiratory System	65,450	54,250	11,200
Larynx	2,850	2,550	350
Lung	61,700	51,200	10,500
Other & Unspecified Respiratory	900	550	350
Breast	30,350	250	30,100
Genital Organs	41,650	18,000	23,650
Cervix Uteri	9,400	—	9,400
Corpus Uteri	3,500	—	3,500
Ovary	9,900	—	9,900
Prostate	17,000	17,000	—
Testis	700	700	—
Other & Unspecified Genital	1,150	300	850
Urinary Organs	15,200	10,000	5,200
Kidney	6,300	3,900	2,400
Bladder & Other Urinary	8,900	6,100	2,800
Skin	5,100	3,000	2,100
Eye	350	150	200
Brain & Central Nervous System	7,900	4,600	3,300
Endocrine Glands	1,550	650	900
Thyroid	1,050	350	700
Other & Unspecified Endocrine	500	300	200
Bone	1,900	1,100	800
Soft-Tissue	1,500	800	700
Leukemia	14,700	8,400	6,300
Lymphomas	17,900	9,950	7,950
Lymphosarcoma & Reticulosarcoma	8,600	4,700	3,900
Hodgkin's Disease	3,700	2,200	1,500
Multiple Myeloma	4,100	2,200	1,900
Other Lymphomas	1,500	850	650
All Other & Unspecified	21,500	11,250	10,250

*) Data from: "1970 Cancer Facts and Figures" by Statistical Research Section, American Cancer Society, New York, N. Y. 10017.

of the incidence, and varies as a function of site of the neoplasm. Numerically, the more important are cancers of the lung, often fatal, and of colon and rectum, where the incidence is actually almost twice as high, but where successful surgery lowers the casualty rate. Also noteworthy are cancers of the endocrine organs, breast, prostate, uterus and ovary, of the liver and pancreas, and leukemias and lymphomas.

What do we know about the causes of disease at these various sites? Despite extensive efforts over the last 50 years we understand amazingly little, and we have only scant hard factual knowledge on the etiology of these main types of neoplasms.

Present concepts suggest that 80 or more percent of cancers of the lung are due to heavy smoking, particularly of cigarettes. Atmospheric pollution, or certain occupations like asbestos mining apparently exacerbate the condition.

Animal experiments supplemented by preliminary suggestive information in man suggest that leukemias and lymphomas may have a viral basis. Even more recently some viral elements have been noted in mammary cancer in human females which is reminiscent of Bittner's mouse mammary tumor virus. In this case, however, the pronounced national differences in incidence on breast cancer (for example, Japan versus most of Western Europe) must be taken into account in developing authoritative views on etiology at this site. Nonetheless it is difficult to visualize environmental factors as playing a major role in the pathogenesis of endocrine cancers.

For primary cancer of the liver, recent developments tend to incriminate, among other factors, mycotoxins like aflatoxin [*24*, *91*], or sterigmatocystin [*67*], cycasin and related plant materials [*47*], and possibly senecio alkaloids [*71*]. In Europe where hepatic cancer is relatively higher than in the United States, the additional enhancing factor of cirrhosis, possibly related to alcoholic beverages, particularly those high in tannins [*42*] or fusel oils [*30*] may also play a role. Interesting proposals yet to be documented, have been made that certain nitrosamines may exist in food or drink as such [*48*], or could conceivably result from the separate consumption of nitrite and certain secondary amines [*70*, *73*].

In this connection, some nitrosamines in experimental animals exhibit a yet poorly understood predilection for esophagus. The contribution of this sort of compound to the occurrence of cancer of the esophagus in man, rather elevated for example in some regions of France or in parts of Africa and Asia, is not clear. The consumption of some alcoholic beverages has also been incriminated [*54*, *69*].

In some areas of the world, local habits like chewing betel, the kangri, kairo, or kang heat and smoke exposure, ultraviolet and solar light exposure, presence of some liver or bladder parasites, explain the presence of special types of cancer in man.

Little can be said about specific etiologic factors responsible for other forms of cancer. Considerably more effort needs to be exerted to delve into this important problem so as to be capable of preventing the occurrence and development of those cancers, which now account for the major part of cancer in the world, in future generations. Because these known types of cancer arise under situations where the industrial and developmental status of nations are such that modern civilization cannot possibly be incriminated, it would seem that certain naturally occurring factors would need to be considered seriously. In addition to mycotoxins, plant products such as cycasin, bracken fern, heat or air modified lipids, possible agents from the intestinal microflora, or chemicals secreted into the bile as conjugates and liberated in the lower intestine by bacterial enzymes, abnormal endocrine metabolites, and many other such materials are subject to speculation. Probably complex mixtures of agents are really involved.

On the other hand, certain types of cancer have been definitely connected with the modern environment, mostly in an occupational situation. Because of the ever increasing industrialization of the world and because of the rapid and efficient means of transportation leading to a more widespread use of many materials around the world, it is also important and relevant to examine industrial products entering the environment for the possible presence of carcinogens. In those instances where carcinogens are identified, a decision must be made whether continued use is really required, is socially acceptable and outweighs the certain risk connected with their controlled use. In the United States, but unfortunately not in some other countries, there is a long history of assessing hazards connected with the entrance of possibly harmful materials into the food chain, and in part into pharmaceutical preparations. Concern with other agents in the environment has been somewhat more spotty depending on the individual circumstances. However, at the present time there fortunately is tremendous public interest and concern in such problems. It is to be expected that much more attention will be brought to bear on assessing the possible carcinogenic potential of environmental factors. Such interest requires investigators not only to utilize existing methods and mechanisms to assess carcinogenic hazards, but to attempt to develop better, quicker and more reliable procedures to examine environmental hazards. It is hoped that such techniques, resulting from these concerted studies, would not only pinpoint those synthetic agents which represent a *carcinogenic hazard now* and which should be removed to *avoid the development of cancer 10, 20 or 30 years from now*, but also assist in delving into the problem of the etiology of important *contemporary types of cancer* such as those in the intestinal tract, breast, prostate, or pancreas, discussed above, *which are due to past exposures to harmful situations*. Such efforts may well be coordinated on an international scale, perhaps through existing agencies like the World Health Organization and its International Agency for Research on Cancer, inasmuch as anything less than a worldwide attack may fall short of expectations and needs. Also, such studies are time-consuming and expensive. Provided precautions are taken to ensure the use of optimal protocols, adequate facilities, and trained individuals, there is no reason why good data generated anywhere in the world should not be used for controlling carcinogenic hazards everywhere else.

Classification of Chemical Carcinogens into Two Broad Classes, Distinguished by their Effectiveness without or with Metabolic Activation by the Host

There are many different types of known chemicals which cause cancer. Nonetheless, contrary to what is sometimes stated, in particular in the lay press and by the public, "not everything can be demonstrated to cause cancer if one is willing to try hard enough". The property of leading to neoplastic change when introduced into a responsive host system is a most specific and delicate property due to the molecular arrangement of a chemical compound. Sometimes even a small change in molecular structure converts a carcinogen to an innocuous compound, or vice versa. It is this property which has been found useful for fundamental studies on the underlying mechanisms. On the other hand, there are other types of compounds, like the nitrosamines, where an entire series bearing specific substituents may be carcinogenic, even though not always to the same target organ under the same conditions. Structure-activity correlations will not be discussed here. Such matters are the subject of several good specialized reviews and general overviews [*1*].

Present concepts distinguish two classes of chemical carcinogens. The first class includes those materials which are often active at the site of application. Many such agents are therefore presumably direct acting, that is the molecules as such are carcinogenic without further metabolic transformation. Examples of this class are alkylating agents such as those derived from the sulfur or nitrogen mustards, the alkyl sulfonates, epoxides, certain lactones and imines, particularly those built on strained rings, or with α, β-unsaturation. Of course, administration by appropriate means where such compounds reach remote sensitive organs in adequate concentration also may lead to tumors at such distant sites.

Because of their lack of specificity and almost ubiquitous activity the carcinogenic polynuclear aromatic hydrocarbons were also thought to belong to the group of direct-acting materials. Recently, however, Brookes and Dipple and their associates [*8*, *15*], supported in part by the biochemical work of Gelboin [*28*] and of Grover and Sims [*32*], developed a new viewpoint. Now it would seem that even these materials, known as carcinogens since the classic work of Kennaway and associates 40 years ago, do require biochemical change of an as yet undefined nature.

The second type of chemicals capable of inducing cancer usually do not do so at the point of application. This fact alone implied that the materials themselves were not carcinogenic but were converted to an active intermediate by the host. At this time polynuclear aromatic hydrocarbons (see above), certain aromatic amines and nitro compounds, nitrosamine derivatives and related compounds such as alkyltriazenes, 1,2-dialkylhydrazines, 1,2-benzylmethylhydrazines, syn. aliphatic azo and azoxy compounds, including cycasin, carcinogenic azo dyes and similar compounds, and perhaps urethane do require such activation. Additionally, there are a number of chemicals with varied structures as for example some mycotoxins, such as aflatoxin, pyrrolizidine alkaloids, the amino acid antagonist ethionine, acetamide, certain halogenated materials such as carbon tetrachloride, and other miscellaneous materials which likewise are subject to specific activation reactions by the host.

A sub-class includes substances which do not require the active participation by the host. Enzymic activation reactions are not necessary, for the materials themselves in the presence of water, or a buffered solution as is available under *in vivo* conditions release the active intermediate. Examples are nitrosomethyl- (or alkyl-) ureas, amides or carbamates, *N*-phenyl-*N*-nitrosourea, and *N*-methyl-*N'*-nitro-*N*-nitrosoguanidine [*78*].

Also, certain metals or derivatives are definitely carcinogenic in experimental animals and in man. These include nickel, titanium, lead, cobalt, chromium, cadmium, beryllium, and perhaps arsenic and manganese. With metals the underlying mechanism is quite obscure.

From a standpoint of biochemical pharmacology, agents of the first type, that is direct or locally acting, show differences in effectiveness based chiefly on their chemical reactivity (or stability) and on the ability of the host to metabolize and detoxify them by reactions which by and large are already well understood. Of course, it is obvious that in addition to control by such biochemical factors many additional host factors impinge on the relative susceptibility of a given experimental or clinical system. This includes endocrine factors, immunological competence, the availability of receptor sites and others, all of which are outside the context of the present discussion.

Biochemical Activation of „Procarcinogens“ of Various Types

Polynuclear Aromatic Hydrocarbons

Let me discuss briefly some of the salient advances in our understanding of the biochemical activation of the second type, the remotely-active compounds. At the outset it must be said that not much is known on systems which activate polynuclear aromatic hydrocarbons. GELBOIN [*28*] visualizes that the active species could be generated during the standard biochemical oxidation of these compounds. WILK and others [*8*, *66*, *81*, *90*] have proposed the transitory existence of a radical cation. Among other theses, the logical formation of epoxides was not really supported by experimental evidence, but then the synthetic epoxides tested may not have been those possibly available through biochemical synthesis in the host [*55*]. The chemical reactivity of the epoxides may also have prevented their reaching a sensitive site [*82*]. Certainly much more information needs to be secured before an authoritative solution is at hand. The system sought must be present in many tissues and in many species inasmuch as the carcinogenic hydrocarbons do cause cancer in many species and in many target sites. In addition to control by activation, the effectiveness of the carcinogenic hydrocarbons is also governed by efficient detoxification mechanisms such as the well known ring-hydroxylation reactions. For example, the sensitivity of mice and rats to subcutaneous injection of benzo(a)pyrene or 7,12-dimethylbenz(a)anthracene, and the relative resistance of rabbits to the same treatment may well be due to differences in rates of hydroxylation, conjugation, and elimination, in addition to possible influence of the activation systems. In this connection, mice and rats usually do not develop liver cancer when treated as adults with carcinogenic hydrocarbons, but do so when injected as newborns. While the difference could be ascribed entirely to relative rates of detoxification, it is also possible that newborns contain the activation enzyme systems which may be repressed in adults. As discussed later, such a behavior has been documented in the case of a β-glucosidase required for the activation of cycasin.

Aromatic Amines, Azo Dyes, and Nitro Compounds

1. Conversion to Hydroxylamino Derivatives. Even though it was known that certain arylamines and azo dyes were carcinogenic and that they would require metabolic activation, it is only recently that the underlying processes have been elucidated at least with respect to those compounds which cause cancer of the liver. As typical aromatic compounds arylamines are extensively hydroxylated on the aromatic ring system. Biologic tests of these hydroxylated metabolites have almost always indicated that these compounds were not the carcinogenic species, for they were not or only weakly active. In contrast, the materials which occur often as only small portions of the overall metabolic conversion products, the *N*-hydroxy derivatives, were found to be more carcinogenic than the parent amines and to be carcinogenic under conditions where the parent amines were not. Thus, *N*-hydroxylation appears to be a most crucial activation process for arylamines and derivatives and the carcinogenic aminoazo dyes. A species like the guinea pig which exhibits only a low capability to carry out *N*-hydroxylation and indeed has a high proclivity for the reverse reaction, is refractory to the carcinogenic effect. Other species where this reaction does occur exhibit variable potentiality. Even in a single species – man – relatively different capacities were noted in the few individuals studied [*18*, *86*].

Also of current interest is 3-aminotriazole. Older studies indicated that this material yielded only tumors of the thyroid, probably by interference with the pituitary-thyroid homeostatic mechanism. However, more recently it has been found that this compound, of commercial importance in agricultural practice, induced liver tumors in mice and rats [*37*, *61*]. It will be useful to determine whether this material undergoes the same type of activation reactions as a more conventional arylamine. Similarly, in studies of the hepatotoxicity of mesidine, LINDSTROM *et al.* [*49*] noted that this compound was converted to an *N*-hydroxy derivative. We are now testing the long-term effect of this compound, of commercial importance, in mice and rats.

The carcinogenicity of certain aminoazo dyes has been known for a long time. A number of hypotheses now only of historic interest were advanced to account for their activity. It is only recently, however, after the mechanism of activation of the aromatic amines was clarified, that like processes were shown to operate also for the azo dyes, typified by *N*, *N*-4-dimethylaminoazobenzene. First, one of the methyl groups is removed oxidatively. Subsequently, *N*-hydroxylation of the amino nitrogen and probable esterification of the hydroxy group yields the reactive intermediate. The only question not yet clear is the need for an *N*-methyl substitution, specifically indicated for this particular series of carcinogens. Other carcinogenic azo dyes such as *o*-aminoazotoluene are active by virtue of the aromatic amino group alone and do not require *N*-methyl substitution.

Nitro analogs of the carcinogenic aromatic amines, as well as the interesting 4-nitroquinoline *N*-oxide are also carcinogenic. There are mammalian and also bacterial enzyme systems which reduce the nitroaryl compounds to the corresponding hydroxylamino derivatives.

Recently, ERTURK, PRICE, BRYAN *et al.* [*19*, *20*, *60*] discovered a series of new chemical carcinogens derived from nitrofurans. While several of these compounds appear to induce tumors specifically in the mammary gland in female Sprague-Dawley rats, other closely related compounds affect many target organs. Although studies on their mode of action will be of keen interest, they may be active after biochemical reduction of the nitro function to a hydroxylamino group and further esterification. These compounds can be visualized as being analogous to aminobiphenyl or benzidine derivatives.

2. Production of Esters of Arylhydroxylamines. N-Hydroxylation is, however, not the last step in the activation of aromatic amines. Male and female rats are quite different in susceptibility to liver cancer formation but the levels of *N*-hydroxy compound derived, for example, from *N*-2-fluorenylacetamide were not sufficient to account for the great variation in biologic response [*84, 85*]. Also, under *in vitro* conditions *N*-hydroxy-*N*-2-fluorenylacetamide failed to interact to a significant extent with certain macromolecular receptors such as DNA, RNA and proteins [*58*]. It was felt that perhaps deacetylation, yielding the corresponding arylhydroxylamine, was the necessary activation step. Indeed, the arylhydroxylamines which were reactive materials especially in the presence of oxygen, or the nitroso derivatives were carcinogenic. Moreover, arylamines are carcinogenic in the dog which of all the common domestic or laboratory animals cannot acetylate aromatic amines. Thus, the *N*-acetyl group certainly is not necessary for carcinogenicity.

Other considerations prompted the MILLER's and their collaborators [*58*] as well as KING and PHILLIPS [*41*] to postulate an esterification of the hydroxylamino or *N*-acetylhydroxylamines via phosphate or sulfate. In addition IRVING [*39*] thought that the glucosiduronic acid deserved consideration. A synthetic ester, *N*-acetoxy-*N*-2-fluorenylacetamide, was highly carcinogenic, mutagenic and reactive *in vitro* with cellular macromolecules. A decision as to which ester was the active intermediate could be made on the basis of earlier somewhat unrelated discoveries. Acetanilide inhibited the carcinogenic effect of *N*-2-fluorenylacetamide mainly because acetanilide interferred with *N*-hydroxylation [*31, 95*]. However, we found that acetanilide also inhibited the carcinogenicity of *N*-hydroxy-*N*-2-fluorenylacetamide. MILLER [*57*] pointed out that it was possible that *p*-hydroxyacetanilide, the major metabolite of acetanilide in the rat, depleted the host of available sulfate, as noted by BÜCH, RUMMEL *et al.* [*9*]. MILLER and colleagues demonstrated that inorganic sulfate enhanced the toxicity of *N*-hydroxy-*N*-2-fluorenylacetamide in the presence or absence of *p*-hydroxyacetanilide [*14, 57*]. We found that addition of exogenous sodium sulfate to the diet of animals receiving *N*-hydroxy-*N*-2-fluorenylacetamide and acetanilide restored the carcinogenic effect inhibited by the treatment with the acetanilide derivative [*88*]. Phosphate or other ions appeared ineffective. Hence the active intermediate, as regards liver carcinogenesis, is a sulfuric acid ester of the aryl hydroxylamine. Of course, additional questions remain to be resolved. Kriek [*43*, *44*] discovered, and Irving *et al.* [*38*, *39*] confirmed that the metabolite bound to DNA of rat liver was chiefly the amino derivative whereas the acetyl group is retained in the RNA adduct. Also whether this mechanism operates in organs other than the liver remains to be documented. Preliminary reports indicate that sulfotransferase required for sulfuric ester formation is low in organs other than the liver. Yet, the sulfate ester is so unstable in aqueous media that it is inconceivable that it could be transported to a remote target organ. It is not even carcinogenic upon subcutaneous injection. Thus, it is only realistic to assume that the active "ultimate" carcinogen is synthesized biochemically in close vicinity to the specific target in the cell.

The recent demonstration that certain purine *N*-oxides are carcinogenic not only at the site of injection but also systemically relates these materials to the carcinogenic aromatic amines [*79*]. While there is now no evidence that *N*-oxidation of purines occurs *in vivo* to constitute an abnormal metabolic pathway accounting for cancer in man, it is nonetheless wise to consider such possibilities. It would seem that purine *N*-oxides, tautomeric with hydroxylamino compounds, do undergo activation reactions, probably by sulfate ester formation as do the aromatic amines. Incorporation into nucleic acids to yield a fraudulent macromolecule is less likely. Along these lines we failed to demonstrate that certain purine and pyrimidine antimetabolites, incorporated into nucleic acids, are carcinogenic [*33*]. There are numerous modulating factors affecting the efficiency with which arylamines and aminoazo dyes are converted to the *N*-hydroxy derivatives. In addition to species, such elements as strain, sex, age, nutritional situation, inducing and inhibiting agents, the structure of the arylamine itself or any substituent on the nitrogen, and the like, operate to control the effective level of *N*-hydroxy derivative produced and available at crucial cellular and molecular receptors.

Among many other factors modifying the carcinogenicity of aromatic amines, nitrosamines and related agents, those that alter the available level of detoxification systems have received thorough study [*29*]. Indeed, the concept of enzyme induction, so well known in pharmacology today, was originally discovered in the laboratory of the Miller's [*56*] in connection with the biochemical analysis of the then curious inhibition of liver cancer formation by carcinogenic azo dyes (4-dimethylaminoazobenzene) or aromatic amines (*N*-2-fluorenylacetamide) when the polynuclear aromatic hydrocarbon 3-methylcholanthrene was fed at the same time. The explanation, now classic, is that the hydrocarbon increases azo dye reductase in the case of the azo dye, and enzymes leading to less carcinogenic ring-hydroxylated products in the case of the aromatic amines. Thus, less of the active *N*-hydroxylated products are formed. The system works thus, however, only in rats. In hamsters, methylcholanthrene tends to increase *N*-hydroxylation relatively more than ring-hydroxylation. In this species therefore, as expected, the yield of tumors is higher [*17*]. On the other hand, phenobarbital induces enzyme sytems in part different from those obtained with the hydrocarbons and yields higher levels of *N*-hydroxy derivative from aromatic amines like *N*-2-fluorenylacetamide in the rat. Interestingly though, there is lower binding of carcinogen to macromolecules like DNA, RNA, proteins in liver (MATSUSHIMA, WEISBURGER, and WEISBURGER, unpublished experiments), and lower tumor yields [*89*]. It is probable that in this case the sulfotransferase system leading to the ultimate carcinogen, the sulfuric acid ester of the *N*-hydroxy derivative is decreased. Phenobarbital also lowers the yield of tumors with diethylnitrosamine consequent to a decreased oxidative dealkylation of this agent [*45*].

Nitrosamines. Many nitrosamine derivatives are carcinogenic, as discovered initially by MAGEE and BARNES [*52*], and documented subsequently on an extensive scale by DRUCKREY, PREUSSMANN, SCHMÄHL *et al.* [*16*]. These compounds show exquisite organotropic behavior. Biochemically, a nitrosamine can be organized into three classes – symmetric dialkyl, unsymmetric alkyl or aryl, and cyclic or heterocyclic nitrosamines. With the first two types, where there is usually an *N*-methyl or an *N*-ethyl group, present concepts indicate that biochemical oxidation of such groups on the endoplasmic reticulum results eventually in the production of an active carbonium ion. This appears to be the specific molecular species responsible for the conversion of a normal to a potential tumor cell. During the established procedures of subcellular fractionation the activity is found in the microsome fraction. Many epithelial cells in virtually all species have this potential accounting possibly for the diversity of the tissues and species susceptible to this type of compound. Thus, nitrosamines constitute severe hazards to most animal species and man. Whereas cancer induction in primates, for example, has been a most challenging task O'GARA *et al.* [*40*] were successful in achieving liver cancer induction in rhesus monkeys in less than 2 years with diethylnitrosamine. Nonetheless, the curious organotropic property of the nitrosamines is not yet clear, and requires additional diligent efforts. The explanation probably will be found to reside in the biochemical and pharmacological properties of the host-substrate interaction.

Related to the active carcinogens derived from the nitrosamines are the aryl triazeno compounds developed by PREUSSMANN, DRUCKREY, *et al.* [*64*]. Just as the nitrosamines, these chemicals yield active carbonium ions after simple biochemical oxidation. These compounds, some of which are intermediates in the dyestuffs industry, are powerful carcinogens for sites not normally affected by the more classic compounds such as brain, the nervous system, or the kidneys. Thus, these materials provide useful tools for studies of the mechanism of formation of tumors occasionally seen in man, and induced with difficulty by other means.

Also in this field is a naturally occurring agent found in the cycad nut, cycasin, possibly connected with the occurrence of liver cancer in man in some areas of the world. This compound, identified as β-glucoside of methylazoxymethanol interestingly undergoes metabolic activation not by mammalian enzyme systems, absent in adult animals, but is split readily into the active aglycone by a β-glucosidase from the bacterial flora in the gut. Thus, this compound is completely inactive in germ-free rats [*46*]. Interestingly, however, it was active in germ-free *newborn* animals which apparently do possess a β-glucosidase, which is subsequently repressed with increasing age [*74*].

Considering the fact that the carcinogenicity of the simplest of the nitrosamines was discovered a mere 16 years ago, amazing progress in unraveling problems of pathogenesis has been made with this series of compounds.

Urethan. The same cannot be said for the simple chemical ethyl carbamate, or urethan, even though the carcinogenicity of this compound was discovered almost 30 years ago. This compound is most potent in inducing alveolar adenocarcinomas in the lungs of susceptible mice. However, it also affects some other tissues and other species, but compared to other carcinogens, urethan does not rate among the most potent. This compound is metabolized very quickly. By analogy with the arylamines it was thought that the *N*-hydroxy derivative of ethyl carbamate could be the active intermediate [*59*]. However, while this compound is effective as a mutagen in microbiological systems, whereas ethyl carbamate itself is not, in mammalian systems the *N*-hydroxy derivative was very quickly converted to the amino compound. Because of the high structural specificity of the ethyl ester for the carcinogenicity of this compound (which should be noted since a large number of other carbamates are useful as insecticides, pesticides, or drugs) Boyland *et al.* directed their attention to the carbethoxy function [*6*]. The carbethoxy portion of ethyl carbamate was attached to cytosine when nucleic acids were examined for the presence of metabolites [*62*]. While more information is required to specifically delineate the mechanism of transformation of and by ethyl carbamate, the production of an active entity from the ester part of the molecule appears plausible.

Ethionine. That the amino acid antagonist ethionine causes liver cancer in rats has been known for approximately 20 years. Much of our information on the mode of action of this material comes from the laboratories of E. Farber [*22, 23, 77*]. As do most other pharmacologically active molecules, ethionine exerts a number of biologic effects which in turn are based on possibly distinct biochemical reactions. In acute or short-term tests ethionine appears to possess the very interesting property of leading to a dramatic lowering of ATP levels. Ethionine seems to be metabolized initially by pathways similar to those for the normal analog, methionine. Thus, ethionine is converted to an activated molecule, S-adenosylethionine. However, in contrast to the other "ultimate" carcinogens described like the carbonium ions and other electrophilic reagents derived from other types of chemical carcinogens which are themselves chemically reactive, S-adenosylethionine requires either additional enzyme steps to yield a chemically reactive intermediate, or more likely the last step in the carcinogenic process with ethionine is enzymically mediated. This interesting feature requires further exploitation. Also whereas almost all chemical carcinogens combine with the known macromolecules in the cells such as DNA, RNA and proteins, ethionine fails to do so with DNA, at least measured by the sensitivity of the methods employed (as does tricycloquinazoline [*2*]). This focuses attention specifically on transfer-RNA with which reaction has been demonstrated and which conceivably could lead to abnormal translation properties, eventually transmitted to the genome by this indirect technique. Such views have also been proposed by NOVELLI *et al.* [*63*] and WEINSTEIN [*83*] for other carcinogens. Considering the recent discoveries in the area of viral biochemistry where RNA viruses controlled a DNA polymerase and thus indirectly modulated the synthesis of cellular genome [*3, 75, 80*], it is entirely within the realm of possibility that such indirect pathways can operate under the impulse of smaller chemical carcinogens. Another instance of this type, by the way, may well be in the example we have recently studied. On the basis of inhibition of the carcinogenicity of acetamide by arginine, we concluded, in a preliminary way to be sure, that acetamide could be carcinogenic because of intracellular liberation of excess ammonium ions [*87*]. It is hard to visualize any direct action on the genome by this scheme but an indirect effect is not too impossible.

Senecio Alkaloids. As with urethan, the hepatotoxicity and possible carcinogenicity of certain of the pyrrolizidine alkaloids may be based on an oxidative step from a pyrrole ring followed by release of portions of an exocyclic ester from the molecule [*13*]. SCHOENTAL [*71*] recently proposed an alternative mechanism based on the oxidation of the Δ-1,2 double bond to an epoxide. Even through these molecules may be potentially quite important in relation to the etiology of liver disease in man, there have been relatively few fundamental studies. Much more work needs to be done to further document the activation processes with these interesting compounds.

Aflatoxin; Mycotoxins; Plant Carcinogens. Another class of natural products which have assumed increasing importance in fundamental studies as well as with respect to their relative importance in cancer in man are mycotoxins such as aflatoxin or sterigmatocystin. Structure-activity studies have indicated that deletion of parts of the molecule results in loss of activity. Thus, both the 2 furan rings as well as the lactone portion are required. One might feel that the α, β-unsaturated lactone ring is the function conferring reactivity and carcinogenicity to the compound, even though this group is in a relatively non-stressed stable configuration. However, species differences, activities related to sex and endocrine function, led to newer views suggesting that aflatoxin also requires metabolic activation. One of the metabolites, aflatoxin M_1, isolated from milk of cattle fed aflatoxin [*36*, *53*] or from humans [*11*] appears to be carcinogenic, but not more so than the parent compound. SCHOENTAL [*71*] postulated an epoxide as the active intermediate. This most interesting structure is one we also feel deserves serious consideration. Hopefully, the synthesis, identification, and bioassay of this intermediate can receive early experimental attention.

Along these lines, the recent finding that a compound isolated from bracken fern may be the active principle contained therein, is of considerable value inasmuch as this material causes tumors in the digestive tract, particularly in the stomach and intestine, as well as in the bladder in laboratory and domestic animals [*21*, *65*]. The prompt clarification of the responsible agent may throw light on cancer induction at these target organs so important in man.

Thioamides. A number of thio derivatives like thiouracil, thioacetamide, thiourea, affect not only thyroid function but are severely hepatotoxic and carcinogenic to the liver. Relatively few studies have been done on the underlying biochemical mechanism. Because of the activity of these materials at relatively low dosages, compared to acetamide, it is quite certain that their mode of action is different. In view of the common thio function of these compounds, it would seem that the key to an understanding of their mode of action lies in considering the fate of the thiogroup.

Carbon Tetrachloride. That carbon tetrachloride is hepatotoxic in virtually all species is well known. Although its carcinogenicity in mice was discovered many years ago, hamsters also develop hepatocellular carcinoma with this agent. Recently REUBER demonstrated that apparent earlier failure of carbon tetrachloride to induce cancer in rats was strain related. The Sprague-Dawley rat readily develops fatal cirrhosis before liver tumors have sufficient time to develop. Strains of rats less susceptible to cirrhosis eventually did exhibit liver tumors [*68*]. Phenobarbital and other conditions leading to higher levels of processing enzymes enhanced the hepatotoxicity of carbon tetrachloride [*27*]. It can be assumed therefore that a metabolite is the active carcinogen.

Inorganic Chemicals. Certain inorganic chemicals can also cause cancer Among them are certain derivatives of beryllium, lead, cadmium, manganese, nickel, cobalt, chromium, and arsenic. Their mechanism of action is not clear at all and certainly deserves further examination. This is especially true as they constitute some of the few chemicals which have affected not only experimental animals but also man during occupational exposure [*26*]. Furthermore the carcinogenicity of certain types of asbestos is also of considerable interest.

Promoting Agents, Cocarcinogens. A paper delivered in Heidelberg cannot fail to mention the contributions made by HECKER and his associates [*35*] in isolating and identifying the active components of croton oil, the classic tumor promoter used by BERENBLUM and SHUBIK to divide the carcinogenic process, at least in mouse skin, into a number of distinct steps amenable to study. While the evidence is at this time tenuous, it stands to reason that cancer in man, at least at the sites most commonly affected such as lung and intestinal tract, may not be due to the sole operation of a single carcinogen. Instead, it may be the result of a number of entities in our complex environment some of which have carcinogenic effects while others act as powerful promoters. Removal of the promoting agents from the environment, after their identification, would assist in reducing in no mean way the carcinogenic hazard of other chemicals, present possibly in such minute amounts in essential materials that their total elimination might be impractical.

Comments and Concluding Remarks

First of all, many important, timely and contemporary studies on the specific interactions of the ultimate forms of carcinogens with proposed cellular and molecular receptors have not been discussed. Yet, this is the area which will permit eventually a molecular explanation of the processes of cancer induction. Once the specific targets are identified, a number of problems now awaiting solution will be resolved on the basis of such a rational approach. *1.* It should become easier and quicker to assess the carcinogenicity of agents in the environment utilizing as endpoint precise and specific information derived from molecular biology. *2.* Knowledge of the potential and actual targets in the cell should generate means of blocking such targets with innocuous compounds as realistic preventive measures.

In the present paper we have briefly discussed in a very general and perhaps superficial way some of the types of known chemical carcinogens and the direct or indirect active forms of such chemicals. Also mentioned were certain of the steps by which an inactive precursor, a procarcinogen, is converted to the ultimate active form. Such activation reactions may be single or multistep. Under the right circumstances, knowledge of the nature of such activation reactions likewise permits inhibition of the carcinogenic process by blocking or minimizing the pathways leading towards active intermediates.

Many of the types of chemical carcinogens known today have demonstrated activity in animal systems. It will be recalled, however, that the entire field of chemical carcinogenesis rests on the discovery of cancer in man which was judiciously related to occupation and exposure to specific chemicals. The list of chemicals known to induce cancer *in man* is relatively short. It encompasses no more than some 20–30 pure chemicals or mixtures. With the curious exception of inorganic arsenic, every-one of those chemicals known to cause cancer in man has also caused cancer in animals. In our opinion, and indeed with conviction, it can be said that the reverse is also true. Chemicals reliably carcinogenic in animals would also be active in man. It is the business of contemporary and future cancer research to avoid enlarging the list of agents which cause cancer in man by suitable preventive measures. The easiest of these seems to be to avoid introduction into the environment of chemicals with demonstrated capability to cause cancer in animals.

Considerable progress, therefore, is at hand in preventing the so-called occupational cancers. Nonetheless, achieving preventive measures in occupational situations, while certainly desirable, unfortunately involves only a relatively small number of individuals. What to do about the hundreds of thousands or even millions of cases of cancer seen in the world today? Some factors which may be causative were discussed in the introduction. For example, cancer in man may be the result of consumption of food, beverage, or primitive medicines, of mycotoxins or plant toxins such as aflatoxin, sterigmatocystin, pyrrolizidine alkaloids, the active agents from bracken fern, and the like. While not one of these has been definitely and unambiguously related to cancer in man at this time, there is substantial evidence that all of these materials are carcinogenic in animals. Thus, it would seem the better part of prudence even now to take active measures on a worldwide scale to insure that such agents are definetely absent from products entering the human environment.

We visualize that future endeavors need to concentrate very heavily on a serious and deliberate examination of those areas, possibly neglected today, which might fruitfully attack the problem of the major types of cancer seen in man. While present efforts relative to a possible viral etiology may well resolve certain of these problems, it is equally certain that others will find an answer only by the identification and elimination of chemicals other than viruses. It is hoped that such approaches will bear fruit and that the desirable and established trend of a decreasing incidence of gastric cancer in the United States and in Western Europe will find counterparts in the many other types of cancer afflicting mankind.

References

1. ARCOS, J. C., ARGUS, M. F.: Molecular geometry and carcinogenic activity of aromatic compounds. New perspectives. Advanc. Cancer Res. **11**, 305 (1968).
2. BALDWIN, R. W., MOORE, M., PARTRIDGE, M. W.: Tricycloquinazoline carcinogenesis: Interaction of carcinogen with mouse skin proteins. Int. J. Cancer **3**, 244 (1968).
3. BALTIMORE, D.: RNA-dependent DNA polymerase in virions of RNA tumour viruses. Nature **226**, 1209 (1970).
4. BAUER, K. H.: Das Krebsproblem. 2. Aufl. Berlin-Göttingen-Heidelberg: Springer 1963.
5. BOURKE, J. B., GRIFFIN, J. P.: Blood-groups in benign and malignant prostatic hypertrophy. Lancet **1962 II**, 1279.
6. BOYLAND, E.: The biochemistry of aromatic hydrocarbons, amines and urethane. In BERGMANN, E. D., PULLMAN, B. (Eds.): Jerusalem Symposia on Quantum Chemistry and Biochemistry I., p. 25. Jerusalem: 1969.
7. — The correlation of experimental carcinogenesis and cancer in man. Progr. exp. Tumor Res. **11**, 222 (1969).
8. BROOKES, P., DIPPLE, A.: On the mechanism of hydrocarbon carcinogenesis. In BERGMANN, E. D., PULLMAN, B. (Eds.): Jerusalem Symposia on Quantum Chemistry and Biochemistry I., p. 139. Jerusalem: 1969.
9. BÜCH, H., RUMMEL, W., PFLEGER, K., ESCHRICH, C., TEXTER, N.: Ausscheidung freien und konjugierten Sulfates bei Ratte und Menschen nach Verabreichung von *N*-Acetyl-*p*-Aminophenol. Naunyn-Schmiedeberg's Arch. exp. Path. Pharmak. **259**, 276 (1968).
10. BURDETTE, W. J.: Causality, casuistry and clinical carcinogenesis. Progr. exp. Tumor Res. **11**, 395 (1969).
11. CAMPBELL, T. C., CAEDO, J. P., Jr., BULATAO-JAYME, J., SALAMAT, L., ENGEL, R. W.: Aflatoxin M_1 in human urine. Nature **227**, 403 (1970).
12. CORREA, P., CUELLO, C., DUQUE, E.: Carcinoma and intestinal metaplasia of the stomach in Colombian migrants. J. nat. Cancer Inst. **44**, 297 (1970).
13. CULVENOR, C. C. J., DOWNING, D. T., EDGAR, J. A.: Pyrrolizidine alkaloids as alkylating and antimitotic agents. Ann. N. Y. Acad. Sci. **163**, 837 (1969).
14. DEBAUN, J. R., SMITH, J. Y. R., MILLER, E. C., MILLER, J. A.: Reactivity *in vivo* of the carcinogen *N*-hydroxy-2-acetylaminofluorene: Increase by sulfate ion. Science **167**, 184 (1970).
15. DIPPLE, A., LAWLEY, P. D., BROOKES, P.: Theory of tumour initiation by chemical carcinogens: Dependence of activity on structure of ultimate carcinogen. Europ. J. Cancer **4**, 493 (1968).
16. DRUCKREY, H., PREUSSMANN, R., IVANKOVIC, S., SCHMÄHL, D.: Organotrope carcinogene Wirkungen bei 65 verschiedenen *N*-Nitroso-Verbindungen an BD-Ratten. Z. Krebsforsch. **69**, 103 (1967).
17. ENOMOTO, M., MIYAKE, M., SATO, K.: Carcinogenicity in the hamster of simultaneously administered 2-acetamidofluorene and 3-methylcholanthrene. Gann **59**, 177 (1968).

18. Enomoto, M., Sato, K.: *N*-Hydroxylation of the carcinogen 2-acetylaminofluorene by human liver tissue *in vitro*. Life Sci. **6**, 881 (1967).

19. Ertürk, E., Cohen, S. M., Price, J. M., Bryan, G. T.: Pathogenesis, histology, and transplantability of urinary bladder carcinomas induced in albino rats by oral administration of *N*-[4-(5-nitro-2-furyl)-2-thiazolyl]formamide. Cancer Res. **29**, 2219 (1969).

20. — — — von Esch, A. M., Crovetti, A. J., Bryan, G. T.: The production of hemangioendothelial sarcoma in rats by feeding 5-acetamido-3-(5-nitro-2-furyl)-6H-1, 2, 4-oxadiazine. Cancer Res. **29**, 2212 (1969).

21. Evans, I. A.: The radiomimetic nature of bracken toxin. Cancer Res. **28**, 2252 (1968).

22. Farber, E.: Ethionine carcinogenesis. Advanc. Cancer Res. **7**, 383 (1963).

23. — Biochemistry of carcinogenesis. Cancer Res. **28**, 1859 (1968).

24. Feuell, A. J.: Types of mycotoxins in foods and feeds. In Goldblatt, L. A. (Ed.): Aflatoxin: Scientific background, control, and implications, p. 187. New York: Academic Press 1969.

25. Fischer, B.: Die experimentelle Erzeugung atypischer Epithelwucherungen und die Entstehung bösartiger Geschwülste. Münch. med. Wschr. **53**, 2041 (1906).

26. Furst, A., Haro, R. T.: A survey of metal carcinogenesis. Progr. exp. Tumor Res. **12**, 102 (1969).

27. Garner, R. C., McLean, A. E. M.: Increased susceptibility to carbon tetrachloride poisoning in the rat after pretreatment with oral phenobarbitone. Biochem. Pharmacol. **18**, 645 (1969).

28. Gelboin, H. V.: A microsome-dependent binding of benzo(a)pyrene to DNA. In Bergmann, E. D., Pullman, B. (Eds.): Jerusalem Symposia on Quantum Chemistry and Biochemistry I., p. 175. Jerusalem: 1969.

29. — Conney, A. H.: Antagonism and potentiation of drug action. In Boyland, E., Goulding, R. (Eds.): Modern Trends in Toxicology I., p. 175. London: Butterworths 1968.

30. Gibel, W., Wildner, G. P., Lohs, K.: Untersuchungen zur Frage einer kanzerogenen und hepatotoxischen Wirkung von Fuselöl. Arch. Geschwulstforsch. **32**, 115 (1968).

31. Grantham, P. H., Mohan, L., Yamamoto, R. S., Weisburger, E. K., Weisburger, J. H.: Alteration of the metabolism of the carcinogen *N*-2-fluorenylacetamide by acetanilide. Toxicol. appl. Pharmacol. **13**, 118 (1968).

32. Grover, P. L., Sims, P.: Enzyme-catalysed reactions of polycyclic hydrocarbons with deoxyribonucleic acid and protein *in vitro*. Biochem. J. **110**, 159 (1968).

33. Hadidian, Z., Fredrickson, T. N., Weisburger, E. K., Weisburger, J. H., Glass, R. M., Mantel, N.: Tests for chemical carcinogens. Report on the activity of derivatives of aromatic amines, nitrosamines, quinolines, nitroalkanes, amides, epoxides, aziridines, and purine antimetabolites. J. nat. Cancer Inst. **41**, 985 (1968).

34. Haenszel, W., Kurihara, M.: Studies of Japanese migrants. I. Mortality from cancer and other diseases among Japanese in the United States. J. nat. Cancer Inst. **40**, 43 (1968).

35. Hecker, E.: Co-carcinogenic principles from the seed oil of *Croton tiglium* and from other Euphorbiaceae. Cancer Res. **28**, 2338 (1968).

36. Holzapfel, C. W., Steyn, P. S., Purchase, I. F. H.: Isolation and structure of aflatoxins M_1 and M_2. Tetrahedron Letters **1966**, 2799.

37. INNES, J. R. M., ULLAND, B. M., VALERIO, M. G., PETRUCELLI, L., FISHBEIN, L., HART, E. R., PALLOTTA, A. J., BATES, R. R., FALK, H. L., GART, J. J., KLEIN, M., MITCHELL, I., PETERS, J. A.: Bioassay of pesticides and industrial chemicals for tumorigenicity in mice: A preliminary note. J. nat. Cancer Inst. **42**, 1101 (1969).
38. IRVING, C. C., RUSSELL, L. T.: Synthesis of the O-glucuronide of *N*-2-fluorenylhydroxylamine. Reaction with nucleic acids and with guanosine 5′-monophosphate. Biochemistry **9**, 2471 (1970).
39. — VEAZEY, R. A., RUSSELL, L. T.: Possible role of the glucuronide conjugate in the biochemical mechanism of binding of the carcinogen *N*-hydroxy-2-acetyl-aminofluorene to rat-liver deoxyribonucleic acid *in vivo*. Chem.-biol. Interactions **1**, 19 (1969).
40. KELLY, M. G., O'GARA, R. W., ADAMSON, R. H., GADEKAR, K., BOTKIN, C. C., REESE, W. H., KERBER, W. T.: Induction of hepatic cell carcinomas in monkeys with *N*-nitrosodiethylamine. J. nat. Cancer Inst. **36**, 323 (1966).
41. KING, C. M., PHILLIPS, B.: *N*-Hydroxy-2-fluorenylacetamide. Reaction of the carcinogen with guanosine, ribonucleic acid, deoxyribonucleic acid, and protein following enzymatic deacetylation or esterification. J. biol. Chem. **244**, 6209 (1969).
42. KORPÁSSY, B.: Tannins as hepatic carcinogens. Progr. exp. Tumor Res. **2**, 245 (1961).
43. KRIEK, E.: Difference in binding of 2-aectylaminofluorene to rat-liver deoxyribonucleic acid and ribosomal ribonucleic acid *in vivo*. Biochim. biophys. Acta **161**, 273 (1968).
44. — On the mechanism of action of carcinogenic aromatic amines. I. Binding of 2-acetylaminofluorene and *N*-hydroxy-2-acetylaminofluorene to rat-liver nucleic acids *in vivo*. Chem.-biol. Interactions **1**, 3 (1969).
45. KUNZ, W., SCHAUDE, G., THOMAS, C.: Die Beeinflussung der Nitrosamincarcinogenese durch Phenobarbital und Halogenkohlenwasserstoffe. Z. Krebsforsch. **72**, 291 (1969).
46. LAQUEUR, G. L.: Carcinogenic effects of cycad meal and cycasin, methylazoxymethanol glycoside, in rats and effects of cycasin in germfree rats. Federation Proc. **23**, 1386 (1964).
47. — MICKELSEN, O., WHITING, M. G., KURLAND, L. T.: Carcinogenic properties of nuts from Cycas circinalis L. indigenous to Guam. J. nat. Cancer Inst. **31**, 919 (1963).
48. LIJINSKY, W., EPSTEIN, S. S.: Nitrosamines as environmental carcinogens. Nature **225**, 21 (1970).
49. LINDSTROM, H. V., BOWIE, W. C., WALLACE, W. C., NELSON, A. A., FITZHUGH, O. G.: The toxicity and metabolism of mesidine and pseudocumidine in rats. J. Pharmacol. exp. Ther. **167**, 223 (1969).
50. MAASS, H., SACHS, H., PAUKA, B.: Epidemiologische Untersuchung bösartiger Neubildungen in Hamburg 1960–1962. Z. Krebsforsch. **73**, 1 (1969).
51. MACDONALD, E. J., WOLF, P. F.: Comparative incidence of cancer in three regions in Texas. In LETTRÉ, H., WAGNER, G. (Hrsg.): Aktuelle Probleme aus dem Gebiet der Cancerologie II. Zweites Heidelberger Symposion, p. 97. Berlin-Heidelberg-New York: Springer 1968.
52. MAGEE, P., N., BARNES, J. M.: Carcinogenic nitroso compounds. Advanc. Cancer Res. **10**, 163 (1967).
53. MASRI, M. S., LUNDIN, R. E., PAGE, J. R., GARCIA, U. C.: Crystalline aflatoxin M_1 from urine and milk. Nature **215**, 753 (1967).
54. MCGLASHAN, N. D.: Oesophageal cancer and alcoholic spirits in central Africa. Gut **10**, 643 (1969).

55. MILLER, E. C., MILLER, J. A.: Low carcinogenicity of the K-region epoxides of 7-methylbenz(a)anthracene and benz(a)anthracene in the mouse and rat. Proc. Soc. exp. Biol. Med. (N. Y.) **124**, 915 (1967).
56. MILLER, E. C., MILLER, J. A., BROWN, R. R., MACDONALD, J. C.: On the protective action of certain polycyclic aromatic hydrocarbons against carcinogenesis by aminoazo dyes and 2-acetylaminofluorene. Cancer Res. **18**, 469 (1958).
57. MILLER, J. A.: Carcinogenesis by chemicals: An overview. Cancer Res. **30**, 559 (1970).
58. — MILLER, E. C.: Metabolic activation of carcinogenic aromatic amines and amides *via* *N*-hydroxylation and *N*-hydroxy-esterification and its relationship to ultimate carcinogens as electrophilic reagents. In BERGMANN, E. D., PULLMAN, B. (Eds.): Jerusalem Symposia on Quantum Chemistry and Biochemistry I., p. 237. Jerusalem: 1969.
59. MIRVISH, S. S.: The carcinogenic action and metabolism of urethan and *N*-hydroxyurethan. Advanc. Cancer Res. **11**, 1 (1968).
60. MORRIS, J. E., PRICE, J. M., LALICH, J. J., STEIN, R. J.: The carcinogenic activity of some 5-nitrofuran derivatives in the rat. Cancer Res. **29**, 2145 (1969).
61. NAPALKOV, N. P.: Peculiarities of experimental liver carcinogenesis in combined action of different carcinogens and antithyroid drugs. Ninth International Cancer Congr., Tokyo 1966, Abstracts, p. 115.
62. NERY, R.: Acylation of cytosine by ethyl *N*-hydroxycarbamate and its acyl derivatives and the binding of these agents to nucleic acids and proteins. J. Chem. Soc. (C) **14**, 1860 (1969).
63. NOVELLI, G. D., ORTWERTH, B. J., DEL MONTE, U., ROSEN, L.: Studies on the alkylation of rat-liver transfer RNA by the hepatocarcinogen ethionine. In: Genetic Concepts and Neoplasia, p. 409. Baltimore: Williams and Wilkins 1970.
64. PREUSSMANN, R., DRUCKREY, H., IVANKOVIC, S., . HODENBERG, A.: Chemical structure and carcinogenicity of aliphatic hydrazo, azo, and azoxy compounds and of triazenes, potential *in vivo* alkylating agents. Ann. N. Y. Acad. Sci. **163**, 697 (1969).
65. PRICE, J. M., PAMUKCU, A. M.: The induction of neoplasms of the urinary bladder of the cow and the small intestine of the rat by feeding bracken fern (Pteris aquilina). Cancer Res. **28**, 2247 (1968).
66. PULLMAN, A., PULLMAN, B.: A quantum chemist's approach to the mechanism of chemical carcinogenesis. In BERGMANN, E. D., PULLMAN, B. (Eds.): Jerusalem Symposia on Quantum Chemistry and Biochemistry I., p. 9. Jerusalem: 1969.
67. PURCHASE, I. F. H., VAN DER WATT, J. J.: Carcinogenicity of sterigmatocystin. Food Cosmet. Toxicol. **8**, 289 (1970).
68. REUBER, M. D., GLOVER, E. L.: Cirrhosis and carcinoma of the liver in male rats given subcutaneous carbon tetrachloride. J. nat. Cancer Inst. **44**, 419 (1970).
69. ROSE, E. F.: The interplay of factors determining a cancer pattern. Progr. exp. Tumor Res. **12**, 95 (1969).
70. SANDER, J., BÜRKLE, G.: Induktion maligner Tumoren bei Ratten durch gleichzeitige Verfütterung von Nitrit und sekundären Aminen. Z. Krebsforsch. **73**, 54 (1969).
71. SCHOENTAL, R.: Hepatotoxic activity of retrorsine, senkirkine and hydroxysenkirkine in newborn rats, and the role of epoxides in carcinogenesis by pyrrolizidine alkaloids and aflatoxins. Nature **227**, 401 (1970).

72. SEGI, M., KURIHARA, M., MATSUYAMA, T.: Cancer mortality for selected sites in 24 countries, Vol. 5 (1964–1965). Sendai: Tohoku Univ. School Med. 1969.
73. SEN, N. P., SMITH, D. C., SCHWINGHAMER, L.: Formation of *N*-nitrosamines from secondary amines and nitrite in human and animal gastric juice. Food Cosmet. Toxicol. **7**, 301 (1969).
74. SPATZ, M.: Toxic and carcinogenic alkylating agents from cycads. Ann. N. Y. Acad. Sci. **163**, 848 (1969).
75. SPIEGELMAN, S., BURNY, A., DAS, M. R., KEYDAR, J., SCHLOM, J., TRAVNICEK, M., WATSON, K.: Characterization of the products of RNA-directed DNA polymerases in oncogenic RNA viruses. Nature **227**, 563 (1970).
76. STASZEWSKI, J., HAENSZEL, W.: Cancer mortality among the Polish-born in the United States. J. nat. Cancer Inst. **35**, 291 (1965).
77. STEKOL, J. A.: Biochemical basis for ethionine effects on tissues. Advanc. Enzymol. **25**, 369 (1963).
78. SUGIMURA, T., FUJIMURA, S., KOGURE, K., BABA, T., SAITO, T., NAGAO, M., HOSOI, H., SHIMOSATO, F., YOKOSHIMA, T.: Production of adenocarcinomas in glandular stomach of experimental animals by *N*-methyl-*N'*-nitro-*N*-nitrosoguanidine. Gann Monograph No. 8, p. 157 (1969).
79. SUGIURA, K., TELLER, M. N., PARHAM, J. C., BROWN, G. B.: A comparison of the oncogenicities of 3-hydroxanthine, guanine 3-N-oxide, and some related compounds. Cancer Res. **30**, 184 (1970).
80. TEMIN, H. M., MIZUTANI, S.: RNA-dependent DNA polymerase in virions of Rous sarcoma virus. Nature **226**, 1211 (1970).
81. TS'O, P. O. P., LESKO, S. A., UMANS, R. S.: The physical binding and the chemical linkage of benzpyrene to nucleotides, nucleic acids and nucleohistones. In BERGMANN, E. D., PULLMAN, B. (Eds.): Jerusalem Symposia on Quantum Chemistry and Biochemistry I., p. 106. Jerusalem: 1969.
82. VAN DUUREN, B. L.: Carcinogenic epoxides, lactones and haloethers and their mode of action. Ann. N. Y. Acad. Sci. **163**, 633 (1969).
83. WEINSTEIN, I. B.: Modifications in transfer RNA during chemical carcinogenesis. In: Genetic Concepts and Neoplasia, p. 380. Baltimore: Williams and Wilkins 1970.
84. WEISBURGER, E. K., GRANTHAM, P. H., WEISBURGER, J. H.: Differences in the metabolism of *N*-hydroxy-*N*-2-fluorenylacetamide in male and female rats. Biochemistry **3**, 808 (1964).
85. — YAMAMOTO, R. S., GLASS, R. M., GRANTHAM, P. H., WEISBURGER, J. H.: Effect of neonatal androgen and estrogen injection on liver tumor induction by *N*-hydroxy-*N*-2-fluorenylacetamide and on the metabolism of this carcinogen in rats. Endocrinology **82**, 685 (1968).
86. WEISBURGER, J. H., GRANTHAM, P. H., VANHORN, E., STEIGBIGEL, N. H., RALL, D. P., WEISBURGER, E. K.: Activation and detoxification of *N*-2-fluorenylacetamide in man. Cancer Res. **24**, 475 (1964).
87. — YAMAMOTO, R. S., GLASS, R. M., FRANKEL, H. H.: Prevention by arginine glutamate of the carcinogenicity of acetamide in rats. Toxicol. appl. Pharmacol. **14**, 163 (1969).
88. — — GRANTHAM, P. H., WEISBURGER, E. K.: Evidence that sulfate esters are key ultimate carcinogens from *N*-hydroxy-*N*-2-fluorenyl-acetamide. Proc. Amer. Ass. Cancer Res. **11**, 82 (1970).
89. WHYATT, P. L., CRAMER, J. W.: Urinary excretion of *N*-hydroxy-2-acetylaminofluorene (N-OH-AAF) by rats given phenobarbital. Proc. Amer. Ass. Cancer Res. **11**, 83 (1970).

90. WILK, M., GIRKE, W.: Radical cations of carcinogenic alternant hydrocarbons, amines and azo dyes, and their reactions with nucleobases. In BERGMANN, E. D., PULLMAN B. (Eds.): Jerusalem Symposia on Quantum Chemistry and Biochemistry I., p. 91. Jerusalem: 1969.
91. WOGAN, G. N.: Naturally occurring carcinogens in foods. Progr. exp. Tumor Res. **11**, 134 (1969).
92. WYNDER, E. L., MANTEL, N.: Some epidemiological features of lung cancer among Jewish males. Cancer **19**, 191 (1966).
93. — KAJITANI, T., ISHIKAWA, S., DODO, H., TAKANO, A.: Environmental factors of cancer of the colon and rectum. II. Japanese epidemiological data. Cancer **23**, 1210 (1969).
94. YAMAGIWA, K., ICHIKAWA, K.: Experimentelle Studien über die Pathogenese der Epithelialgeschwülste. Mitt. med. Fak. Tokyo **15**, 295 (1916).
95. YAMAMOTO, R. S., GLASS, R. M., FRANKEL, H. H., WEISBURGER, E. K., WEISBURGER, J. H.: Inhibition of the toxicity and carcinogenicity of *N*-2-fluorenylacetamide by acetanilide. Toxicol. appl. Pharmacol. **13**, 108 (1968).

Zum Biochemismus carcinogener Nitrosamine

Von

F. W. Krüger

Zusammenfassung

1. An Transplantationstumoren von Ratten und Mäusen wurde die alkylierende und tumorhemmende Wirkung von ^{14}C-Dimethylnitrosamin und ^{14}C-Methylnitrosoharnstoff untersucht. Nach intravenöser Applikation von ^{14}C-Dimethylnitrosamin war keine Bildung von 7-Methylguanin in der Ribonucleinsäure des Tumors nachweisbar. Hingegen kam es nach intravenöser Gabe von ^{14}C-Methylnitrosoharnstoff zu einer gut nachweisbaren Methylierung des Guanins der Tumor-RNS. In Korrelation zu diesen Beobachtungen steht der chemotherapeutische Effekt von Methylnitrosoharnstoff, während Dimethylnitrosamin keine tumorhemmende Wirkung besaß.

2. Die nach Applikation beider Verbindungen beobachtete biologische Inkorporation der ^{14}C-Aktivität in die Purinbasen der Tumor-RNS konnte bei hepatektomierten Ratten nicht mehr beobachtet werden.

3. Untersuchungen der Ribonucleinsäuren aus Leber und Muskulatur von Regenbogenforellen nach Gabe von ^{14}C-Methylnitrosoharnstoff führten zu ähnlichen Ergebnissen, wie sie bei der Analyse der Tumor-Ribonucleinsäuren hepatektomierter Ratten nach Applikation der gleichen Verbindung beobachtet wurden.

4. Es wird für die Bildung des Methylkations aus Methylnitrosoharnstoff und Dimethylnitrosamin als gemeinsame Zwischenstufe die intermediäre Bildung einer Methylnitrosocarbaminsäure angenommen, die auf verschiedenen Reaktionswegen aus DMNA und NMH entsteht. Dies läßt eine Deutung der unterschiedlichen Organotropie der Alkylierung beider Verbindungen zu.

5. Die metabolische Bildung von Formaldehyd läßt sich durch die Oxydation des primär gebildeten Methylalkohols erklären, welcher durch Reaktion des Methylkations mit den OH-Gruppen des Wassers entsteht.

Erschienen in Z. Krebsforsch. **74**, 434–447 (1970).

Zur Synthese neuartiger Nitrosamine

Von

M. Wiessler

Dialkylnitrosamine bilden die hinsichtlich ihrer cancerogenen Wirkung wohl am besten untersuchte chemische Substanzenklasse. Wie von Druckrey et al. [*1*] nachgewiesen wurde, bedingt die Art der Alkylsubstitution in starkem Maße die cancerogenen Eigenschaften. Symmetrisch substituierte Nitrosamine induzieren bei oraler Gabe im wesentlichen Lebertumoren, unsymmetrisch substituierte dagegen hauptsächlich Speiseröhrenkrebs. Cyclische Nitrosamine oder solche mit funktionellen Gruppen zeigen keine einheitliche Organotropie. In Kenntnis dieser Unterschiede stellte sich uns die Frage: Genügt bereits das Vorhandensein eines optisch aktiven Zentrums im Molekül des Nitrosamins, um die cancerogenen Eigenschaften der beiden Antipoden in verschiedener Weise zu beeinflussen? Oder anders formuliert: Sind die Enzyme, die bei der Metabolisierung des Nitrosamins zur cancerogenen Wirkform beteiligt sind, so spezifisch, daß sie die beiden Antipoden unterscheiden können?

Nitrosamine, deren Chiralitätszentrum der Amin-Stickstoff ist, sind bisher nicht bekannt. Um stabile, optisch aktive Nitrosamine zu erhalten, muß das Asymmetriezentrum in die aliphatische Seitenkette verlegt werden. Zur Synthese ist allgemein zu sagen, daß auf der Stufe des Amins die Trennung in die Antipoden vollzogen wird, die dann nach der üblichen Methode in die Nitrosamine übergeführt werden. Aus zwei Gründen wählten wir das α-Pipecolin oder 2-Methylpiperidin aus: Zum ersten ist die Racematspaltung beschrieben [*5*]; sie gelingt mit Hilfe von D- und L-Weinsäure recht einfach, so daß auch größere Mengen zugänglich sind, und zum anderen lassen sich beide Antipoden gewinnen, was zur Bestimmung der optischen Reinheit nicht ohne Bedeutung ist.

Die Trennung wird durchgeführt wie in Abb. 1 angezeigt. Nach Freisetzung der Basen aus den Tartraten zeigt sich, daß die Drehwerte für links- und rechtsdrehendes α-Pipecolin entgegengesetzt gleich sind. Die Drehwerte der daraus dargestellten Nitrosamine steigen durch die Einführung der polaren Nitrosogruppe erwartungsgemäß an, zeigen aber innerhalb der Fehlergrenzen den gleichen Betrag. Die von uns gefundenen Drehwerte für die optisch aktiven Basen stimmen nicht befriedigend

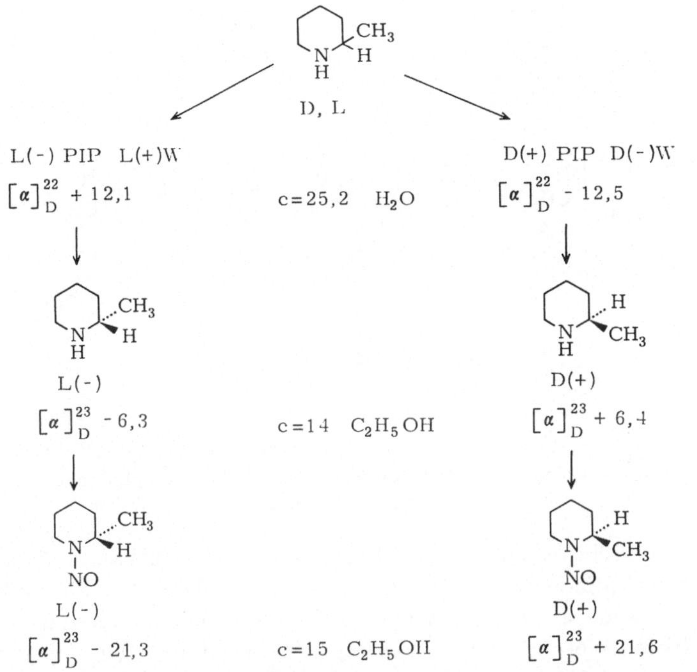

D, L

L(-) PIP L(+)W — $[\alpha]_D^{22}$ + 12,1 — c = 25,2 H_2O — D(+) PIP D(-)W — $[\alpha]_D^{22}$ - 12,5

L(-) $[\alpha]_D^{23}$ - 6,3 — c = 14 C_2H_5OH — D(+) $[\alpha]_D^{23}$ + 6,4

L(-) $[\alpha]_D^{23}$ - 21,3 — c = 15 C_2H_5OH — D(+) $[\alpha]_D^{23}$ + 21,6

Abb. 1. Syntheseschema der optisch aktiven Nitrosamine und Drehwerte der dargestellten Verbindungen

mit Literaturwerten [*3*, *4*, *5*, *6*] überein. Das bedeutet, daß unsere Basen nicht optisch rein sind. Dem entgegen steht ein allgemein anerkannter Befund. Gelingt es nämlich, beide Antipoden so, wie hier ausgeführt, auf unabhängigen Wegen darzustellen, zeigen diese oder ihre Salze bei weiterer Reinigung kein Ansteigen der Drehwerte mehr, und sind diese Drehwerte entgegengesetzt gleich, so gilt dieses schon als ein gutes Kriterium der optischen Reinheit, wenn auch nicht als ein absolutes.

Was ist optische Reinheit? Unter optischer Reinheit eines durch Racematspaltung gewonnenen Materials versteht man den Überschuß des einen Enantiomeren, ausgedrückt in Prozent des gesamten Materials; so beträgt bei einem Verhältnis der Antipoden von 80:20 der optische Reinheitsgrad 60%. Die Frage der optischen Reinheit ist in unserem Falle von Bedeutung. Zeigen die optisch aktiven Nitrosamine Unterschiede in der cancerogenen Wirkung, so können diese im Falle einer ungenügenden optischen Reinheit verwischt werden; ganz verschwinden können sie jedoch nicht. Selbst bei Anlegung kritischer Maßstäbe beträgt der optische Reinheitsgrad unserer Amine mit Sicherheit mehr als 80%.

Um eine sichere Entscheidung in der Frage der optischen Reinheit vornehmen zu können, wollen wir die korrelative Methode anwenden.

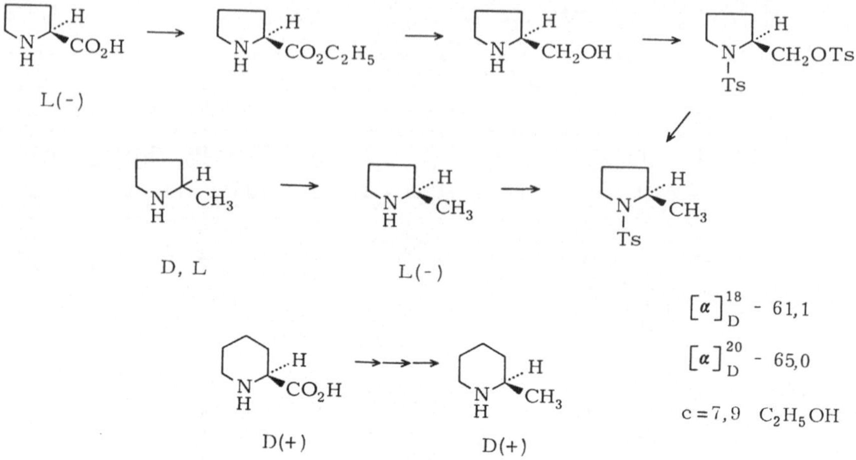

L(−) → → → (N-Ts)

D, L → L(−) → (N-Ts)

$[\alpha]_D^{18}$ − 61,1

$[\alpha]_D^{20}$ − 65,0

c = 7,9 C_2H_5OH

D(+) → → → D(+)

Abb. 2. Syntheseschema zur Bestimmung der optischen Reinheit nach der Korrelations-Methode

Ist die optische Reinheit einer Bezugssubstanz A bekannt, dann kann man einen Mindestwert für die optische Reinheit der Verbindung B angeben, wenn es gelingt, A und B chemisch ineinander umzuwandeln ohne Racemisierung, d. h. Änderung der Anordnung der Substituenten am Asymmetriezentrum. In unserem Falle wäre diese Bezugssubstanz die Pipecolinsäure, deren optische Reinheit bekannt ist und die sich chemisch in das Pipecolin umwandeln ließe (Abb. 2). Es gibt dazu ein Analogiebeispiel von Karrer [2], der diese Reaktionsfolge am Prolin durchgeführt hat. Nach dem in Abb. 2 angegebenem Schema wird das N-tosylierte Amin als Treffpunkt gewählt, das – obwohl auf verschiedenen Wegen gewonnen – in den Drehwerten nur eine geringe Differenz zeigt; d. h., während der Reaktionsabläufe tritt keine nennenswerte Racemisierung ein. Wir sind zur Zeit damit beschäftigt, diese Reaktionsfolge mit der Pipecolinsäure durchzuführen, und hoffen, dann eine präzise Aussage hinsichtlich der optischen Reinheit machen zu können.

Die toxikologischen Befunde der beiden Nitrosamine zeigen geringfügige Unterschiede. Bei oraler Gabe beträgt die DL_{50} für das L(−)-Pipecolin 600 mg/kg, für das D(+)-Pipecolin liegt sie etwas höher. Werden die Substanzen i.p. gespritzt, so sinken die Werte ab; für das L(−)-Pipecolin beträgt die DL_{50} dann 100 mg/kg, für das D(+)-Pipecolin liegt sie wiederum etwas höher. Zum Vergleich: Beim Nitrosopiperidin beträgt die DL_{50} bei oraler Gabe 200 mg/kg.

Obwohl die optische Reinheit der Nitrosamine noch nicht endgültig gesichert ist, haben wir den Tiertest auf cancerogene Wirkung schon begonnen. Dabei wird sich zeigen, ob zwischen optischer Aktivität der Nitrosamine und ihrer cancerogenen Wirkung eine Beziehung besteht.

Literatur

1. DRUCKREY, H., PREUSSMANN, R., IVANKOVIC, S., SCHMÄHL, D.: Organotrope carcinogene Wirkungen bei 65 verschiedenen N-Nitroso-Verbindungen an BD-Ratten. Z. Krebsforsch. **69**, 103 (1967).
2. KARRER, P., EHRHARDT, K.: Überführung optisch aktiver α-Aminocarbonsäuren in optisch aktive Amine mit gleichem Kohlenstoffskelett. Helv. Chim. Acta **34**, 2202 (1951).
3. LADENBURG, A.: Über das Isoconiin und den asymmetrischen Stickstoff. Chem. Ber. **26**, 854 (1893).
4. LEITHE, W.: Über die natürliche Drehung des polarisierten Lichtes durch optisch aktive Basen. Mh. Chem. **50**, 40 (1928).
5. MARCKWALD, W.: Über die optisch aktiven α-Pipecoline und das sogenannte Isopipecolin. Chem. Ber. **29**, 43 (1896).
6. TALLENT, W. K., HORNING, E. C.: The structure of pinidine. J. Amer. Chem. Soc. **78**, 4467 (1956).

Immunsuppression durch Carcinogene

Von

H. R. Scherf

Zahlreiche Untersuchungen aus jüngster Zeit haben gezeigt, daß einige krebserzeugende Substanzen eine immunsuppressive Wirkung besitzen. Die Arbeiten von Stjernswärd [6–8], Stutman [9], Gericke u. Mitarb. [2] und Kearney [4] berichten übereinstimmend, daß nach Gabe von Carcinogenen vom Typ der polycyclischen Kohlenwasserstoffe wie 20-Methylcholanthren, 3,4-Benzpyren und 7,12-Dimethyl-benzanthracen eine deutliche immunsuppressive Wirkung bei Versuchstieren zu beobachten war.

Zur Klärung der Frage, ob carcinogene N-Nitroso-Verbindungen ähnliche immunologische Eigenschaften besitzen, haben wir vier verschiedene Verbindungen dieses Typs oral an Ratten appliziert und auf immunsuppressive Wirkung untersucht: das Dimethylnitrosamin und das N-Nitrosomorpholin (die bei oraler Gabe Leberkrebs hervorrufen), den Methyl-nitrosoharnstoff (der Magencarcinome induziert) und das asymmetrisch gebaute Aethyl-n-butyl-nitrosamin (das vorwiegend zu Ösophaguscarcinomen führt) [1].

Methodik

Als Versuchstiere verwendeten wir männliche Ratten des Stammes Sprague-Dawley, welche bei Versuchsbeginn ca. 250 g schwer waren. Sie wurden mit Altromin-Pellets und Wasser ernährt.

In einem ersten Versuch gaben wir den Versuchstieren eine einmalige Dosis von 40% der DL_{50} der oben genannten Verbindungen per os mit der Schlundsonde, und zwar 16 mg/kg Dimethylnitrosamin, 152 mg/kg Aethyl-n-butyl-nitrosamin, 128 mg/kg N-Nitroso-morpholin und 44 mg/kg Methyl-nitrosoharnstoff.

Eine weitere Untersuchung führten wir nach oraler Applikation einer geringeren Dosis (7% der DL_{50}) dieser vier Nitroso-Verbindungen durch, welche jeweils einmal wöchentlich über 7 Wochen hinweg gegeben wurde. Die Wochendosis betrug demnach beim Dimethylnitrosamin 2,8 mg/kg, beim Aethyl-n-butyl-nitrosamin 26,6 mg/kg, im Falle des N-Nitrosomorpholins 22,4 mg/kg und des Methyl-nitroso-harnstoffs 7,7 mg/kg.

Zur Immunisierung verwendeten wir Schaferythrocyten. Diese wurden nach der letzten Gabe der Testsubstanz intraperitoneal injiziert, und zwar in einer Konzentration von 10^9 Erythrocyten pro Versuchstier in 1 ml physiologischer Kochsalzlösung.

Die Immunreaktion verfolgten wir hierauf über 12 Tage mit Hilfe des Plaque-Tests nach JERNE [*3*]. Das Prinzip dieses Tests besteht darin, daß man Hämolysin-bildende Zellen sichtbar macht. Zu diesem Zweck töteten wir pro Test- bzw. Kontrollgruppe und Versuchstag 5 Tiere, deren Milz wir herauspräparierten und zu einer Milzzellsuspension verarbeiteten. Nach Auszählung der Zellkonzentration dieser Suspensionen in einer Zählkammer wurden zu 2 ml einer 42° C warmen, 0,7%igen Agar-Lösung in Eagle-Earle's Medium, die einen Zusatz von 1 mg DEAE-Dextran enthielt, 0,1 ml einer 25%igen Schaferythrocyten-Suspension und 0,1 ml einer Milzzellsuspension hinzugefügt. Jede 2 ml-Portion wurde gut gemischt und in Petrischalen mit 9 cm Durchmesser ausgegossen, welche tags zuvor mit 20 ml einer 1,4%igen Agarlösung in Eagle-Earle's Medium versetzt worden waren. Nach der Inkubation der Platten für 60 min bei 37° C pipettierten wir 2 ml von frischem, 1:15 verdünntem Meerschweinchenserum als Komplementdonator auf die Testschicht und stellten die Platten für weitere 45 min in den Inkubator. Nach Beendigung der Reaktion wurden die entstandenen Plaques mittels eines Colony-Counters unter dem Stereomikroskop ausgezählt.

Die in den Milzzellen während der Inkubation synthetisierten Hämolysine diffundieren radial in die Umgebung, in der die Erythrocyten liegen, und bilden dort mit diesen Antigen-Antikörper-Komplexe. Durch die Komplementaktivität tritt deshalb in unmittelbarer Umgebung derjenigen Zellen, welche dieses spezifische Immunglobulin bilden, Hämolyse auf.

Die Ergebnisse des Plaque-Tests wurden als Plaques pro 10^6 Milzzellen berechnet und als Funktion von der Zeit nach der Immunisierung dargestellt.

Ergebnisse

Mit dieser Methodik konnten wir feststellen, daß die einmalige hohe Dosis von 40% der DL_{50} der Nitroso-Verbindungen bei den so behandelten Tieren keine deutliche Proliferationshemmung der immunglobulinbildenden Zellen verursacht. Die gegenüber der Kontrollgruppe auftretenden Differenzen kann man eher als primär-toxische Effekte deuten, zumal die Gabe der Nitroso-Verbindungen lediglich zu einem verspätet auftretenden Maximum der Proliferationsrate der Hämolysin-bildenden Zellen führt.

Die Tabelle stellt die Plaque-Bildung nach Gabe von 7% der DL_{50} der Carcinogene einmal wöchentlich über 7 Wochen dar. Sie zeigt,

Tabelle. *Proliferation immunglobulinbildender Zellen in der Milz von Sprague-Dawley-Ratten nach 7 wöchiger Vorbehandlung mit 7% der DL_{50} der vier N-Nitroso-Verbindungen einmal wöchentlich. Die Ergebnisse sind als Plaques pro 10^6 Milzzellen dargestellt (Mittelwerte ± Standardabweichungen von 5 Tieren pro Tag und Gruppe)*

Tag nach der Immunisierung	Kontrolle	Dimethyl-nitrosamin	N-Nitroso-morpholin	Aethyl-n-butyl-nitros-amin	Methyl-nitroso-harnstoff
2	11 ± 7	20 ± 29	10 ± 6	9 ± 3	4 ± 2
3	22 ± 14	44 ± 16	23 ± 4	55 ± 21	32 ± 12
4	174 ± 102	109 ± 67	94 ± 70	98 ± 94	149 ± 62
5	1812 ± 333	434 ± 434	469 ± 442	1302 ± 569	568 ± 225
6	1028 ± 350	752 ± 667	554 ± 404	623 ± 108	526 ± 334
7	142 ± 145	113 ± 92	143 ± 101	87 ± 31	103 ± 45
8	180 ± 117	167 ± 89	197 ± 80	225 ± 90	199 ± 132
9	463 ± 193	126 ± 73	350 ± 106	292 ± 111	171 ± 95
10	239 ± 72	204 ± 115	92 ± 84	131 ± 77	86 ± 36
11	324 ± 152	203 ± 51	196 ± 147	267 ± 55	303 ± 171

daß trotz erheblicher Streuung der Meßwerte, die mehrmalige Gabe der kleineren Dosis bei allen behandelten Tieren im Bereich des Proliferationsmaximums eine deutliche Verminderung der Hämolysin-bildenden Milzzellen bewirkt. Die Zahl der gebildeten Plaques beträgt hier – außer bei mit Aethyl-n-butyl-nitrosamin behandelten Ratten – meist weniger als die Hälfte der Werte bei den Kontrollen.

Diskussion

Unsere Untersuchungen haben gezeigt, daß eine mehrmals applizierte kleine Dosis von Nitroso-Verbindungen zu einer deutlichen Hemmwirkung auf die Bildung von IgM-Hämolysin produzierenden Milzzellen führt, eine einmalige hohe Dosis dagegen nicht.

Inwieweit diese Erscheinung mit der Cancerisierung zusammenhängt, können wir nach diesen vorläufigen Versuchen nicht beurteilen. Zwar könnten die Befunde, welche nach Gabe der polycyclischen Kohlenwasserstoffe gewonnen wurden, die immunsuppressive Wirkung als eine Eigenschaft aller Carcinogene nahelegen; doch mag man bedenken, daß es viele Substanzen gibt, die zwar immunsuppressive, aber keine carcinogenen Eigenschaften besitzen – z. B. einige Antimetabolite [5].

Um hier eindeutige Aussagen machen zu können, müssen weitere Langzeitversuche, insbesondere mit unterschiedlicher Dosierung verschiedener Carcinogene, durchgeführt werden; dabei sollte neben der Wirkung auf die humorale Immunität auch geprüft werden, inwieweit die Immunzellen beeinflußt werden.

Literatur

1. Druckrey, H., Preussmann, R., Ivankovic, S., Schmähl, D.: Organotrope carcinogene Wirkungen bei 65 verschiedenen N-Nitroso-Verbindungen an BD-Ratten. Z. Krebsforsch. **69**, 103 (1967).
2. Gericke, D., Chandra, P., Wacker, A.: Inhibition of immune response after tumor transplantation and chemical carcinogenesis in mice. Z. Krebsforsch. **75**, 85 (1970).
3. Jerne, N. K., Nordin, A. A., Henry, C.: The agar plaque technique for recognizing antibody producing cells. In Amos, B. and Koprowski, H. (Eds.): Cell-bound Antibodies, pp. 109. Philadelphia: Wistar Institute Press 1963.
4. Kearney, R., Hughes, L. E.: The effect of tumour growth on immune competence. A study of DMBA mammary carcinogenesis in the rat. Brit. J. Cancer **24**, 319 (1970).
5. Scherf, H. R., Krüger, C., Karsten, C.: Untersuchungen an Ratten über immunosuppressive Eigenschaften von Cytostatica unter besonderer Berücksichtigung ihrer carcinogenen Wirkung. Arzneimittel-Forsch. **20**, 1467 (1970).
6. Stjernswärd, J.: Effect of bacillus Calmette-Guérin and of methylcholanthrene on the antibody-forming cells measured at the cellular level by a hemolytic plaque test. Cancer Res. **26**, 1591 (1966).
7. Stjernswärd, J.: Age-dependent tumor-host barrier and effect of carcinogen-induced immunodepression on rejection of isografted methylcholanthrene-induced sarcoma cells. J. nat. Cancer Inst. **37**, 505 (1966).
8. Stjernswärd, J.: Studies on host immune status and tumor-host relationships in hydrocarbon carcinogenesis. Stockholm: Balder 1967.
9. Stutman, O.: Carcinogen-induced immune depression: Absence in mice resistant to chemical oncogenesis. Science **166**, 620 (1969).

Neue Aspekte der Aktivierung carcinogener aromatischer Amine und Amide

Von

M. Traut, H. Bartsch und E. Hecker

Zusammenfassung

N-hydroxy-N-acetyl-2-aminofluoren (N-OH-AAF) läßt sich mit $K_3[Fe(CN)_6]$ unter milden Bedingungen zu einem freien Nitroxidradikal oxydieren, das durch UV- und IR-Spektren charakterisiert wird. Das Radikal disproportioniert spontan zu 2-Nitrosofluoren und N-acetoxy-N-acetyl-2-aminofluoren. Derselbe Reaktionstyp läuft im System Peroxidase/H_2O_2/N-OH-AAF ab und wird an Rattenlebermikrosomen untersucht. Der Mechanismus dieser Oxydationsreaktion und seine Bedeutung für die Aktivierung von N-OH-AAF *in vivo* wurde diskutiert.

Ausführliche Darstellung in Bartsch, H., Traut, M., Hecker, E.: Biochim. Biophys. Acta **237**, 556—566 (1971) sowie Bartsch, H., Hekker, E.: Biochim. Biophys. Acta **237**, 567—578 (1971).

Proliferation Control of Normal, Neoplastic and Virus-Transformed Human Glia Cells

By

J. PONTÉN and B. WESTERMARK

Malignant cells in an expanding population have a proliferation rate which exceeds their death rate. The multiplication does not have to be extremely rapid, it is in many instances slower than that of non-neoplastic cells. The single most characteristic feature of malignant cells *in vivo* is their inability to stop dividing rather than a high growth rate *per se*.

A series of observations have suggested that lack of growth control can be assessed *in vitro* [*15*]. Attention has been focused on "loss of contact inhibition". Contact inhibition was originally introduced to denote a specific membrane to membrane interaction among normal cells, which led to paralysis of locomotion. Loss of it was found in certain sarcoma cells [*2*, *3*]. Later the term has been extended to cover lack of proliferation control. The basis for this is the tendency of a variety of normal cells to be confined to monolayered growth and to show strong growth retardation, once the extensive mutual cell contacts of a complete cell sheet have been established. This control can be broken by tumorigenic viruses which induce the formation of multilayered, apparently unrestrained cell multiplication. Cultures of experimental *in vivo* tumors also show signs of a similar disturbed growth control. The phenomenon is referred to as loss of contact (or density dependent) inhibition of cell division [*17*].

The idea that loss of contact inhibition of cell division reflects an essential property of neoplastic cells has not been remained unchallenged. KRUSE and MIEDEMA [*8*] performed extensive experiments where a variety of lines have been perfused with large volumes of medium. All malignant, established, heteroploid lines which, under standard conditions, showed loss of contact inhibition of division also displayed these features under perfusion. The only normal diploid line studied – WI-38 human embryonic lung fibroblasts – did not deviate from this pattern and it was concluded that the apparent controlled growth of WI-38 on a standard regimen was an artefact, "... more a reflection of the *in vitro* culture methods employed than, . . . a property derived from monolayer cell to cell contact . . ." [8]. EAGLE *et al.* [5] did not find a good correlation between loss of contact inhibition of cell division and tumorigenicity in a variety of mammalian cell lines. These studies, taken together, imply that all cells, regardless of their non-neoplastic or neoplastic origin, multiply with little or no restraint *in vitro*. Any separation between normal and malignant cells would be based on arbitrarily chosen culture conditions.

The controversy about the importance of loss of proliferation control *in vitro* can partly be explained by use of incomparable pairs of normal and tumor cells. The main cause is, however, of a technical nature. No method has been described which unequivocally measures growth control and its loss under well defined stable tissue culture conditions.

We approached this problem in a two-fold manner. A search for stable cells led us to human brain cells. With the notable exception of lymphoid tissue [*11*, *12*], all normal human organs give rise to stable lines. By this we mean that they are of a uniform morphologic appearance, diploid and – what is most important – fail to transform spontaneously into heteroploid, pleomorphic, infinitely growing cell lines [*6*]. Human tissues contrast sharply with those of rodent origin which are notoriously unstable in culture. Mouse tissues, for instance, transform spontaneously into permanent, tumorigenic, heteroploid lines with a frequency of 100% within a few months after explantation [*16*].

Normal human brain cells can be compared with neoplastic cells from human gliomas or glia cells transformed by neoplastic viruses (Rous sarcoma virus or simian virus 40).

The second important factor concerns the culture conditions. By employing an excess of medium, it has been possible to create a "steady state" where the effects of environmental factors on cell growth can be checked under stable circumstances. A "steady state" is defined as a condition where the supply of medium is sufficient to maintain the concentration of metabolites and other growth factors within the optimal range for maximally fast growth.

Proliferation Control of Normal Glia-Like Cells

Explants of non-neoplastic adult human brain obtained from operations on aneurysms etc. invariably give rise to serially transferrable cell lines. These are composed of uniform elements of astrocyte-like appearance [*14*]. It has not yet been definitely proved by the identification of a specific cell product that these cells are of glial origin. The star-shaped cells are, however, morphologically distinct and differ from meningocytes and other fibroblasts. Partly by exclusion of other possibilities, we have concluded that they are of astrocytic origin. They are referred to as normal glia-like cells (Fig. 1).

A consecutive series of more than 25 glia-like lines have been studied. They have a total life span *in vitro* corresponding to 15–30 subcultivations at a 1:2 split ratio. During the last 5 passages they show progressive, irreversible, degenerative changes of the same nature as those reported for "phase III" human fibroblasts [*6*, *9*].

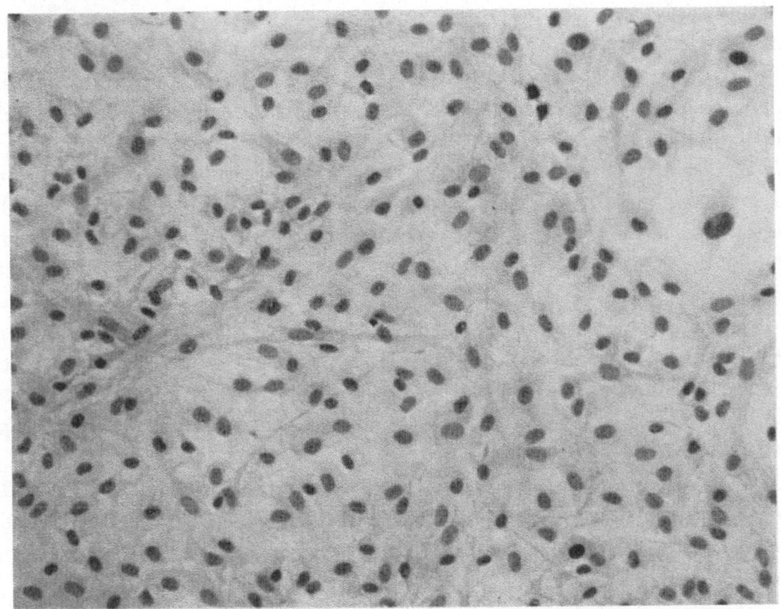

Fig. 1. A complete sheet of normal glia-like cells at a density of about 100,000 cells/cm². Note virtual absence of nuclear overlapping and regularity of growth pattern

Prior to phase III, the glia-like lines have remarkably similar features. A one-step growth curve begins with a latent period of about 24 h after which the cells enter a logarithmic growth phase with a population doubling time of around 20 h. Under a standard regimen with change of medium (Eagle's minimal essential, MEM, with 10% calf serum and antibiotics) twice a week, they will reach a density of $6–7 \times 10^4$ cells/cm² plastic surface. In this phase DNA synthesis and mitotic rate decrease sharply. After 24 h of exposure to tritiated thymidine, 3 days after a medium change, less than 0.5% of the cells will become labelled indicating a strong degree of "contact inhibition of cell division". The inhibition can temporarily be counteracted by addition of fresh medium (an undialyzable serum component is the active factor), which leads to

DNA synthesis in an estimated 5–10% of the cells [*14*], if a short pulse of radioactive thymidine is used as a tracer.

The discontinuous supply of fresh medium under the standard regimen and its effect on cell growth raised the question of the mechanism for the growth restraint. Is it caused by exhaustion of the medium, accumulation of inhibitors or the creation of a special intercellular relationship? Kruse and Miedema have suggested [*8*] that all cells are potentially capable of unrestrained one-step growth, provided that they are abundantly supplied with new nutrient fluid. This implies that "contact inhibition of cell division" may be an artefact imposed by an insufficient medium supply. In order to test this the following experiment was set up as described in detail elsewhere [*19*]. Glia-like cells were seeded onto small (3 cm ∅) punched-out plastic disks. These were then incubated (37° C; 5% CO_2 in air) in a large Petri dish containing 50 ml of MEM with different concentrations of calf serum. The cells were immersed at the same depth as in a 50 mm ∅ Petri dish with 5 ml of fluid, ensuring the same conditions of gaseous exchange as under the standard regimen. Medium was changed at 24 h intervals.

A special set of experiments showed that increasing the frequency of medium change over one per day did not lead to any enhanced cell growth. Medium harvested from these cultures was as efficient as fresh medium in stimulating cell growth. The large volume and frequent change of medium, therefore, met our criteria for a "steady state".

Cell growth curves were constructed from glia-like cells under steady state conditions. An assembly of such curves is given in Fig. 2. It is seen

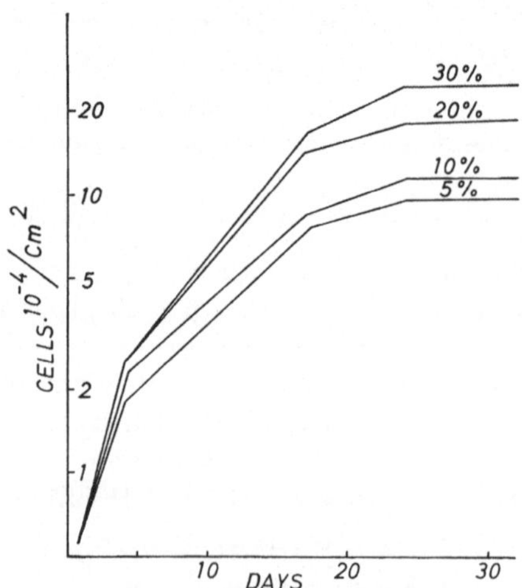

Fig. 2. Growth curves of normal glia-like cells under steady state conditions at various concentration of serum

that they retain the basic shape already established under the standard regimen. A post-logarithmic phase commencing around day 20 with only very slow or no growth can clearly be identified. The density at which this is reached increased with the serum concentration. The steady level at 10% calf serum (12×10^4 cells/cm^2) was about twice that seen under the standard regimen. It corresponds to a dense monolayer with little nuclear (but considerable cytoplasmic) overlapping.

The most important inference from this experiment is that glia-like cells have a mechanism for growth restraint which cannot be explained by exhaustion of the medium or secretion of inhibitors. In both these instances, an increase in the frequency of medium change would enhance growth – an effect which was not observed. Instead, special intercellular relations seem to be responsible for cessation of proliferation.

Simultaneously with the present studies, DULBECCO [*4*] introduced the term "topoinhibition" to denote topographical factors which inhibit DNA synthesis in a cell layer. He investigated the response of different cell types to wounding, i.e., the creation of a defect by scratching of a cell layer [*10*]. Depending on the concentration of serum and type of cells, a varying stimulation of DNA synthesis was obtained along the wound. The labelling index in the wound minus the labelling index (tritiated thymidine) in the unscored layer is divided by the first parameter and the quotient is used as a numerical expression for topoinhibition. The analysis was not carried out during steady state conditions, but at such a low serum concentration that any effect of serum would be minimal. As our inhibition most probably reflects the same phenomenon, we adopted DULBECCO's terminology.

The establishment of topoinhibition under steady state conditions is unexpected in the light of the findings of KRUSE and MIEDEMA [*7*, *8*]. These authors *inter alia* studied one normal diploid line – WI-38 embryonic lung fibroblasts. It can be compared with our glia-like cells, since it has been derived from normal tissue and did not undergo spontaneous transformation. The WI-38 line showed but a relative growth inhibition and it was considered likely that contact inhibition phenomena were unimportant in checking cell multiplication even in dense cultures. KRUSE and MIEDEMA's experiments lasted 8 days only and the density (50×10^4 cells/cm^2) at which the perfusion was stopped was not maximal for embryonic lung fibroblasts. It was not excluded that a continuation of the perfusion would have led to complete cessation of growth, *albeit* at a higher level than that reached by the glia-like cultures. Another interesting feature is that our rate of fluid renewal on a per cell basis exceeded that of KRUSE and MIEDEMA by a factor of about 7.

The establishment of topoinhibition is important because it makes further studies possible with a defined quantifiable parameter. It can be measured in our system as a function of the difference in slope of the growth curve during the postexponential and exponential phase respectively.

Topoinhibition in Mixtures of Normal Cells

Dulbecco's and our own method are suitable only for assessment of topoinhibition within a uniform cell population. It would, however, also be desirable to be able to measure topoinhibition between different types of cells.

To make this possible, we utilized the unusual capacity of glia-like cells to form almost perfectly stationary monolayers under medium conditions which permit rapid exponential growth (MEM/10% calf serum). The principle of the experiment is outlined in Fig. 3. Test cells are seeded onto preformed stationary glia-like cells and bare plastic surfaces. The proliferation of the test cells is then monitored by electronic cell counting. Control experiments with autoradiography of test or bottom cells labelled with tritiated thymidine have shown that the computed growth is only ascribable to test cell multiplication in this system, because the bottom cell layer is not influenced by the addition of the test cells. If no test cell proliferation is seen in the mixed cultures, total inhibition exists. If the proliferation is equally rapid in the presence and absence of the stationary glia-like cells, no inhibition has been established. Intermediate values can be calculated as percent growth inhibition.

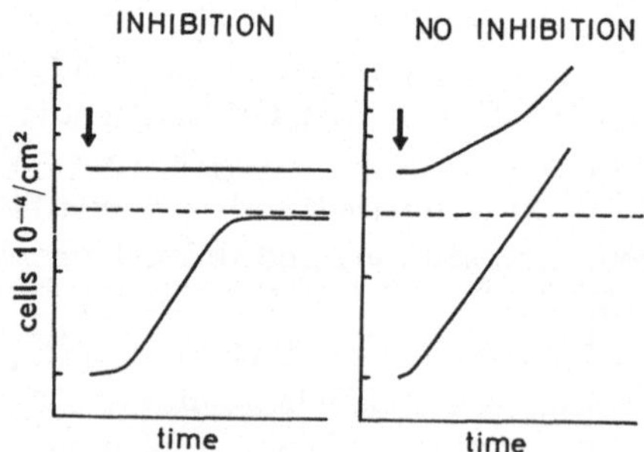

Fig. 3. Growth of test cells seeded on top of stationary monolayers. The dotted lines indicate growth in the bottom layer. The lower uninterrupted curves symbolize multiplication of test cells grown in isolation. The two upper curves exemplify proliferation of the respective test cells after seeding on top of stationary monolayers

The multiplication of the following test cells was found to be completely curtailed: syngeneic or allogeneic glia, allogeneic adult meningocytes or skin fibroblasts, embryonic chicken or quail fibroblasts. From this we concluded that topoinhibition exerted by adult human glia-like cells may cross species, tissue and histocompatibility barriers.

One exception to the rule that normal glia-like cells inhibit other normal cells has been found. Human embryonic lung fibroblasts showed 85% growth inhibition in contrast to 100% found with the other cell types. The reason for the aberrant behaviour of these cells has not been understood. It may be due to synthesis of insulating sheets of collagen or to an unusually high sensitivity to serum stimulation.

Proliferation Control of Glioma Cells

Extensive experience with unselected series of malignant human tumors has shown that more than 99% of them have a short life span after explantation *in vitro* [*10*]. The literature only contains a few documented instances of establishment of permanent tumor lines derived from solid neoplasms.

We have explanted a consecutive series of biopsies from brain tumors during the last 4 years [*13, 18*]. From malignant gliomas grade III-IV 11 permanent lines have been obtained which corresponds to a success rate of about 15%. This seems to be the highest figure observed in any human tumor material and our collection of glioma lines is the largest reported from a consecutive unselected series of biopsies.

Two characteristics are used to define the glioma lines as being of neoplastic origin. The first is the presence of an infinite growth potential. A large number of human cell lines have been tested in our laboratory and elsewhere for their long term growth capacity. With the exception of normal lymphoid tissue [*12*], every variety of normal organs or cells has only given rise to mortal lines, i.e., after a variable number of passages the cells stopped multiplying and deteriorated. Our 11 glioma lines differ from this pattern being capable of an endless number of divisions.

The second characteristic is heteroploidy. Normal glia cells remain diploid prior to phase III in contrast to the tumor-derived cells which have shown varying types of departure from a normal chromosomal pattern during their entire life span *in vitro* [*18*].

The morphology of the glioma lines has been extremely variable, ranging from rather monomorphic spindle cells to larger somewhat epithelial-like pleomorphic elements. In certain lines an astrocyte-like appearance can be discerned [*18*].

The growth pattern, cytology and chromosomes are sufficiently different to give each line its individual profile (see Figs. 4 and 5).

The reasons why most gliomas do not give established lines are unknown. It does not seem to be due to maltreatment of the biopsy

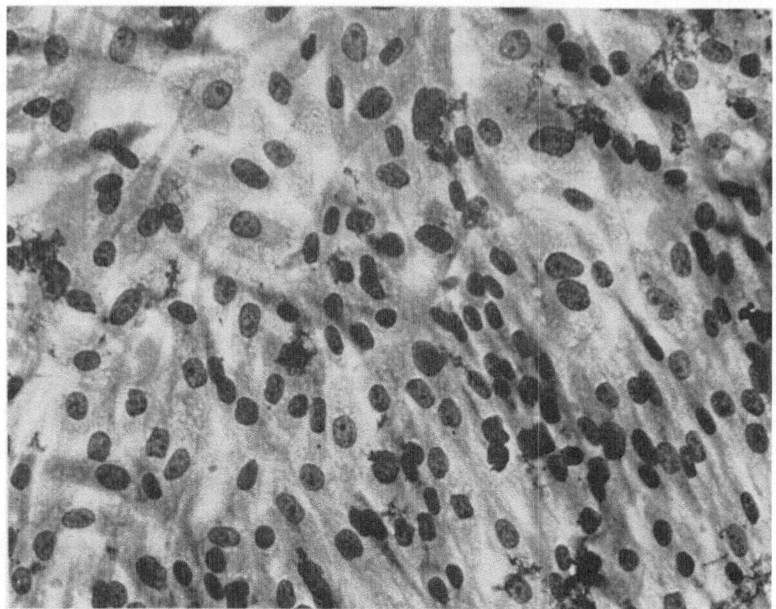

Fig. 4. An established glioma cell-line. Note irregular overlapping growth pattern and nuclear pleomorphism in contrast to Fig. 1

because, in most instances, temporary growth of glioma cells is obtained which is later superseded by multiplication of normal looking glia.

Seven of the established glioma lines have been tested under the same conditions as the mixtures of normal cells. Four of the lines did not respond to the presence of stationary normal glia-like cells by any inhibition. The remainder ranged from 85–100% inhibition. The line with the strongest degree of inhibition did not differ significantly from the embryonic lung fibroblast in this test.

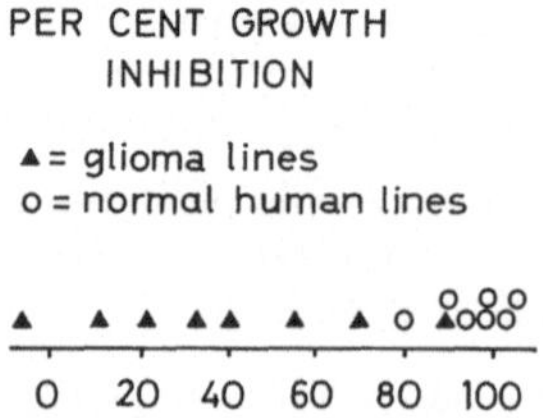

PER CENT GROWTH
INHIBITION

▲ = glioma lines
o = normal human lines

0 20 40 60 80 100

Fig. 5. Growth inhibition among test cells seeded on top of the stationary glia-like cells. Per cent inhibition is calculated by comparing multiplication rates according to Fig. 3

The use of a panel of glioma lines could thus show that the degree of manifest inhibition may vary over a wide spectrum. The most significant common feature was a failure to ever show the perfect inhibition of all normal lines (except embryonic lung fibroblasts).

Discussion

Two findings of this presentation seem to be of particular significance. The first concerns the mechanism for proliferation restraint of normal cells. Multiplication declined sharply in a predictable manner at a defined density in spite of the abundant supply of fresh medium created by the frequent renewal of large volumes. This would seem to rule out the possibility that secretion of inhibitory soluble molecules by the cells played a decisive role in their growth retardation because such substances would be expected to be washed out. There was also no evidence of any exhaustion of the medium with respect to non-specific metabolites or specific growth promoting macromolecular serum factors. Our interpretation of the growth inhibition is based on the special topographical relations which exist among glia cells at terminal density. Our knowledge about these relations is still fragmentary but two major hypotheses have been formulated. One postulates that specific cell to cell interactions are of importance [*2*]. When normal cells come in close mutual contact, plasma membrane movement ("ruffling") is completely curtailed along the line of contact. The cells may then receive no signals to initiate DNA synthesis and, therefore, remain stationary in the G1 phase [*15*]. Support for this hypothesis was derived from a study where time-lapse cinematography showed cessation of ruffling to coincide with a sharp decline in DNA synthesis in normal glia-like cells [*14*]. This may, however, have been coincidental and the cited experiments do not prove a cause and effect relationship.

The other hypothesis assumes that uptake of serum factor from the medium has a strong influence on cell growth. Zetterberg and Auer [*20*] found a direct linear correlation between cell surface area and labelling index (tritiated thymidine) in mouse embryo kidney epithelium which, to a large extent, was independent of the presence or absence of lateral cell to cell contacts. They proposed that the size of the cell surface available for growth factor uptake from the medium determines the length of the cell cycle. A small area will automatically lead to slow growth. A normal cell in culture will have a finite minimal surface area below which a given serum concentration is insufficient to permit uptake of enough growth factor. This will lead to a complete arrest in G1. Our results are compatible with both these explanations and it is thus not known if topoinhibition is a reflection of the establishment of stable lateral cell to cell contacts or the altered cell form which follows cell crowding and leads to a diminished cell surface area or a combination of both. Further exploration of the dynamics of a steady state should permit a distinction between the two possibilities.

The results with the glioma cells strongly suggest that it should be possible to define a specific proliferation control defect among neoplastic elements at least at the level of the cell population. All glioma lines were characterized by deficient growth inhibition after contact with stationary normal cells. The degree of this deficiency varied within wide limits. The growth rate of a few glioma lines was reduced considerably, but 3 of 7 showed no reduction. Unpublished observations indicated that virus-transformed cells fall in the latter category.

The variability among the glioma lines has proved a stable property. It is not known if all cells in a population are equally susceptible to inhibition or constitute a stabilized mixture between cells of different degrees of sensitivity to topoinhibition by normal cells.

Previous attempts to demonstrate a consistent difference between normal and neoplastic cells in vitro have not been entirely successful. In certain mouse lines a correlation was found between terminal density and tumorigenicity [*1*]. This relation cannot, however, be generalized because in other systems considerable overlapping occurs. Normal embryonic human lung fibroblasts will, for instance, reach a considerably higher density than certain of our glioma lines.

Some virus-transformed cells never show any inhibition of cell division at high densities in contrast to normal cells of the same origin [*15*].

References

1. Aaronson, S., Todaro, G. J.: Basis for the acquisition of malignant potential by mouse cells cultivated in vitro. Science **162**, 1024 (1968).
2. Abercrombie, M., Heaysman, J. E. H., Karthauser, H. M.: Social behaviour of cells in tissue culture. III. Mutual influence of sarcoma cells and fibroblasts. Exp. Cell Res. **13**, 276 (1957).
3. Abercrombie, M., Ambrose, E. J.: The surface properties of cancer cells: a review. Cancer Res. **22**, 525 (1962).
4. Dulbecco, R.: Topoinhibition and serum requirement of transformed and untransformed cells. Nature **227**, 802 (1970).
5. Eagle, H., Foley, G. E., Koprowski, H., Lazarus, H., Levine, E. M., Adams, R. A.: Growth characteristics of virus-transformed cells. Maximum population density, inhibition by normal cells, serum requirement, growth in soft agar, and xenogeneic transplantability. J. exp. Med. **131**, 863 (1970).
6. Hayflick, L., Moorhead, P.: The serial cultivation of human diploid cell strain. Exp. Cell Res. **25**, 585 (1961).
7. Kruse, P. F., Jr., Miedema, E. J.: Production and characterization of multiple layered populations of animal cells. J. Cell Biol. **27**, 273 (1965).

8. Kruse, P. F., Whittle, W., Miedema, E. J.: Mitotic and nonmitotic multiple-layered perfusion cultures. J. Cell Biol. **42**, 113 (1969).
9. Macieira-Coelho, A., Pontén, J., Philipson, L.: The division cycle and RNA-synthesis in diploid human cells at different passage levels *in vitro*. Exp. Cell Res. **42**, 673 (1966).
10. Moore, C. E., Koike, A.: Growth of human tumour cells in vitro and in vivo. Cancer **17**, 11 (1964).
11. Moore, G. E., McLimans, W. F.: The life span of the cultured normal cell: Concepts derived from studies of human lymphoblasts. J. theor. Biol. **20**, 217 (1968).
12. Nilsson, K., Pontén, J., Philipson, L.: Development of immunocytes and immunoglobulin production in long-term cultures from normal and malignant human lymph nodes. Int. J. Cancer **3**, 183 (1968).
13. Pontén, J., Macintyre, E.: Long term culture of normal and neoplastic human glia. Acta path. microbiol. scand. **74**, 465 (1968).
14. Pontén, J., Westermark, B., Hugosson, R.: Regulation of proliferation and movement of human glia-like cells in culture. Exp. Cell Res. **58**, 393 (1969).
15. Pontén, J.: Spontaneous and virus-induced transformation in cell culture. Wien-New York: Springer 1971.
16. Sanford, K. K.: Malignant transformation of cells in vitro. Int. Rev. Cytol. **18**, 249 (1965).
17. Stoker, M., Rubin, H.: Density dependent inhibition of cell growth in culture. Nature **215**, 171 (1967).
18. Westermark, B., Pontén, J., Hugosson, R.: Determinants for establishment of permanent tissue culture lines from malignant human glioma. To be published.
19. Westermark, B.: Results to be published.
20. Zetterberg, L., Auer, G.: Proliferative activity and cytochemical properties of nuclear chromatin related to local cell density of epithelial cells. Exp. Cell Res. **62**, 262 (1970).

Genetische Eigenschaften des Herpesvirus hominis

Von

KL. MUNK und G. LUDWIG

Seit der Beobachtung des Epstein-Barr-Virus in Zellen des Burkitt-Tumors und seitdem dieses Virus als herpesähnlich identifiziert wurde [*2*], ist bei der Suche nach einer möglichen Virusätiologie menschlicher Tumoren die besondere Aufmerksamkeit auf die Herpesvirusgruppe gelenkt worden. Auch das Herpesvirus hominis (HVH) wurde in den Kreis der Virusarten einbezogen, die möglicherweise onkogene Eigenschaften besitzen.

In früheren Untersuchungen [*3–5*] haben wir verschiedene Merkmale beschrieben, mit denen sich aus genitaler Lokalisation isolierte HVH-Stämme von solchen unterscheiden, die aus Effloreszenzen von Lippe, Haut oder Cornea stammen. Die genitalen Stämme zeigen charakteristische plaquemorphologische Eigenschaften. Sie bilden im Plaquetest nach DULBECCO u. VOGT [*1*] neben den kleinen Plaques, wie sie auch die nicht-genitalen Stämme produzieren, Plaques mit einem dreimal größeren Durchmesser.

In neueren Untersuchungen haben wir [*6*] dieses plaquemorphologische Merkmal genauer untersucht. Wir isolierten Virusklone aus den Plaques der beiden verschiedenen Größenordnungen. Dabei zeigte es sich, daß Virusklone, die von einem großen Plaque abgeleitet worden waren, auch nach wiederholtem Plaque-Klonen jedesmal Plaques sowohl vom großen als auch vom kleinen Typ produzierten. Es war niemals möglich, einen Virusklon zu erhalten, der nur große Plaques zeigt. Demgegenüber produzierten die Virusklone, die aus einem Plaque vom kleinen Typ isoliert worden waren, auch nach wiederholtem Isolieren von Klonen aus einer Klonlinie immer nur Plaques vom kleinen Plaquetyp.

Dieses Phänomen könnte so gedeutet werden, daß das Virus, welches das genetische Merkmal „Großplaque" besitzt, dieses Merkmal nur in Gegenwart des Genoms mit dem Merkmal „Kleinplaque" ausdrücken kann. Es könnte sich also beim „Großplaque"-Genom um ein defektes Virusgenom handeln.

Um diese Hypothese experimentell zu bestätigen, haben wir Versuche im Sinne eines „marker rescue experiment" unternommen.

Material und Methoden

Virus: Für diese Versuche wurde Virusmaterial der Klonlinien „Großplaqueklon" und „Kleinplaqueklon" des Virusstammes HOF verwendet, der aus genitaler Lokalisation isoliert worden war [*3*]. Die hier verwendeten Klone waren durch 7mal wiederholtes Isolieren von Plaqueklonen gewonnen worden [*6*]. Die Bestimmung des Virustiters erfolgte im Plaquetest nach Dulbecco u. Vogt [*1*].

Zellkultur: Für Versuche, Plaquetests und Viruspassagen wurden HeLa-Zellkulturen in Hanks'scher Lösung mit 0,5% Lactalbuminhydrolysat, 5% bzw. 10% Kälberserum und Antibiotica benutzt. Die Viruspassagen erfolgten in Vierkantflaschen und die Plaqueversuche in 6 cm ∅ Plastik-Petri-Schalen. Beim Plaquetest wurde dem Nährmedium 0,8% Agar zugefügt und als Vitalfarbstoff Jodnitrotetrazolium-Chlorid verwendet.

UV-Inaktivierung des Virus: Das für das „marker rescue experiment" verwendete Virusmaterial, dessen Infektionstiter vorher bestimmt worden war, wurde in Hanks'scher Lösung suspendiert und davon 1 ml in 6 cm ∅ Plastik-Petri-Schalen – in einer Schichtdicke von ca. 0,5 mm – während einer Dauer von 1 min bzw. 2 min bei einem gleichbleibenden Lampenabstand von 5 cm mit der Quarzlampe (Fa. Hanau, Modell Original Hanau Sterisol F 1137) inaktiviert. Diese Dauer und Intensität der UV-Bestrahlung wurde in Vorversuchen als ausreichend ermittelt, um eine Reduzierung des Infektionstiters von 2 bzw. 3 Zehnerpotenzen zu erreichen.

Versuchsansatz: In unserem Versuchsansatz verwendeten wir als inaktiviertes Virus das Material, bei dem durch die UV-Inaktivierung eine Titerreduktion um 2 bzw. 3 Zehnerpotenzen erreicht worden war. Das UV-inaktivierte Virusmaterial vom „Kleinplaqueklon" wurde mit dem nicht inaktivierten Virusmaterial vom „Großplaqueklon" zusammengebracht, und der daraus resultierende Titer im Plaquetest zugleich mit dem Plaquetiter der beiden Komponenten ermittelt. Aus der Addition der Plaquezahlen der beiden Komponenten ergab sich der theoretische Wert, der als Vergleich zu dem im Versuch erhaltenen Wert diente.

Ergebnis und Diskussion

Das „marker rescue experiment" sollte klären, ob das partiell UV-inaktivierte Virusgenom mit dem Merkmal „Kleinplaque" die Ausprägung des „defekten" Virusgenoms mit dem Merkmal „Großplaque" begünstigt.

Es erbrachte folgendes Ergebnis: In einer Reihe von Versuchsansätzen wurde dem Virus vom „Großplaqueklon" das UV-inaktivierte

Tabelle. *Ergebnisse des Marker Rescue Experiments (Einzelheiten s. Text)*

I	II			III			IV		
HOF/KLEIN inaktiviert	HOF/GROSS nicht inaktiviert			HOF/GR + HOF/KL nicht inaktiv. inaktiv.			THEORET. WERT HOF/GR + HOF/KL nicht inaktiv. inaktiv.		
Anzahl der Plaques									
KL	GES	GR	KL	GES	GR	KL	GES	GR	KL
24	92	35	57	194	106	88	116	35	81
12	92	35	57	172	98	74	104	35	69
12	45	14	31	118	67	51	57	14	43

Material vom „Kleinplaqueklon" zugefügt. Wie aus der Tabelle zu ersehen ist, zeigte sich im Versuchsergebnis eine etwa dreifach höhere Zahl von *großen* Plaques (Spalte III) als der theoretische Wert (Spalte IV) erwarten ließ, der sich aus der Addition der effektiven Plaquezahlen des UV-inaktivierten Virusmaterials (Spalte I) und des nicht inaktivierten Virusmaterials (Spalte II) ergibt. Die Zahl der kleinen Plaques war nicht wesentlich erhöht.

Aus diesem Experiment ist zu erkennen, daß sich die Ausprägung des „Großplaque"-Merkmals durch Zufügen von „Kleinplaque"-Genomen aktivieren läßt. Das bestätigt, daß das „Großplaque"-Genom defekt sein muß und zu seiner genetischen Funktion die Hilfe des „Kleinplaque"-Genoms benötigt. Bemerkenswert ist es, daß diese besondere Eigenschaft, ein defektes Genom zu enthalten, unter den von uns untersuchten HVH-Stämmen nur die Stämme besitzen, die aus genitaler Lokalisation isoliert worden waren. Es handelt sich also hierbei um eine besondere genetische Eigenschaft dieser HVH-Stämme.

Literatur

1. Dulbecco, R., Vogt, M.: Plaque formation and isolation of pure lines with poliomyelitis viruses. J. exp. Med. **99**, 167 (1954).
2. Epstein, M. A., Achong, B. G., Barr, Y. M.: Virus particles in cultured lymphoblasts from Burkitt's lymphoma. Lancet **1964**, I, 702.
3. Munk, K., Donner, D.: Cytopathischer Effekt und Plaque-Morphologie verschiedener Herpes-simplex-Virusstämme. Arch. ges. Virusforsch. **13**, 529 (1963).
4. Munk, K., Fischer, H.: Fluoreszenzimmunologische Unterschiede bei Herpes-simplex-Virus-Stämmen. Arch. ges. Virusforsch. **15**, 539 (1965).
5. Munk, K., Waldeck, C.: Kernrandveränderungen bei Herpes-simplex-Virus-infizierten HeLa-Zellen. Naturwissenschaften **11**, 567 (1969).
6. Munk, K., Ludwig, G.: In Vorbereitung.

Die Kontrolle der Tumorvirus-Genaktivität

Von

G. Sauer

Die kleinen DNS-Tumorviren können eine Zelle auf verschiedene Weise beeinflussen: Der Kontakt einer Zelle mit einem DNS-Tumorvirus kann entweder zu einer produktiven Infektion oder aber zur Transformation führen. In einer produktiv infizierten Zelle findet Virusvermehrung statt, eine neue Generation infektiöser Virusteilchen reift heran, und die Zelle wird lysiert. Im Gegensatz dazu läuft in einer transformierten Tumorzelle keine Virusvermehrung ab. Solche transformierten Zellen sind weiterhin teilungsfähig und bleiben frei von infektiösem Virus.

In einer produktiv infizierten Zelle sind alle Gene des Virusgenoms aktiv [*4*]. Alle Virusfunktionen werden in diesem Falle für die Herstellung von Virusnachkommenschaft benötigt. Andererseits beruht der Umstand, daß in einer durch das Virus transformierten Tumorzelle die Virusvermehrung unterbleibt, darauf, daß in einer solchen Zelle nur ein Teil des Virusgenoms in Funktion ist.

Wieviele der auf der Virus-DNS befindlichen Gen-Funktionen in einer Zelle aktiv sind, läßt sich anhand der von der Virus-DNS kopierten Messenger-RNS analysieren. Man bedient sich dazu der DNS-RNS-Hybridisierungstechnik. Da die Virus-Messenger-RNS der Virus-DNS komplementär ist, vermag sich auch die Virus-Messenger-RNS unter geeigneten Reaktionsbedingungen an die Virus-DNS zu binden und einen DNS-RNS-Hybridkomplex zu bilden: Sind sämtliche Gene des Virus in einer Zelle aktiv, so wird auch die in der Zelle enthaltene Virus-Messenger-RNS zu 100% mit der Virus-DNS homolog sein. Die Frage, ob während eines Virusvermehrungscyclus alle Virusgene zugleich funktionieren oder ob sie im Laufe der Zeit in einer bestimmten Reihenfolge aktiviert werden, konnte bereits vor einiger Zeit entschieden werden [*1*, *5*, *6*]. Abb. 1 zeigt die schematische Darstellung der am Beispiel des SV40-Tumorvirus gewonnenen Ergebnisse. Während der produktiven Infektion werden die Virusgene schrittweise nacheinander, und zwar in zwei Gruppen, abgelesen. In der frühen Phase der Infektion, kurz nachdem das Virus in die Zelle eingedrungen ist, werden nur etwa 25% der Virus-DNS in Messenger-RNS übersetzt. Man spricht von sogenannter „früher“ Messenger-RNS. Erst in einer späteren, fortgeschrittenen Phase der Infektion, wenn die Virus-DNS-Replikation begonnen hat, werden außer „frühen“ auch die restlichen „späten“ Sequenzen der Virus-DNS abgelesen. Die Aktivierung solcher später Virusgene hängt ausschließlich davon ab, ob sich die Virus-DNS in der Zelle vermehren kann. Dies ist durch Verwendung einer Hemmsubstanz, eines Inhibitors der DNS-Synthese, nachgewiesen. Prüft man die nach Arabinofuranosylcytosin (ARA-C) in der Zelle synthetisierte Messenger-RNS, so stellt sich heraus,

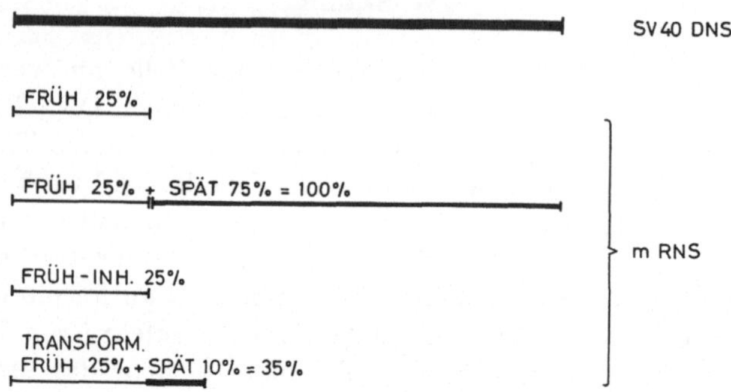

Abb. 1. Homologien zwischen SV40-DNS und SV40-Messenger-RNS. Die obere Linie gibt schematisch die relative Länge eines SV40-DNS-Stranges an. Die aus produktiv infizierten Zellen isolierte SV40-Messenger-RNS besitzt, abhängig vom Zeitpunkt nach der Infektion, verschiedene Homologien (komplementäre Basensequenz) mit der SV40-DNS. Vor dem Einsetzen der Virus-DNS-Replikation werden „frühe“ SV40-Messenger-RNS Sequenzen synthetisiert. Nach dem Beginn der SV40-DNS-Vermehrung kommen zu den „frühen“ noch neue, „späte“ SV40-Messenger-RNS Sequenzen hinzu. Die Synthese von „später“ Messenger-RNS bedarf der Virus-DNS-Replication: Inhibitoren der DNS-Synthese verhindern auch die Bildung „später“ Messenger-RNS in produktiv infizierten Zellen. In transformierten Zellen wird ein größerer Abschnitt der SV40-DNS abgelesen als „früh“ im produktiven Cyclus, jedoch fehlt ein großer Teil „später“ Messenger-RNS-Sequenzen

daß nur frühe Sequenzen abgelesen werden. Warum dies so ist, läßt sich zur Zeit noch nicht beantworten. Allerdings konnte die wichtige Frage, wieviele der Virusgene in einer durch das Virus transformierten Tumorzelle aktiv sind, bereits geklärt werden [*1*, *5*, *6*]. Es stellte sich heraus, daß außer den sog. frühen Genen nur einige der späten Gene aktiv sind. In einem solchen Falle ließ sich nachweisen, daß lediglich 35% des gesamten Virusgenoms abgelesen werden. Hier sind also über die 25% der frühen Gene hinaus auch 10% der späten Gene beteiligt.

Aus dieser Beobachtung stellt sich die Frage, ob auch unter Verwendung eines Inhibitors der DNS-Synthese die 10% der späten Gene in einer transformierten Zelle weiterhin abgelesen werden oder ob – wie im Falle der produktiven Infektion – nur die frühen Gene bei gehemmter Virus-DNS-Vermehrung aktiv bleiben. Eine Beantwortung dieser Frage würde klären, ob die Aktivierung des Virusgenoms in einer produktiven Infektion bzw. in einer transformierten Zelle verschiedenen Gesetzmäßigkeiten gehorcht.

Das Ergebnis unserer Untersuchungen ist in Abb. 2 zusammengefaßt. Werden in einer produktiv infizierten Zelle bei gehemmter Virus-DNS-Synthese nur 25% der Virus-DNS – nämlich frühe Gene – kopiert, so

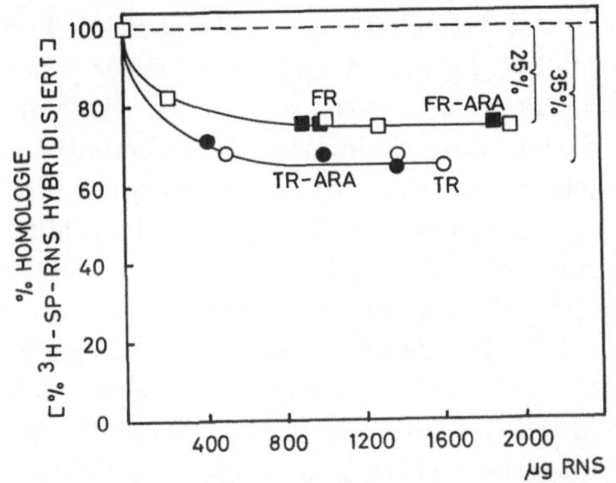

Abb. 2. Hybridisierungs-Kompetitionsexperiment. Jedes Reaktionsgemisch enthielt 0,05 µg immobilisierter SV40-DNS und 200 µg (^{3}H) „später" SV40-Messenger-RNS. Diese RNS-Menge sättigt die homologen DNS-Sequenzen zu 100%. Außerdem wurden den Hybridisierungsexperimenten verschiedene unmarkierte RNS-Präparationen in zunehmender Menge zugesetzt, um zu prüfen, inwieweit Homologien mit der (^{3}H) „späten" Messenger-RNS bestanden. Die Technik des Experiments wurde bereits beschrieben [*6*]. FR: RNS 16 Std nach der Infektion (p. i.) von CV-1 Zellen isoliert. FR-ARA: RNS 19,5 Std p. i. aus CV-1 Zellen isoliert, die während dieser Zeit mit 12,5 µg ARA-C/ml behandelt worden waren. TR: RNS aus SV40-transformierten Affennierenzellen (GMK-EVa). TR-ARA: RNS aus SV40-transformierten GMK-EVa-Zellen, die für 26 Std mit 12,5 µg ARA-C/ml behandelt worden waren

spielt es keine Rolle, ob man in der transformierten Zelle die DNS-Synthese selbst für mehr als einen Tag mit Hilfe von ARA-C hemmt oder nicht. In jedem Falle werden 35% des Virusgenoms kopiert. „Späte" Messenger-RNS-Sequenzen werden trotzdem synthetisiert. Offenbar unterliegt also in der transformierten Zelle die Aktivierung der Virusgene anderen Gesetzmäßigkeiten als im produktiven Vermehrungscyclus.

Die Interpretation dieser Ergebnisse ist schwierig, jedoch lassen sich verschiedene Möglichkeiten diskutieren. Die Transkription der Virus-DNS geschieht mit Hilfe eines Enzyms – der DNS-abhängigen RNS-Polymerase –, welches die Synthese von Messenger-RNS katalysiert. Dabei muß die Polymerase bestimmte, möglicherweise auf der DNS befindliche Stop-Start-Signale erkennen. Diese Signale müssen symbolisieren, welche Gene abgelesen werden und welche Gene nicht aktiviert werden. In jüngerer Zeit sind bei Bakterien bestimmte Faktoren entdeckt worden, welche einen kontrollierenden Einfluß auf die Polymerase ausüben [*2*, *7*]. Ob sie jedoch bei Säugetierzellen und bei transformierten Zellen eine Rolle spielen, ist noch nicht bekannt.

Andererseits könnte auch die physikalische Konfiguration der Virus-DNS selbst bestimmte Stop-Start-Signale freigeben. Diese Möglichkeit ist nicht auszuschließen, da die Virus-DNS in verschiedenen Konfigurationen auftreten kann. Innerhalb der Viruspartikel kommt sie als ein geschlossener Doppelstrangring in eng geknäuelter Superhelix-Konfiguration vor. In produktiv infizierten Zellen, in welchen sich die Virus-DNS vermehrt, findet man replikative Intermediate mit bestimmten Verzweigungsstellen im Molekül [*3*]. Zwar ist noch nicht bekannt, wie die Replikation im einzelnen vor sich geht; jedoch läßt sich vorstellen, daß dabei bestimmte Signale gegeben werden, welche die Polymerase erkennt. Ganz anders scheint die Virus-DNS in transformierten Krebszellen vorzuliegen. Hier ist die geschlossene, infektiöse Form nicht mehr nachweisbar; vielmehr muß die Virus-DNS als ein geöffnetes Molekül vorhanden sein. Möglicherweise ist diese lineare Form der Virus-DNS in die Zell-DNS integriert, so daß sich auf diese Weise vielleicht neue Anfangs- und Endstellen für die Ablesung ergeben. Ob dies jedoch der Fall ist, bedarf noch des Beweises.

Literatur

1. Aloni, Y., Winocour, E., Sachs, L.: Characterization of the simian virus 40-specific RNA in virus-yielding and transformed cells. J. mol. Biol. **31**, 415 (1968).
2. Burgess, R. R., Travers, A. A., Dunn, J. J., Bautz, E. K. F.: Factor stimulating transcription by RNA polymerase. Nature **221**, 43 (1969).
3. Levine, A. J., Kaug, H. S., Billheimer, F. E.: DNA replication in SV40 infected cells. J. mol. Biol. **50**, 549 (1970).
4. Martin, M. A., Axelrod, D.: SV40 activity during lytic infection in a series of SV40 transformed mouse cells. Proc. nat. Acad. Sci. **64**, 1203 (1969).
5. Oda, K., Dulbecco, R.: Regulation of transcription of the SV40 DNA in productively infected and in transformed cells. Proc. nat. Acad. Sci. **60**, 525 (1968).
6. Sauer, G., Kidwai, J. R.: The transcription of the SV40 genome in productively infected and transformed cells. Proc. nat. Acad. Sci. **61**, 1256 (1968).
7. Travers, A. A.: Positive control of transcription by a bacteriophage. Nature **225**, 1009 (1970).

The Abortive Transformation of Monkey Kidney Cells by SV40

By

E. C. Hahn

In the model systems which are used experimentally to study the development of malignancy, viral oncogenesis has the advantage that a genetic entity induces specific cellular alterations. These induced alterations are called "transformation". Viral transformation is characterized by the acquisition of growth and morphological changes, a new nuclear tumor antigen (T antigen) and surface antigens which are specific for the transforming virus, and, where it can be measured, an increased resistance to the inducing agent [*1*]. Current interest has been focused on whether the process is reversible.

Stoker [*7*] has reported that the initial alterations of transformation in the non-permissive cell system using polyoma virus and BHK21 hamster cells are not permanent in all cells. His criterion for transformation, the ability of transformed but not normal cells to form colonies in agar, was progressively lost from a portion of the originally altered cells after various numbers of divisions. Stoker has called this transiency of acquired properties "abortive transformation". Smith *et al.* [*6*] have reported similar observations using SV40 and the non-permissive host cell Balb/3T3.

African green monkey (AGMK) cells are permissive for SV40 and are, therefore, used generally as the assay system. The interaction of SV40 with these cells is lytic and results in cell death. However, the virus can interact infrequently with the result that cells become resistant to further infection and acquire the characteristics of transformed cells. These alternative fates, lysis or survival, depend on whether the cells are in stationary phase during the early stage of infection or growing [*2*]. The requirements for resistance development [*3*] are the same as the requirements for transformation [*8*].

Results from this laboratory have concerned the emergence of resistant cell colonies during the initial cycles of SV40 infection in cultures of growing AGMK cells [*3*]. The methods have been reported [*3*, *5*]. In this system, cells which are progressing to the transformed state are completely selected from the normal, susceptible cells. During the initial infection, large amounts of virus are produced by the majority of the cells. A small proportion of the cells grow to form colonies. The colonies withstand the high titers of progeny virus produced during the first week after infection and are able to grow at cell densities which are too low for establishment of normal, uninfected cells. Later, after repeated renewal of the culture medium, the level of virus in the culture drops. Loss of cells due to infection of virus-free cells would be expected to occur only during the initial cycles of replication when cells are exposed to large quantities of virus. The experimental results show, in contrast, that the initial number of surviving colonies continues to decrease during subsequent weeks in spite of decreasing concentrations of SV40.

In an experiment designed to quantitate the fate of the resistant colonies appearing after infection, CV-1 cells were infected, trypsinized, and seeded in 60 mm plastic Petri dishes where renewed growth could take place. With time after infection, decreasing numbers of the surviving colonies continued growth; many cells divided a few times and then ceased. During the 5 weeks observation period, the average number of colonies per plate decreased exponentially.

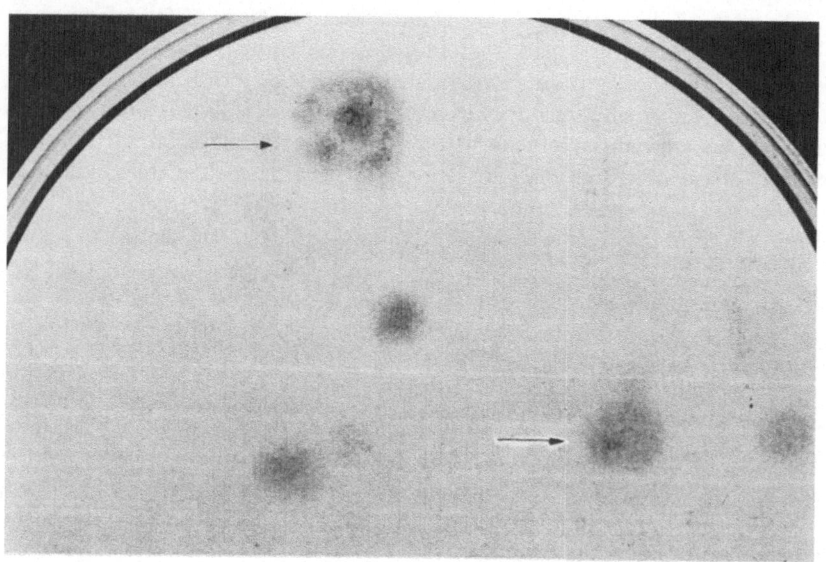

Fig. 1. Colonies of resistant CV-1 cells. 100,000 infected cells were seeded per 60 mm plastic Petri dish and incubated for 5 weeks before haematoxylin staining. Arrows show areas of secondary growth

A plate containing surviving colonies at 5 weeks after infection is shown in Fig 1. The colonies display different morphology and pattern of growth. Two colonies (arrows) contain areas where new growth of cells with morphology different from the remainder of the colony can be seen. In the upper example, renewed growth occurred at the periphery of the entire colony. The other example shows a segmented pattern. These modifications suggest that secondary genetic changes took place after the initial alteration from susceptibility to resistance.

In an attempt to monitor the appearance of the specific SV40 tumor antigen, coverslips were stained two weeks after infection and again several weeks later after the resistant cells had been transferred twice. At 2 weeks after infection, counts of several fields showed that an average of 20% of the cells were positive for T antigen. Cells after two passages exhibited almost 80% positive fluorescence for T antigen. Fully transformed cells are 100% T positive. Figs. 2a and b show a typical field in a 2 weeks old resistant colony as seen with both UV and phase optics. Of the T-positive nuclei, several are enlarged (arrows) and display a distribution of chromatin similar to that first described by HSIUNG and GAYLORD [*4*] for lytically infected AGMK cells. These swollen nuclei are presumably those in which lytic virus production is taking place. In the lower micrographs, after 2 passages (Figs. 2c, d), a higher percentage of positive cells can be seen. Here is also an absence of swollen nuclei; the cells are more homogenous.

The question arises as to whether the abortive transformation of permissive cells results from lytic virus production and cell death or from the fact that the density of cells is too low for their survival. Since many small colonies remain but do not grow, abortive transformation is in part due to loss of the initial growth stimulation by SV40. However, there is also virus production by cultures containing the resistant colonies and many nuclei appear lytic. With CV-1 cells this virus production continues for a long time. The results of infectious center assays have shown that not all cells produce virus at any one time. Virus production can be caused by either a few lytic cells which produce normal yields (in which case the cells would be killed) or by many cells which produce small amounts of virus (in which case they might survive).

A virus-shedding culture was examined by electron microscopy with the purpose of finding whether the occasional producing cells contained normal yields of virus. Fig. 3 is an electron micrograph of a cell whose nucleus is full of complete SV40 particles. This is exactly what is seen at the end of the infectious cycle just before lysis [*4*]. It indicates that some resistant cells which are producing virus can probably produce normal yields and are certainly killed in the process.

To summarize, when permissive cells are in exponential growth phase, a portion of the cells upon infection resist the lytic potential of the virus. All other cells are eliminated. Initially, the virus can be repressed to a greater extent than what is seen in later cultures of transformed cells,

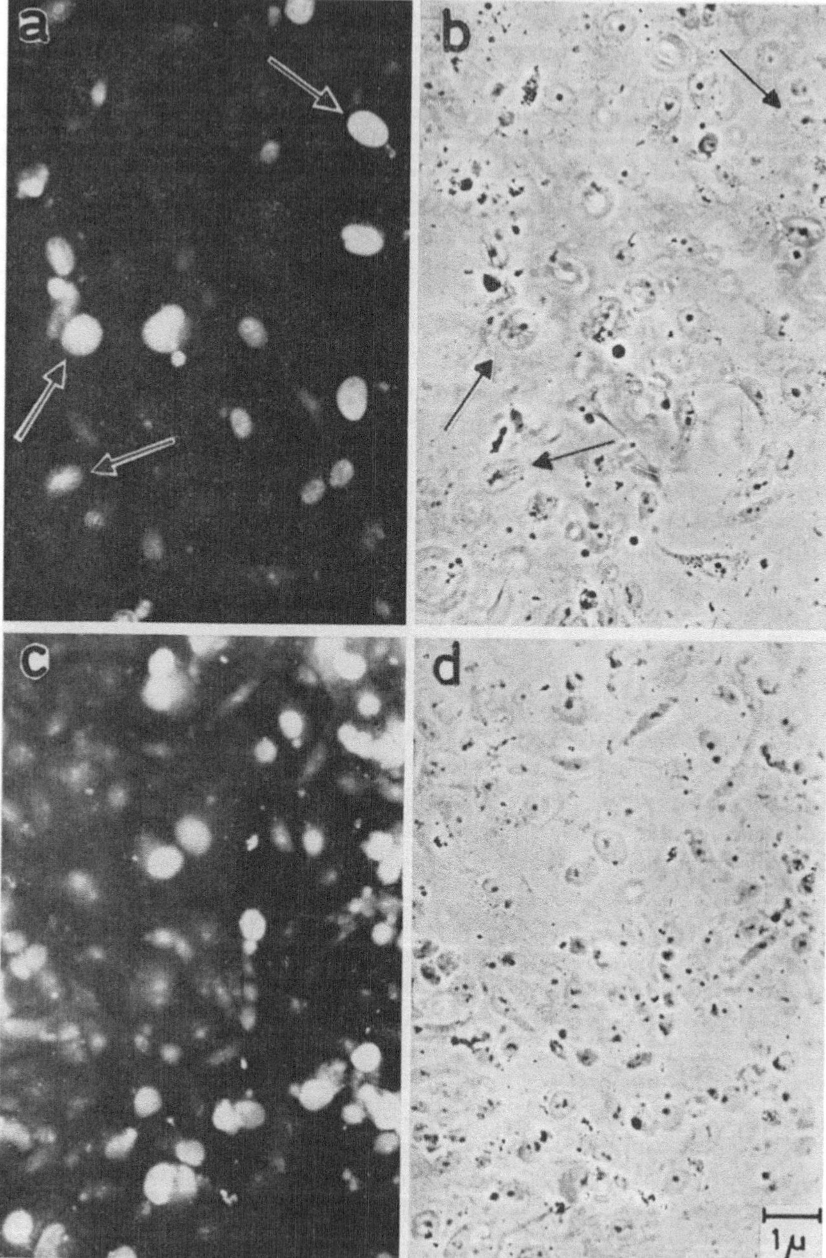

Fig. 2. Fluorescent and phase micrographs of surviving AGMK cells. (a and b): A portion of a colony, 2 weeks after infection. Examples of enlarged, positive nuclei are indicated with arrows. (c and d): Cells after 2 passages

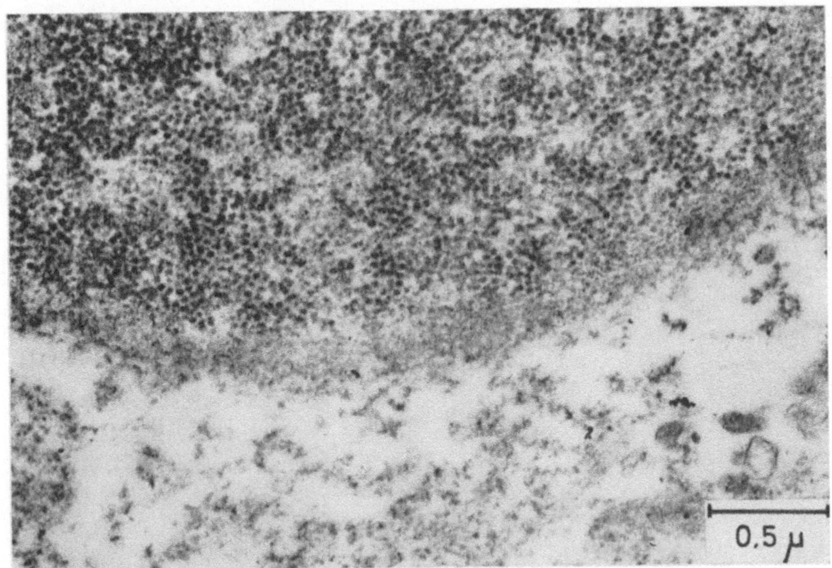

Fig. 3. Electron micrograph of a CV-1 cell, 45 passages after infection. A portion of the cell nucleus is shown containing mature SV40 particles in non-crystalline array

since in resistant colonies, many cells contain no detectible T antigen. Both resistance of the cells and the increased ability to grow in small numbers are initially reversible. In addition to changes back to the phenotype of susceptibility and limited cloning efficiency, resistant cells also undergo secondary genetic changes. These changes produce the more stable phenotype of the transformed cell.

In non-permissive systems, abortive transformation has been characterized as the loss of newly acquired growth potential. In the permissive system studied in this laboratory, where the initial resistance is critical for cell survival, abortive transformation results from the loss of initial resistance superimposed upon the loss of increased growth potential.

References

1. Black, P. H.: The oncogenic DNA viruses: A review of *in vitro* transformation studies. Ann. Rev. Microbiol. **22**, 391 (1968).
2. Carp, R. I., Gilden, R. V.: A comparison of the replication cycles of simian virus 40 in human diploid and African green monkey kidney cells. Virology **28**, 150 (1966).
3. Hahn, E. C., Sauer, G.: Initial stage of transformation of permissive cells by SV40: Development of resistance to productive infection. J. Virology **8**, 7 (1971).

4. Hsiung, G.-D., Gaylord, W. H.: The vacuolating virus of monkeys. I. Isolation, growth characteristics, and inclusion body formation. J. exp. Med. **114**, 975 (1961).
5. Sauer, G., Hahn, E.: The interaction of SV40 with SV40-transformed and non-transformed monkey kidney cells. Z. Krebsforsch. **74**, 40 (1970).
6. Smith, H. S., Scher, C. D., Todaro, G. J.: Abortive transformation of Balb/3T3 by simian virus 40. Bact. Proc. 1970. Abstracts of the 70th Annual Meeting Amer. Soc. for Microbiology, p. 187. Washington, D.C. 1970.
7. Stoker, M.: Abortive transformation by polyoma virus. Nature **218**, 234 (1968).
8. Todaro, G. J., Green, H.: Cell growth and the initiation of transformation by SV40. Proc. nat. Acad. Sci. **55**, 302 (1966).

Kinetik der Proteinsynthese in SV40-infizierten Affennierenzellen

Von

H. Fischer

Unser Modell für die Untersuchung der viralen Onkogenese ist die Reaktion einer Wirtszelle auf die Infektion mit dem onkogenen Virus SV40. Durch die Infektion wird eine Zellyse [*6*] oder eine Zelltransformation [*1*] herbeigeführt. In beiden Fällen kommt es zur Depression bzw. Induktion von Enzymen [*3*, *4*] und Antigenen [*5*], d. h. das Proteinmuster im Inneren der Zelle und an der Zelloberfläche erfährt eine wesentliche Änderung. Die grundlegenden Fragen sind: 1. wie verändert sich das Proteinmuster der normalen Zelle beim Übergang zur transformierten Zelle? 2. stammt die genetische Information vom Genom des Virus oder der Wirtszelle, oder kommt sie durch das Zusammentreffen beider zustande?

Wir haben die Änderungen im Proteinmuster einer SV40-infizierten Zelle im Vergleich zur normalen, nicht infizierten Zelle verfolgt [*2*]. Diese sind dann besonders interessant, wenn man mit SV40-transformierten Zellen vergleicht. Zu solchen Untersuchungen eignet sich die Methode der Polyacrylamidgel-Elektrophorese.

Für die Proteinaufarbeitung gibt es zwei Möglichkeiten: Man kann erstens mit Detergentien behandeln und erfaßt auf diese Weise auch einen großen Teil der zellulären Strukturproteine. Dabei gehen aber wesentliche biologische Eigenschaften der Proteine verloren, wie z. B. ihre enzymatische und serologische Aktivität. Nach dieser Aufarbeitung können die Proteine nur mit Hilfe ihrer elektrophoretischen Wanderung charakterisiert werden.

In unseren Versuchen haben wir uns für die zweite Aufarbeitungsmöglichkeit entschieden, bei der die löslichen Proteine mit Ammoniumsulfat ausgefällt werden und die biologische Aktivität erhalten bleibt. In allen Experimenten wurden CV-1-Zellen – ein Affennieren-Dauer-Zellstamm – mit 20 Plaque-bildenden Einheiten SV40-Virus beimpft. Die nicht infizierten Kontrollkulturen wurden in gleicher Weise mit gebrauchtem Medium behandelt. Zu verschiedenen Zeiten nach der Infektion wurden die SV40-infizierten und die nicht infizierten Zellen geerntet. Dann wurden die Zellen gefroren, getaut und beschallt. Die löslichen Proteine der Zellen wurden in 0,05 M KH_2PO_4 (pH = 7,5) aufgenommen und bei 60% Ammoniumsulfatsättigung gefällt.

Die Proteine wurden dann auf eine 7,5%ige Polyacrylamidgelsäule aufgesetzt. Ein charakteristisches Disc-Muster, das nach der eben beschriebenen Methode erhalten wurde, zeigt die Abb. 1. Hier ist der Zeitpunkt 48 Std p. i. am Ende des einstufigen Vermehrungscyclus gewählt worden.

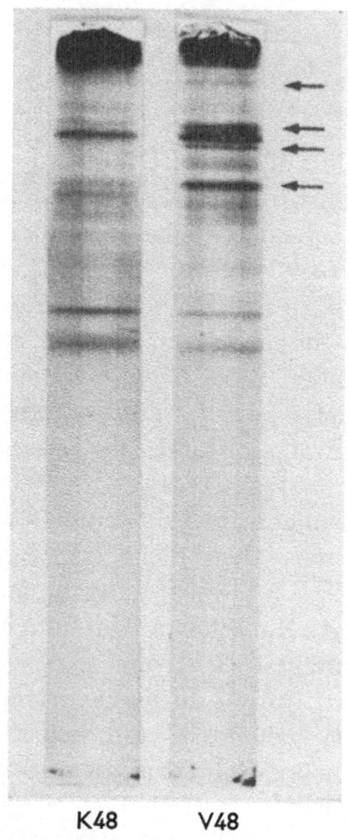

Abb. 1. Polyacrylamidgelelektrophorese von Proteinen aus nicht infizierten und SV40-infizierten CV-1-Zellen (48 Std p.i.). Coomassie-blue-Färbung

Um diese Änderungen im Proteinmuster, die durch die SV40-Infektion hervorgerufen werden, noch exakter zu erfassen, kann man die Polyacrylamidgele densitometrisch auswerten (Abb. 2). Auch hier sind deutliche Unterschiede zwischen der nicht infizierten CV-1-Kontrolle und den infizierten Zellen 72 Std p. i. als neue Gipfel und Schultern zu sehen.

Durch Inkubation der Proteine mit spezifischem Antiserum läßt sich weiterhin unterscheiden, ob durch die Infektion virus-spezifische Proteine (v) synthetisiert oder zelluläre Proteine induziert (i) werden. Die

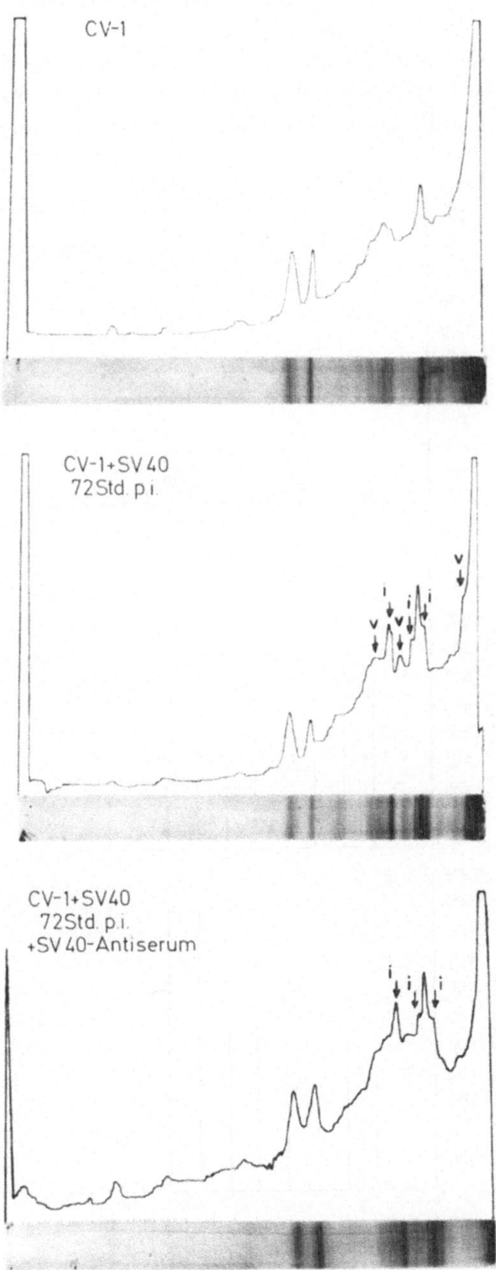

Abb. 2. Densitometerkurven von Coomassie-blue-gefärbten Polyacrylamidgelen

beiden unteren Densitometerkurven zeigen einen solchen Versuch. Hier wurden die Proteine, die noch ihre serologische Aktivität besitzen, mit Anti-SV40-Cercopithecus-Serum inkubiert und dann die Elektrophorese durchgeführt. Die Gipfel, die auf diese Weise eliminiert werden können, sind virusspezifische Proteine. Dabei könnte es sich entweder um Proteine

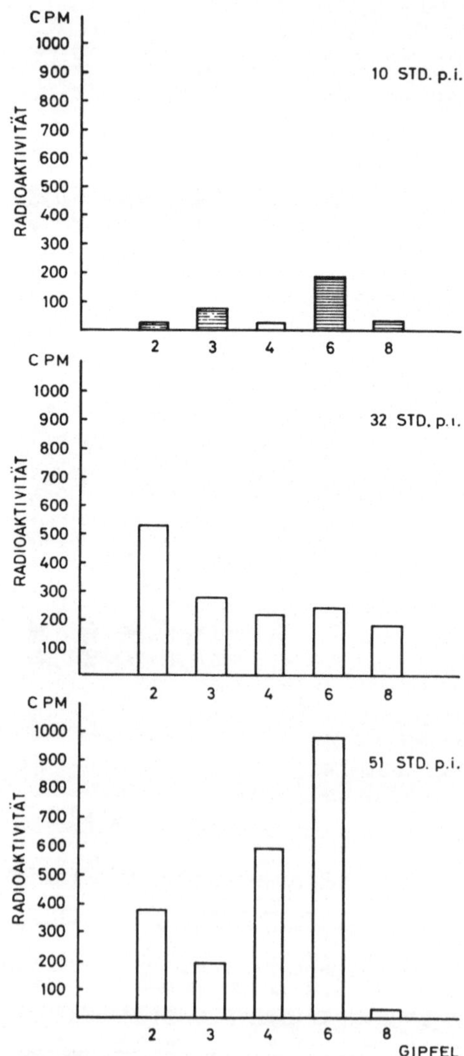

Abb. 3. Syntheseaktivität der Fraktionen 2, 3, 4, 6, 8, 10, 32 und 51 Std p. i. Abgetragen ist die Differenz zwischen Kontrolle und infizierten CV-1-Zellen. ≡ verminderte Syntheseaktivität, □ erhöhte Syntheseaktivität

handeln, die vom Virus codiert wurden (z. B. Komponenten des T-Antigens oder Hüllproteine), oder solche, die durch eine virusbedingte Induktion oder Derepression von den Wirtszellen gebildet wurden.

Verfolgt man die Proteinsyntheserate durch Pulsmarkierung mit ^{14}C-Aminosäuren zu verschiedenen Zeitpunkten p. i., so treten die Unterschiede noch deutlicher hervor.

Zu diesem Zweck wurden die Disc-Säulen in 1 mm-Scheibchen zerlegt und die Radioaktivität im Flüssigkeits-Scintillationszähler gemessen. Die Proteinfraktionen zeigen zu verschiedenen Zeiten p. i. eine verschieden starke Syntheseaktivität. Zur Vereinfachung sind aus dem sehr komplexen Synthesemuster 5 Gipfel ausgewählt und in Abb. 3 dargestellt. Abgetragen ist die Verminderung oder Steigerung der Syntheseaktivität im Vergleich zur Kontrolle.

10 Std p. i. finden wir in fast allen Gipfeln, mit Ausnahme von 4, eine Hemmung der Proteinsynthese. 32 Std p. i. zeigen die Gipfel 2, 3 und 8 ihre höchste Syntheseleistung, wohingegen in Gipfel 4 und 6 erst am Ende des Vermehrungscyclus (51 Std p. i.) die höchste Syntheseaktivität erreicht wird. Auf diese Weise läßt sich die Zeitfolge neuer Proteine bestimmen. Besonders interessant sind solche Proteine, die im frühen Vermehrungscyclus auftreten, da sie auch bei der Tumorgenese eine Rolle spielen.

Analoge Untersuchungen wollen wir auch an transformierten Zellen durchführen; doch war es zuerst notwendig, Informationen über das lytische Virus-Wirtszellverhältnis zu erhalten. Proteine aus dem frühen lytischen Vermehrungscyclus und Proteine aus den transformierten Zellen werden mit den geschilderten Methoden genau erfaßt und sind somit einer präparativen Aufarbeitung zugänglich.

Literatur

1. Fernandes, M. V., Moorhead, P. S.: Transformation of African green monkey kidney cultures infected with simian vacuolating virus (SV40). Tex. Rep. Biol. Med. **23** (Suppl. 1), 242 (1965).
2. Fischer, H., Munk, K.: The pattern of protein synthesis in SV40-infected CV-1 cells. Int. J. Cancer **5**, 21 (1970).
3. Kit, S., Dubbs, D. R., Frearson, P. M., Melnick, J. L.: Enzyme induction in SV40-infected green monkey kidney cultures. Virology **29**, 69 (1966).
4. Kit, S., Dubbs, D. R., Piekarski, L. J., de Torres, R. A., Melnick, J. L.: Acquisition of enzyme function by mouse kidney cells abortively infected with papovavirus SV40. Proc. nat. Acad. Sci. **56**, 463 (1966).
5. Rapp, F., Kitahara, T., Butel, J. S., Melnick, J. L.: Synthesis of SV40 tumor antigen during replication of simian papovavirus (SV40). Proc. nat. Acad. Sci. **52**, 1138 (1964).
6. Sweet, B. H., Hilleman, M. R.: The vacuolating virus SV40. Proc. Soc. exp. Biol. (N. Y.) **105**, 420 (1960).

B.

2. Wissenschaftliche Sitzung am Donnerstag, den 24. 9. 1970

Vorsitz: E. Hecker und Kl. Goerttler

Die Carcinogenese der Hautepidermis aus dynamischer Sicht

Von

O. H. Iversen

Bei der Erörterung der Carcinogenese der Haut erscheint es notwendig, eine dynamische Betrachtungsweise einzunehmen. Die Haut ist kein „establishment" starr-statischer Einheiten; sie ist vielmehr ein sehr dynamisches Gewebe, das sich aus vielen verschiedenen und stets sich ändernden Bestandteilen zusammensetzt.

Der wichtigste Teil der Haut ist die Epidermis mit ihren Anhangsgebilden. Sie ist ein sehr schnell regenerierendes Gewebe und steht in dauernder inniger Beziehung zum Corium, dessen Gefäßen und Nerven und somit auch zur Homöostase des Kreislaufs, Nervensystems und des Endokriniums. Bei der Auslegung von Ergebnissen, die die Hautcarcinogenese betreffen, sollte man sich dieser Tatsache immer erinnern.

Viele der alten Ideen über die Hautcarcinogenese waren im Grunde statisch. Dies mag davon herrühren, daß die morphologische Methode für viele Jahre im makroskopischen wie auch im mikroskopischen Bereich die fast alleinige Forschungsweise war. Auf Grund kinetischer Untersuchungen über die Frühstadien der Carcinogenese der Epidermis nahm man zum Beispiel an, daß eine einmalige Applikation eines Carcinogens auf die Oberfläche der Haut einen beträchtlichen Zelluntergang hervorruft (Iversen and Evensen [*10*]). Ein sehr erfahrener Forscher auf diesem Gebiet erhob dagegen Einspruch, weil er „Tausende histologische Präparate der Epidermis gesehen habe, die mit Carcinogenen vorbehandelt waren, aber nie tote Zellen". Er hatte nicht daran gedacht, daß tote Zellen in der Epidermis oft Oberflächenzellen sind, die im Schuppungsvorgang sehr schnell verloren gehen. Es ist natürlich unmöglich, „nicht vorhandene" Zellen zu sehen. Daß man sie nicht sieht, ist noch kein Beweis dafür, daß sie nicht doch verlorengegangen sind. Eine dynamische Betrachtungsweise löst derartige Probleme.

Unser Versuchsmodell ist die haarlose Mäusehaut. Die Haut haarloser Mäuse hat eine Epidermis mit einigen Krypten und Talgdrüsen. Im Corium – und manchmal auch in der Subcutis – finden sich viele Cysten, die wahrscheinlich degenerierte Haarfollikel darstellen. In manchen dieser Cysten ist eine entzündliche Reaktion mit Fremdkörperriesenzellen nachweisbar. Das Corium selbst ist dem normalen Mäusecorium sehr ähnlich. Die interfollikuläre Epidermis ist geringfügig dicker als bei behaarten Mäusen. Sie besteht aus einer basalen Schicht, einer Schicht sich differenzierender Zellen und einer darüber liegenden Hornschicht (Abb. 1).

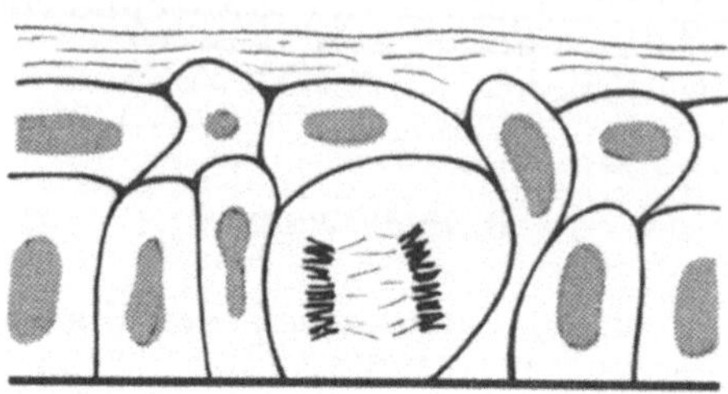

Abb. 1. Aufbau der interfollikulären Epidermis. Eine in Teilung befindliche Zelle drängt eine andere Zelle in die Differenzierungs-Zellschicht

Das Stratum granulosum ist nicht sehr deutlich; bei Fällen von Hyperplasie kann es jedoch stark hervortreten. Die Zellpopulation insgesamt setzt sich hauptsächlich aus Keratinocyten zusammen; daneben werden auch einige Melanocyten und Langerhans-Zellen gefunden. Der Vorgang der Zellerneuerung läuft normalerweise nur in den Basalzellen ab. Zu jedem Zeitpunkt lassen sich diese in zwei „Familien" unterteilen, nämlich diejenigen, die sich wieder teilen und jene, welche in die sich differenzierende Schicht ausgestoßen werden, noch bevor sie sich geteilt haben. Die erste Familie hat man die *Progenitor*- und die zweite die *Non-progenitor-Zellen* genannt. 60% der Basalzellen sind im Durchschnitt Progenitor- und 40% Non-progenitor-Zellen. Die mittlere Generationszeit für eine Progenitor-Zelle ist 3–5 Tage. Die Non-progenitor-Zellen bleiben im Durchschnitt 2,5 Tage an der Basalmembran, bevor sie ausgestoßen werden. Das Auswechseln der Epidermiszellen dauert ungefähr 6 Tage; hinzu kommt die Hornschicht, die für 4–6 Tage bestehen bleibt (Iversen, Bjerknes und Devik [*9*]).

Papillome und Carcinome können in der Haut dieser Mäuse mit einer einzigen Methylcholanthrenapplikation (MCA) erzeugt werden (Iversen u. Iversen [*11*]). Mehr als 50 μg Methylcholanthren rufen zahlreiche, 30 μg Methylcholanthren und weniger rufen nur einzelne Papillome hervor.

Wir wollen uns nun mit den Vorgängen befassen, die eintreten, wenn ein Tropfen einer Lösung von Methylcholanthren in Benzol auf die Oberfläche der Epidermis appliziert wird. Eine der wesentlichen Folgen ist ein *Zellschaden*, der zu Zelltod und Zellverlust führt. Der erste Hinweis auf eine Beeinträchtigung sind pyknotische Kerne, die man nach einigen Stunden sieht. Mit der Tetrazolium-Methode wurde versucht, den Zellschaden quantitativ zu erfassen. Dies führte zu der Entdeckung, daß in den ersten Stunden nach der Einwirkung auf die Haut viele chemische Carcinogene sowie ionisierende Strahlen eine erhöhte Ablagerung von Formazan in der Epidermis hervorrufen. Nichtkrebserzeugende Reizmittel führten zu einer verminderten Ablagerung von Formazan in derselben Zeitspanne (IVERSEN [7]; Abb. 2). Der diesen Befunden zugrunde liegende Mechanismus ist noch keinesfalls klar, doch scheint es so zu sein, daß die Zerstörung der Mitochondrien durch Carcinogene verschieden ist von dem Schaden, der durch ein Nicht-Carcinogen hervorgerufen wird. Es ist möglich, daß der Unterschied nur quantitativ ist und nur den Zeitverlauf betrifft. Die Reaktion ist nicht vollkommen spezifisch und ist bei schwach carcinogenen Substanzen nicht eindeutig. Ich bin jedoch der Ansicht, daß dies ein interessanter Befund ist, der die Grundlage für den sogenannten Tetrazolium-Test bildet. Es ist von Interesse, daß dieser Test für höhere Methylcholanthrenkonzentrationen als $^1/_8$% positiv ist, während er bei Konzentrationen unter $^1/_{32}$% negativ ausfällt.

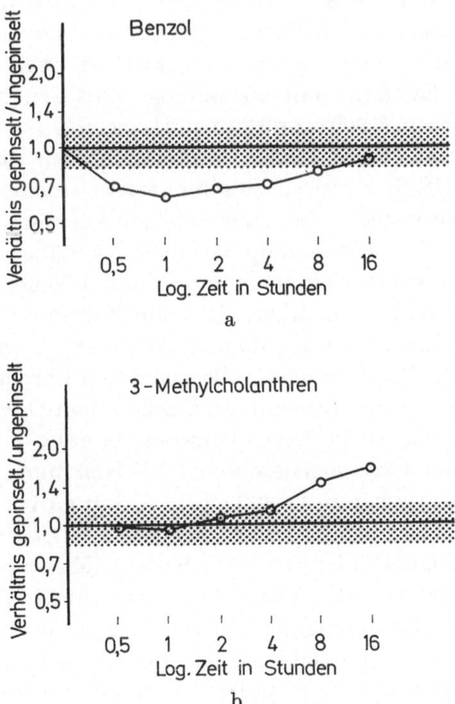

Abb. 2. Ergebnisse des Tetrazolium-Tests in der Haut haarloser Mäuse während der ersten Stunden nach (a) Benzol- und (b) 1% Methylcholanthren-Applikation (in Benzol)

Nach einer einmaligen Applikation von 50 Mikrogramm Methylcholanthren in Benzol haben wir einen Zellverlust von 21% der Zellen am ersten Tag, von 35% der Zellen am zweiten Tag und 18% der Zellen am dritten Tag errechnet. Dieser Zellverlust bedeutet insgesamt eine 80%ige Erhöhung des normalen Zellverlustes. Dies hat uns veranlaßt, das Vorhandensein und das Ausmaß dieses Zellverlustes mit anderen Methoden zu untersuchen (Skjaeggestad [*17*]). Die Existenz des Zellverlustes konnten wir bestätigen; aber er ist sicher kein spezifisches Phänomen, das nur bei Carcinogenen auftritt. Alle Hautreizmittel, die später eine epidermale Hyperplasie bewirken, haben eine solche initiale Reaktion zur Folge. Carcinogene Substanzen zerstören jedoch im allgemeinen mehr Zellen und haben eine viel länger dauernde Zellen-zerstörende Wirkung als die untersuchten Nicht-Carcinogene. Wir wissen nicht, ob die längere Dauer der Zellen-zerstörenden Wirkung mit der Carcinogenese etwas zu tun hat.

Untersuchungen über die Veränderungen der kinetischen Parameter zeigen, daß die erste Wirkung der Applikation eines Carcinogens in einem sofortigen Block der DNS-Synthese und der Mitoserate besteht. Die Blockierung tritt bei höheren Methylcholanthren-Dosen auf und erscheint bei Konzentrationen unter $^{1}/_{32}\%$ nicht mehr (Evensen [*3*]). Dieser Block wurde 1961 von Evensen mit autoradiographischen Methoden festgestellt und vor kurzem (1969) von Paul u. Hecker [*14*] mit biochemischen Methoden bestätigt. Diese beiden Verfasser stellen die Frage, ob die Hemmung der DNS-Synthese spezifisch mit der Carcinogenese verbunden sein könnte. Beweise zugunsten einer solchen Annahme stützen sich auf die Beobachtung, daß alle Zellpopulationen gegenüber chemischen Carcinogenen (β-Propiolactone ausgenommen) empfindlicher sind (Hennings, Bowden u. Boutwell [*5*]), wenn sich zum Zeitpunkt der Applikation viele Zellen in DNS-Synthese befinden (Iversen, Iversen, Hennings u. Bjerknes [*12*]). Zwar hemmen alle geprüften Carcinogene die DNS-Synthese; eine eindeutige Beziehung zwischen dem Grad der Hemmung und der Anzahl der ausgelösten Tumoren besteht jedoch nicht. Die Beziehung zwischen Carcinogenese und DNS-Hemmung ist daher immer noch unklar (Hennings u. Boutwell [*4*]). Aufgrund von Beobachtungen an anderen Geweben sind andere Autoren (Shimkin, Gruenstein, Thatcher u. Baserga [*15*]; Shimkin, Sasaki, McDonough, Baserga, Thatcher u. Wieder [*16*]; und Tominaga, Libby u. Dao [*18*]) der Meinung, daß die Hemmung der DNS-Synthese als toxischer Nebeneffekt zu werten ist, und nicht als das Schlüsselereignis in der Carcinogenese. Wir haben auch eine ähnliche Hemmung schon beim Abziehen von Tesafilm beobachtet (Hennings u. Elgjo [*6*]). Eine derartige anfängliche Hemmung der DNS-Synthese nach Abziehen von Tesafilm oder nach Applikation eines Carcinogens dauert einige wenige Stunden (vielleicht 4–12), und dann wird ein schneller Anstieg in der zellulären Proliferation ausgelöst (Abb. 3 und 4). Je nach der Dosis hat dieser Anstieg seinen Gipfel 2–3 Tage nach der Applikation. Die Zahl der Mitosen ist sehr hoch. Dies ist nicht nur auf eine Erhöhung der *Mitoserate* zurückzuführen, denn es besteht außerdem eine signifikante Verlängerung der *Mitosedauer* von normalerweise 60 bis auf maximal 120 min. Eine derartige Verlängerung der Mitosedauer wird auch nach der Applikation von Nicht-Carcinogenen beobachtet; sie ist dabei jedoch weniger deutlich

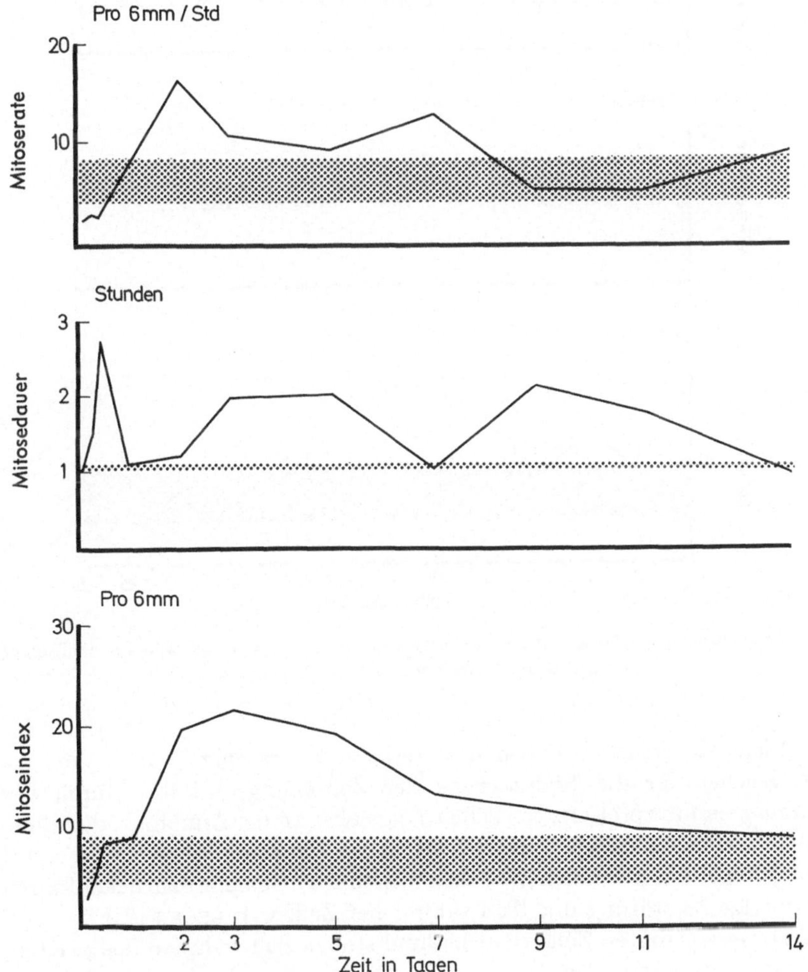

Abb. 3. Mitoserate, Mitosedauer und Mitoseindex während der einer einzelnen Methylcholanthren-Applikation folgenden 2 Wochen

und dauert viel kürzere Zeit (Abb. 5). Es mag von Bedeutung sein, daß bei Carcinogenen die verlängerte Mitosedauer über eine viel längere Zeit bestehen bleibt (ELGJO [*1*, *2*]). Der Grund hierfür könnte darin bestehen, daß kleine Mengen des Carcinogens in den Zellen der Epidermis verhältnismäßig lange vorhanden sind.

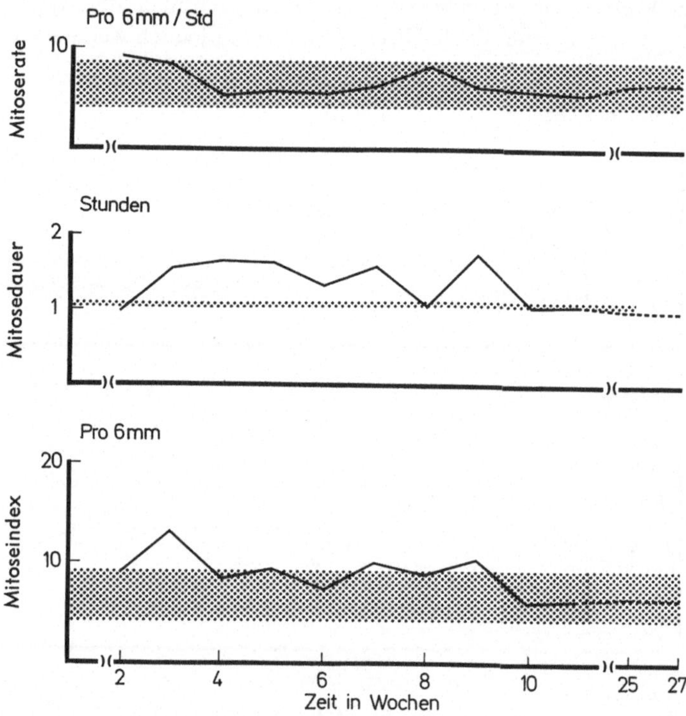

Abb. 4. Mitoserate, Mitosedauer und Mitoseindex von der 3.–27. Woche nach einer einmaligen Methylcholanthren-Applikation

Viele Untersucher haben die Periode des raschen Wachstums als ein Zeichen für die *Stimulierung* der Zellteilungsaktivität durch das Carcinogen interpretiert. Ich selber neige eher zu der Annahme, daß diese „Wachstumsexplosion“ eine regenerative Reaktion darstellt, die auf den Mangel der normalen Wachstumshemmer (Chalone) zurückzuführen ist infolge Zerstörung und Tod zahlreicher Zellen (IVERSEN [*7*]).

Die geschädigten Zellen sterben und stoßen sich während des zweiten, dritten und vierten Tages ab, und die Epidermis ergänzt sich mit jungen Zellen von der Basalschicht her. Die mittlere Lebenserwartung der ganzen Zellpopulation verlängert sich erheblich infolge dieser Verschiebung der Population zugunsten jüngerer Zellen. Mit anderen Worten: die Applikation eines Hautreizmittels bewirkt eine Gleichschaltung der kinetischen Parameter der Epidermis. Dies läßt sich auch am schubartigen Rhythmus der Schuppung beobachten, der nach der Applikation auftritt.

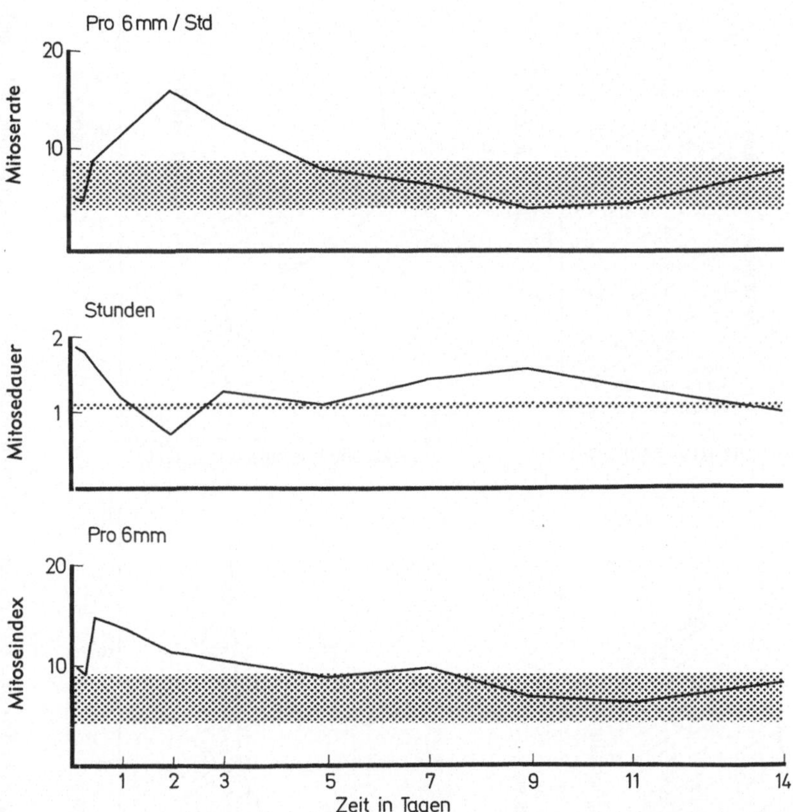

Abb. 5. Mitoserate, Mitosedauer und Mitoseindex während der ersten 14 Tage nach einer einzelnen Cantharidin-Applikation

Die Anzahl der Zellen bleibt bis zum dritten Tag im Normbereich, dann setzt eine vorübergehende Hyperplasie ein. Diese erreicht ihren Höhepunkt am 5.–7. Tag, je nach der verabreichten Dosis. Diese Hyperplasie ist nicht gleichmäßig und besteht an verschiedenen Stellen aus 3–5 Zellagen. Im Durchschnitt findet sich in der behandelten Epidermis eine Erhöhung der Zellzahl um etwa 30%. Diese Hyperplasie nimmt später ab, und nach ungefähr 3 Wochen ist die Dicke der Epidermis

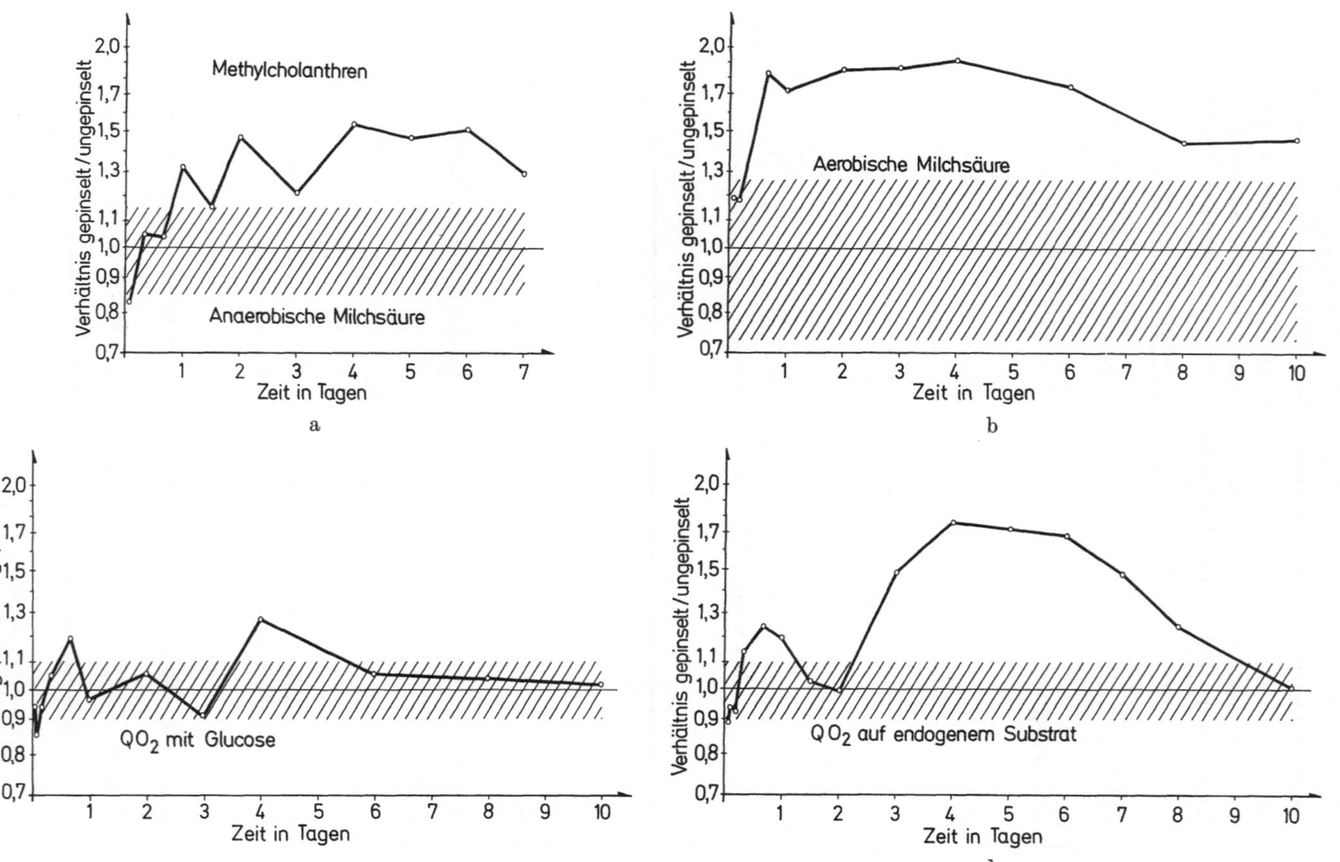

Abb. 6a-d. Die Darstellung einiger Stoffwechselparameter in der Mäusehaut nach einer einzelnen Methylcholanthren-Applikation

wieder normal. Die gleiche Art einer hyperplastischen Reaktion wurde bei vielen Carcinogenen gefunden. Sie ist auch bei nicht-krebserzeugenden Reizmitteln sowie nach Abhebung oberflächlicher Epidermis-Zellschichten mittels aufgeklebten Tesafilms zu beobachten. Wenn man den Mechanismus einer indirekten Rückkoppelung für die Wachstumsregulation als richtig ansieht, dann läßt sich diese vorübergehende Hyperplasie ohne weiteres als eine rein regenerative dynamische Reaktion auf den akuten Zelltod erklären (Elgjo [*1*, *2*]).

Die einmalige Applikation eines Carcinogens auf die Haut führt in der Epidermis zu rasch wechselnden Veränderungen des Sauerstoffverbrauchs und der Milchsäureproduktion (Laerum [*13*]; Abb. 6). Man unterscheidet eine Initialphase von etwa 4 Std Dauer, die durch eine merkbare Senkung der Atmung und der Glycolyse gekennzeichnet ist. Dann folgt eine Intermediärphase, die von der 4. bis zur 36. Std nach Applikation dauert. Diese Phase ist gekennzeichnet durch einen Anstieg des Sauerstoffverbrauchs und der Glycolyse. Diese Wirkung scheint allein vom Lösungsmittel Benzol hervorgerufen zu werden, da sie nach Pinselung mit Benzol allein auch beobachtet wird. Dann kommt die von uns als „Wachstumsphase" bezeichnete Zeitspanne, die von der 36. bis zur 48. Std dauert. In dieser Phase zeigen die Zellen der Epidermis einen niedrigen Sauerstoffverbrauch, während die aerobe und anaerobe Milchsäureproduktion hoch sind. Schließlich läßt sich eine hyperplastische Phase beobachten, die vom 2. bis zum 21. Tag nach der Behandlung dauert und durch eine mäßig verringerte Atmung und Glycolyse gekennzeichnet ist. Nichtkrebserzeugende Stoffe – wie zum Beispiel Benzol allein – rufen einen schnell auftretenden Anstieg in der Atmung, eine hohe aerobe Glycolyse und einen hohen Sauerstoffverbrauch hervor (Abb. 7). Das Bild normalisiert sich jedoch schnell wieder.

Wir fassen zusammen: Eine einmalige Applikation eines Carcinogens ruft dramatische dynamische Veränderungen in der Epidermis hervor. Wir unterscheiden eine initiale „Schock-Phase" oder toxische Phase, die einige Stunden dauert. In dieser Phase sind die DNS-Synthese und die mitotische Aktivität vollständig aufgehoben, Glycolyse und Sauerstoffverbrauch sind gleichermaßen gedrosselt. Mit der Tetrazolium-Methode werden die Zeichen eines irreversiblen Zellschadens durch erhöhte Formazan-Ablagerungen mit einem Maximum 16 Std nach der Applikation beobachtet. Dieser Zellschaden führt zu einer erhöhten Absterberate der Zellen vom 2. bis zum 4. Tag. Es ist zu vermuten, daß während dieser Zeit auch die Chalon-Produktion zum Stillstand kommt und so der normalerweise vorhandene Wachstumshemmstoff verschwindet. Ein anderer denkbarer Mechanismus wäre, daß Chalonspaltende Enzyme freigesetzt werden, z. B. infolge Zerstörung von Lysosomen. Wenn sich die Zellen vom ersten „toxischen Schock" er-

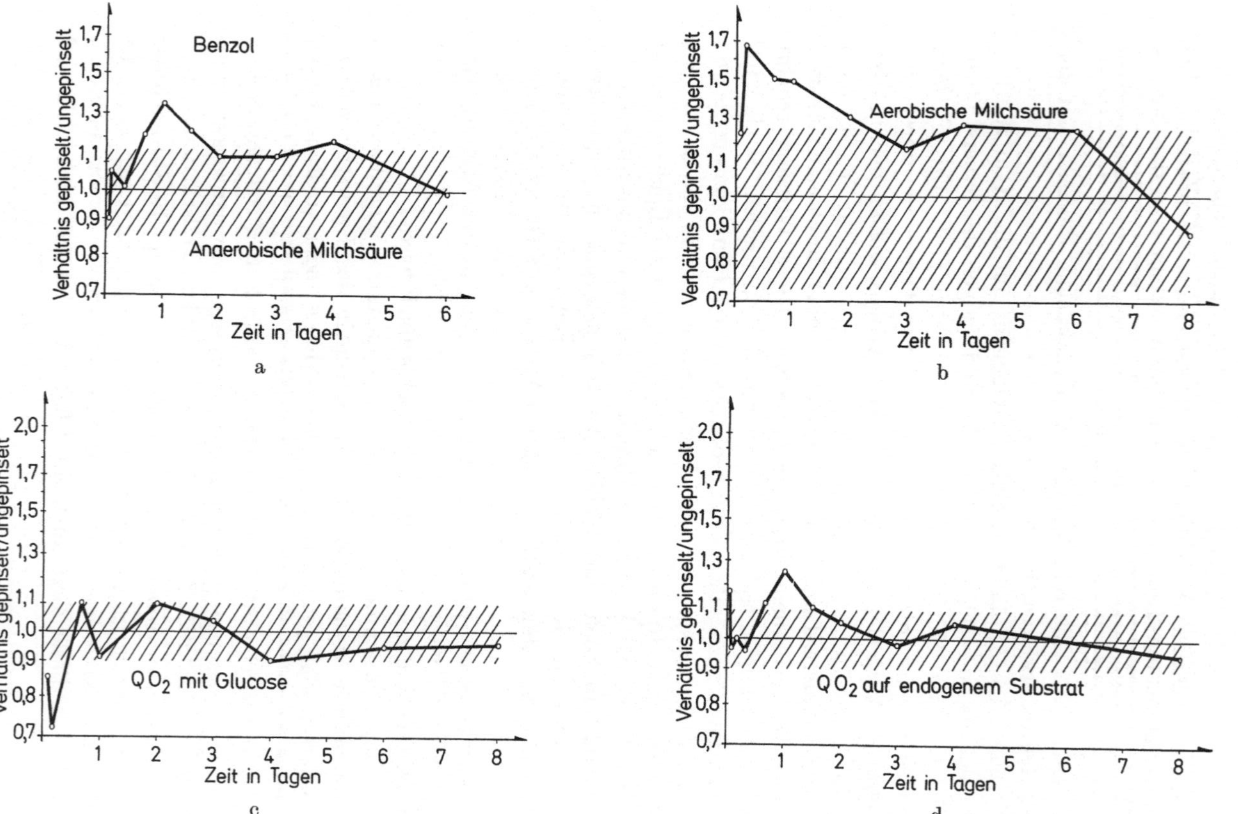

Abb. 7a-d. Die Veränderung einiger Stoffwechselparameter in der Mäusehaut nach einer einmaligen Applikation von Benzol

holen, wird ein erhöhtes Wachstum vorbereitet während einer intermediären „Erholungsphase", in der auch eine signifikante Erhöhung des Sauerstoffverbrauchs und der Glycolyse besteht. Es folgt eine proliferative oder „Wachstumsphase", in der die DNS-Synthese und die mitotische Aktivität bis zum Fünffachen über den Normalwert ansteigen. Für eine lange Zeit ist die Zahl der Mitosen vermehrt. Die Mitoserate ist geringer als vermutet, weil auch die Mitosedauer merklich verlängert ist. In dieser dritten Phase des Wachstums findet man einen niedrigen Sauerstoffverbrauch, jedoch eine hohe Produktion aerober und anaerober Milchsäure. Am Ende der Wachstumsphase zeigt die Tetrazolium-Reaktion eine abnehmende Menge an Formazan-Bildung, die während der ganzen hyperplastischen Phase niedrig bleibt. Dies ist wahrscheinlich allein darauf zurückzuführen, daß junge Zellen weniger Mitochondrien und eine niedrige oxydative Phosphorylierung aufweisen. Die vierte hyperplastische Phase ist gekennzeichnet durch einen geringen Sauerstoffverbrauch und eine niedrige Glycolyse, ein weiterer Hinweis auf die verhältnismäßig niedrige metabolische Aktivität junger Zellen.

Nichtkrebserzeugende Hautreizmittel rufen eine ähnliche dynamische Reaktion hervor. Es bestehen jedoch Unterschiede. Die erhöhte initiale Ablagerung von Formazan dürfte auf einen spezifischen Schaden der Zellen durch Carcinogene hinweisen. Dabei dürfte der signifikanten Drosselung der DNS-Synthese eine besondere Bedeutung zukommen. Die betonte und lang anhaltende Verlängerung der Mitosedauer könnte wichtig sein. Eine starke und lang andauernde zellschädigende und zellvernichtende Wirkung scheint auf die Carcinogenapplikation zu folgen. In der Wachstumsphase ähneln die metabolischen Parameter sehr dem klassischen Tumorstoffwechsel Warburgs, aber diese Phase dauert nur kurze Zeit und könnte vollständig oder zumindest teilweise durch die Anwesenheit junger, neu gebildeter Zellen in der Epidermis bedingt sein. Einige dieser Reaktionen haben ein Dosis/Wirkungs-Verhältnis, das demjenigen während der Tumorerzeugung nach einer einzelnen Carcinogenapplikation entspricht.

Wir haben somit augenblicklich keinen Beweis, daß auch nur eine einzige der beobachteten dynamischen Veränderungen wirklich mit der Carcinogenese *an sich* zusammenhängt. Aber dieses Gebiet ist natürlich offen für sehr interessante Spekulationen.

Abschließend möchte ich noch einmal betonen, daß kein Ergebnis in der experimentellen Carcinogenese auf statische Weise erörtert werden sollte. Biochemische Versuche kann man nur verstehen, wenn sie zu den wechselnden Parametern der Zellkinetik in Beziehung gebracht werden. Eine dynamische Interpretation in einem vielschichtigen System zu geben, ist aber sehr schwierig. Das menschliche Gehirn scheint für derartige Arbeit nicht gebaut zu sein. Wir müssen uns deshalb helfen durch Aufstellen von Modellen und durch den Gebrauch elektronischer Rechner. Uns steht heute ein nützliches Modell der Epidermis zur Verfügung (Iversen u. Bjerknes [8]). Viele werden solch ein Modell als Spielerei ansehen. Obwohl ich diese Ansicht verstehen kann, sollten wir jedoch bedenken, daß hinter dem Spiel eines Kindes immer ein vernünftiger Gedanke steckt.

Literatur

1. Elgjo, K.: Epidermal cell population kinetics after a single application of some hyperplasia-producing substances. Europ. J. Cancer **3**, 519 (1968).
2. Elgjo, K.: Epidermal cell population kinetics after repeated applications of some hyperplasia-producing substances. Europ. J. Cancer **4**, 183 (1968).
3. Evensen, A.: Changes in the synthesis of deoxyribonucleic acid (DNA) and in mitotic count in epidermis of hairless mice after a single application of one per cent 3-methylcholanthrene in benzene. A preliminary report. Acta path. microbiol. scand. Suppl. **148**, 43 (1961).
4. Hennings, H., Boutwell, R. K.: The inhibition of DNA synthesis by initiators of mouse skin tumorigenesis. Cancer Res. **29**, 510 (1969).
5. Hennings, H., Bowden, G. T., Boutwell, R. K.: The effect of croton oil pre-treatment on skin tumor initiation in mice. Cancer Res. **29**, 1773 (1969).
6. Hennings, H., Elgjo, K.: Epidermal regeneration after cellophane tape stripping of hairless mouse skin. Cell Tissue Kinet. **3**, 243 (1970).
7. Iversen, O. H.: Effects of carcinogens on mitochondrial function. In Iversen, O. H., and Evensen, A. (Eds): Experimental skin carcinogenesis in mice. Acta path. microbiol. scand. Suppl. **156**, 29 (1962).
8. Iversen, O. H., Bjerknes, R.: Kinetics of epidermal reaction to carcinogens. Acta path. microbiol. scand. Suppl. **165**, 1 (1963).
9. Iversen, O. H., Bjerknes, R., Devik, F.: Kinetics of cell renewal, cell migration and cell loss in the hairless mouse dorsal epidermis. Cell Tissue Kinet. **1**, 351 (1968).
10. Iversen, O. H., Evensen, A.: Experimental skin carcinogenesis in mice. Acta path. microbiol. scand. Suppl. **156**, 7 (1962).
11. Iversen, O. H., Iversen, U.: A study of epidermal tumourigenesis in the hairless mouse with single and with repeated applications of 3-methylcholanthrene at different dosages. Acta path. microbiol. scand. **62**, 305 (1964).
12. Iversen, U., Iversen, O. H., Hennings, H., Bjerknes, R.: Diurnal variation in susceptibility of mouse skin to the tumorigenic action of methylcholanthrene. J. nat. Cancer Inst. **45**, 269 (1970).
13. Laerum, O. D.: Studies of respiration and glycolysis of epidermal cells in relation to early skin carcinogenesis. Thesis. Oslo: Universitetsforlaget 1969.
14. Paul, D., Hecker, E.: On the biochemical mechanism of tumorigenesis in mouse skin. Z. Krebsforsch. **73**, 149 (1969).
15. Shimkin, M. B., Gruenstein, M., Thatcher, D., Baserga, R.: Tritiated thymidine labelling of cells in rats following exposure to 7,12-dimethylbenz(a) anthracene. Cancer Res. **27**, 1494 (1967).
16. Shimkin, M. B., Sasaki, T., McDonough, M., Baserga, R., Thatcher, D., Wieder, R.: Relation of thymidine index to pulmonary tumor response in mice receiving urethan and other carcinogens. Cancer Res. **29**, 994 (1969).
17. Skjaeggestad, Ø.: Experimental epidermal hyperplasia in mice. Relation to carcinogenesis. Acta path. microbiol. scand. Suppl. **169**, 1 (1964).
18. Tominaga, T., Libby, P. R., Dao, T. L.: An early effect of 7,12-dimethylbenz(a)-anthracene on rat mammary gland DNA synthesis. Cancer Res. **30**, 118 (1970).

Zur Kultivierung von Mäuse-Epidermiszellen in vitro

Von

N. E. Fusenig

Die Untersuchung der chemischen Carcinogenese an der Mäusehaut mit biochemischen Methoden ist wegen der Heterogenität dieses Gewebes mit erheblichen Schwierigkeiten verbunden. Wir versuchen deshalb – wie vor uns schon andere Untersucher [*1*, *2*, *3*] – ein *In-vitro*-Modell der Mäuse-Epidermis aufzubauen, um an diesem Modell die Transformation mit chemischen Carcinogenen studieren zu können. Eine solche „Epidermis *in vitro*" sollte ohne Bindegewebe in der Kultur wachsen und Differenzierungsleistung aufweisen.

Da die biologischen und biochemischen Experimente zur chemischen Carcinogenese in unserem Institut an der Haut 6–8 Wochen alter Mäuse durchgeführt werden [*4*], versuchten wir zunächst, die Epidermiszellen erwachsener Tiere zu isolieren und zu kultivieren.

Die Angaben in der Literatur zur Kultivierung von Epidermiszellen [*2*, *5*, *6*] beziehen sich überwiegend auf menschliche Haut. Sie waren, ebenso wie andere bekannte Methoden zur Isolierung von Hautzellen (Literatur siehe bei [*3*]) für unsere Fragestellung nicht brauchbar. Die Menge der nach diesen Methoden isolierten Zellen war entweder zu gering oder ihre Vitalität zu niedrig oder die Reinheit der epidermalen Population war nicht hoch genug.

Wir isolierten die Epidermiszellen nach folgender Methode: Epilierte und kleingeschnittene Hautstückchen werden für 90–120 min in 0,2% Trypsin vorsichtig gewirbelt. Dabei findet eine Trennung von Epidermis und Dermis statt. Nach Beginn der Epidermisablösung (ca. 30–45 min) werden im Abstand von 5–10 min 30 ml-Fraktionen der Suspension mit den jeweils isolierten Zellen durch Nylongaze abfiltriert. Die gleiche Menge an frischem Ferment wird wieder zu den Hautstücken zu weiteren Isolierungen zugegeben. Die Isolierung wird fortgesetzt, bis die Epidermiszellen überwiegend abgelöst sind.

Die Ausbeute dieser Isolierungsmethode lag bei 7×10^6 Zellen/20 cm^2 Rückenhaut. Die Trypanblau-Anfärbbarkeit lag bei 5%. Der ^3H-Thymidineinbau in frisch isolierte Epidermiszellen in Suspension stieg über 4 Std linear an.

Obwohl diese Ergebnisse auf eine gute Vitalität der isolierten Zellen schließen lassen, blieb die Zahl der in Kultur wachsenden Zellen äußerst gering. Das Wachstum erfolgte nur nach einer Aggregierung der Einzelzellen. Ähnliches wird von Epidermiszellen aus menschlicher Haut berichtet [*2*]. Fibroblasten wurden in den Kulturen der normalen Hautzellen nicht beobachtet.

Die Epidermis-Kulturen zeigten nur geringe Proliferationstendenz, konnten aber in teilungsfähigem Zustand bis zu 10 Wochen am Leben erhalten werden. Abb. 1 zeigt ein Beispiel einer 10 Wochen alten Kultur mit deutlich epithelialem Charakter.

Es gelang nicht, die Ausbeute an wachsenden Zellen zu erhöhen, so daß wir uns entschlossen, dieses Modell vorläufig aufzugeben, da es zum Studium der chemischen Carcinogenese *in vitro* wenig geeignet erschien.

Erfolgreicher waren die Versuche mit Epidermiszellen embryonaler Mäuse. Die meisten in der Literatur angegebenen Modelle zur Carcinogenese *in vitro* [*1, 7*] sind von embryonalen Geweben abgeleitet, oft ohne nähere cytologische Charakterisierung der Kulturen. Voraussetzung für die Realisierung eines *In-vitro*-Modells der Epidermis aus Mäuseembryonen war die Reinisolierung von Epidermiszellen, d. h. ihre Trennung von Fibroblasten.

Im folgenden werden die Methode der Isolierung und die ersten Ergebnisse der Kultivierung beschrieben.

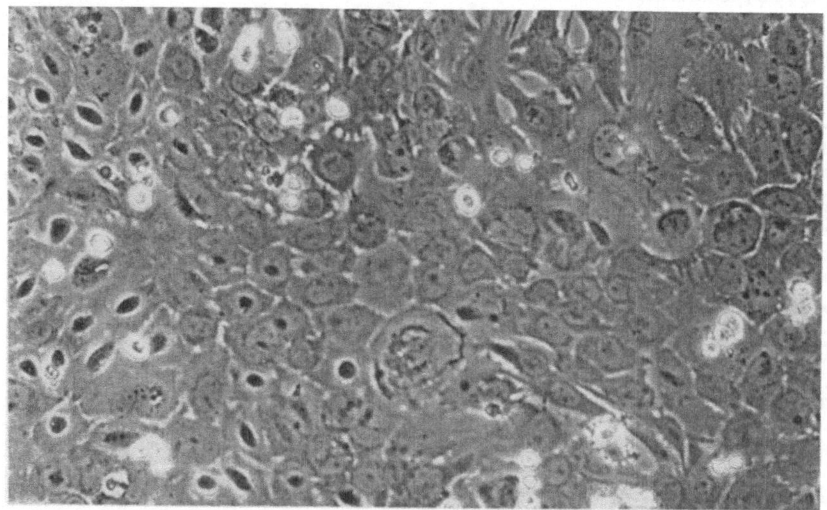

Abb. 1. 8 Wochen alte epitheliale Monolayer-Kultur aus isolierten Zellen der Epidermis 7 Wochen alter Mäuse (Phasen-Kontrast, × 180)

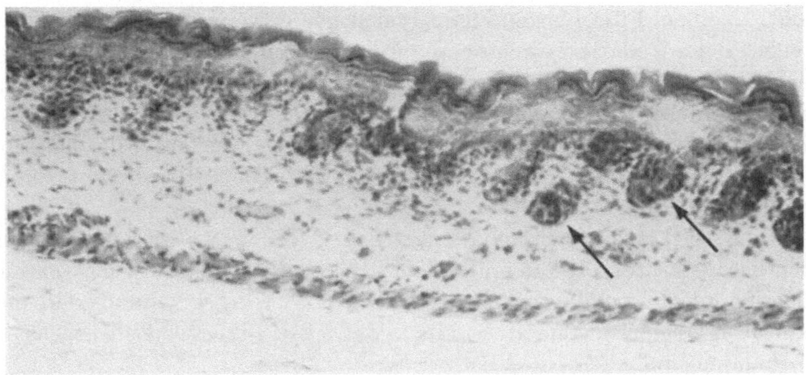

Abb. 2. Histologischer Schnitt durch die Haut 18–20 Tage alter Mäuse-Embryonen (HE; × 40) Pfeil: Beginnende Zellsprossen der Haaranlagen

Die Kultivierung der Zellen erfolgte in der Regel in Falcon-Schalen und Eagles Minimal Medium, angereichert mit 20% foetalem Kalb-Serum, unter Luft/CO_2(95/5%)-Atmosphäre.

Trypsiniert man Häute von 18–20 Tage alten Embryonen und kultiviert die so gewonnenen Zellen, dann sieht man nach 24 Std folgendes

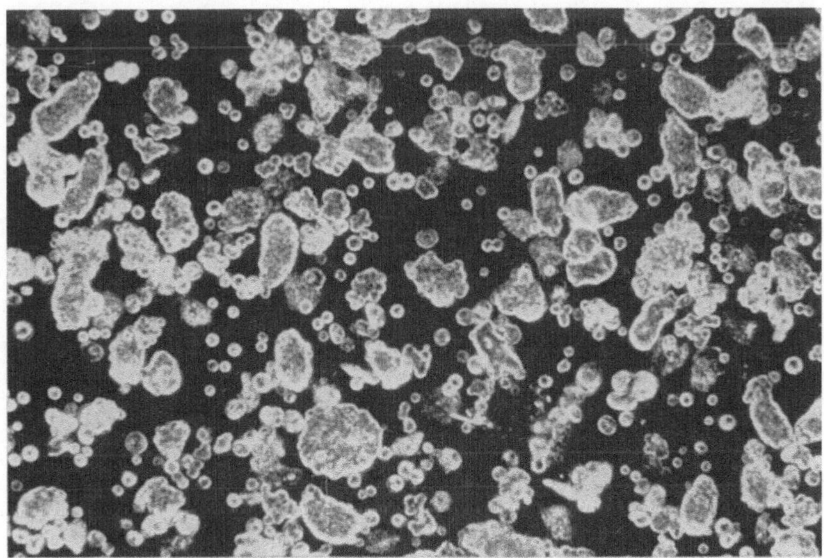

Abb. 3. Isolierte Epidermis-Zellklumpen aus der Haut 18–20 Tage alter Embryonen nach Aussaat in der Petrischale (Phasen-Kontrast; × 60)

Bild: In einem Fibroblasten-Monolayer liegen einzelne Inseln epithelialer Zellen. Beide Zellarten wachsen, die Fibroblasten jedoch ungleich schneller. Nach einigen Tagen überwuchern die Fibroblasten die Epithelinseln. Eine Trennung der beiden konkurrierenden Zellarten nach dem Anwachsen in der Kultur ist nur unvollständig möglich. Geringe Fibroblastenverunreinigungen reichen aus, die abgetrennten Epithelinseln von neuem zu überwuchern.

Eine selektive Gewinnung epidermaler Zellen wurde möglich, als sich herausstellte, daß die epithelialen Inseln aus Zellklumpen wachsen, die sich nicht wie die Zellen erwachsener Tiere erst sekundär in der Kultur aggregieren, sondern bereits in der frisch isolierten Zellsuspension vorhanden sind.

Es dürfte sich dabei im wesentlichen um Epithelzellen von Haaranlagen handeln, die bei 18–20 Tage alten Embryonen im histologischen Schnitt als Zellsprossung zu erkennen sind (Abb. 2), zum geringeren Teil um verklumpte Zellen des interfollikulären Stratum basale.

Eine zufriedenstellende Trennung dieser Zellklumpen von den Einzelzellen konnte über diskontinuierliche Ficoll-Gradienten erreicht werden, wie die Präparation nach dem Aussäen in der Petrischale zeigt (Abb. 3).

Nach 15 Std sind die Zellklumpen zu Inseln ausgewachsen (Abb. 4), die sich dann vergrößern und schließlich zu einem Monolayer zusammenwachsen. Abb. 5 zeigt einen Ausschnitt einer Kultur nach 2 Tagen mit der charakteristischen perinucleären Granulation.

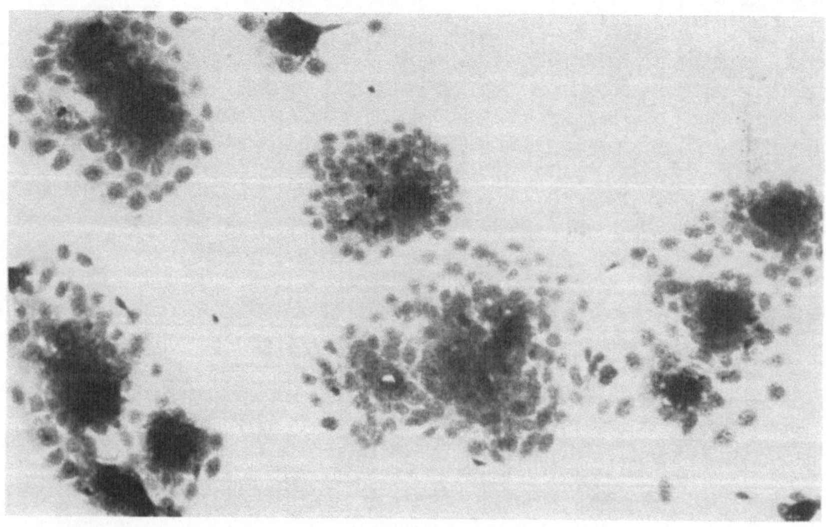

Abb. 4. 24 Std alte Kultur. Epidermis-Zellinseln aus der Haut 18–20 Tage alter Mäuse-Embryonen (C 57Bl/6J) (May Grünwald/Giemsa; $\times$ 110)

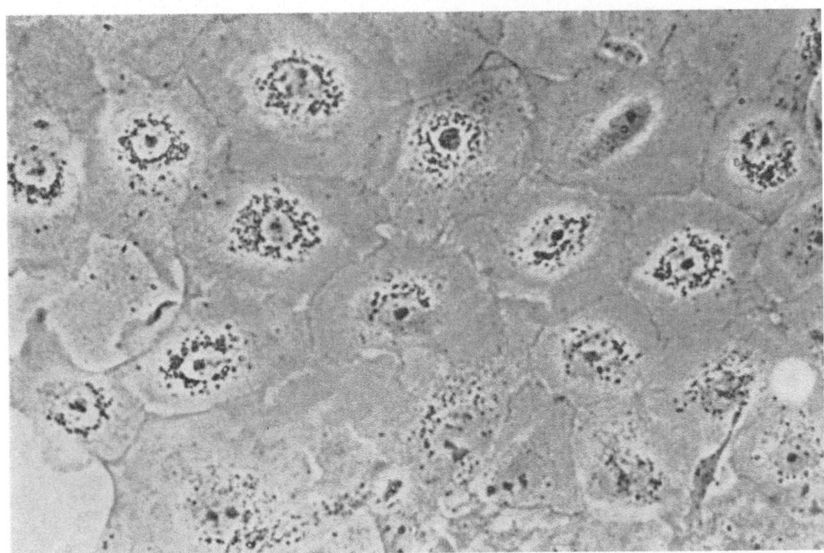

Abb. 5. 2 Tage alte Kultur. Epidermis-Zellen aus der Haut 18–20 Tage alter Mäuse-Embryonen (Phasen-Kontrast; × 380)

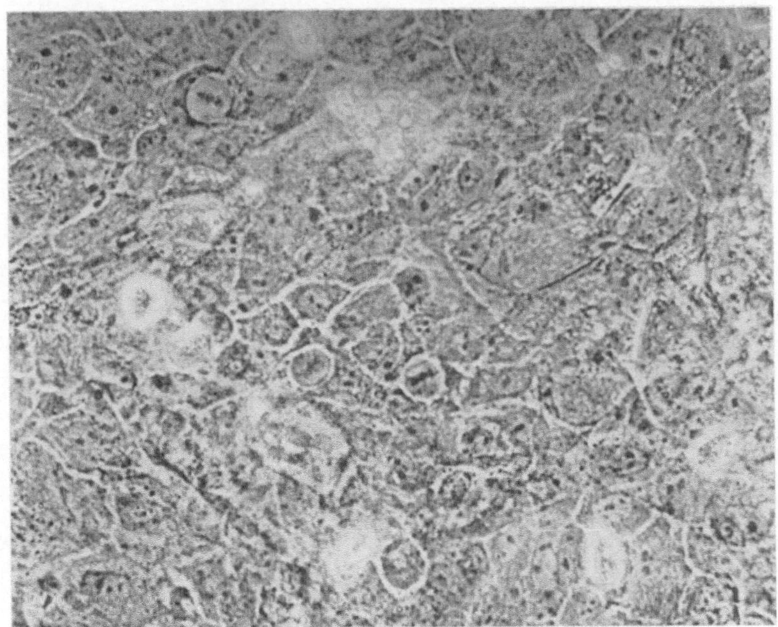

Abb. 6. 3 Tage alte Kultur. Epidermis-Zellen aus der Haut 18–20 Tage alter Mäuse-Embryonen. Beginn der streifig-granulären Zeichnung. 3 Metaphasen-Zellen. (Phasen-Kontrast; × 180)

Der Thymidineinbau in diesen Kulturen ist bereits nach 10 Std nachweisbar und zeigt nach 30 Std ein erstes Maximum. Die ersten Mitosen erscheinen nach 15 Std und erreichen nach ca. 36 Std ein deutliches Maximum. Die Generationszeit des ersten Proliferationsschubes dürfte bei 24 Std liegen. Die Mitosedauer beträgt ca. 1 Std.

Bereits nach 3 Tagen tritt eine markante Veränderung der Zellmorphologie in Form einer streifig-granulären Zeichnung des Zellplasmas auf (Abb. 6). Sie kann nur schwer im Sinne einer Degeneration interpretiert werden, da die mitotische Aktivität der Zellen unvermindert anhält.

Nach 4–6 Tagen ist ein 2–3schichtiger Zellrasen mit streifiger, granulierter Oberschicht auf einer generativen Unterlage entstanden. Das ist besonders gut zu sehen, wenn es, wie in Abb. 7, zu einer kuppelförmigen Abhebung der oberen Zellage kommt.

Nach 10–12 Tagen sind die Zellkerne in der Oberschicht bereits pyknotisch (Abb. 8). Die Zellmembran ist deutlich verdickt. Das Plasma ist stark granuliert. Unter dieser Zellschicht sind noch kleine Inseln

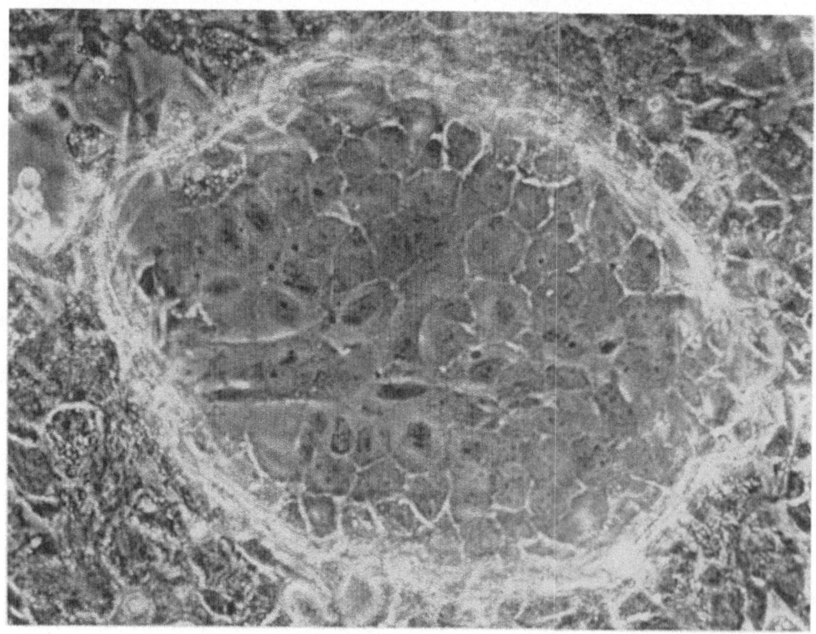

Abb. 7. 6 Tage alte Kultur. Epidermis-Zellen aus der Haut 18–20 Tage alter Mäuse-Embryonen. Zwei Zellschichten-Stadium. Die obere „granulierte" Schicht hat sich kuppelförmig angehoben und gibt den Blick frei auf die untere, „generative" Zellage (Phasen-Kontrast; $\times$ 180)

nicht differenzierter Zellen zu erkennen; Mitosen sind aber zu diesem Zeitpunkt nur noch selten zu sehen.

Papanicolaou-Färbungen von abgelösten Oberschichten – ebenso wie positive Rhodamin-B-Fluoreszenz der Hornzellen – lassen den Schluß zu, daß es sich bei diesen Veränderungen um eine Art Keratose handelt.

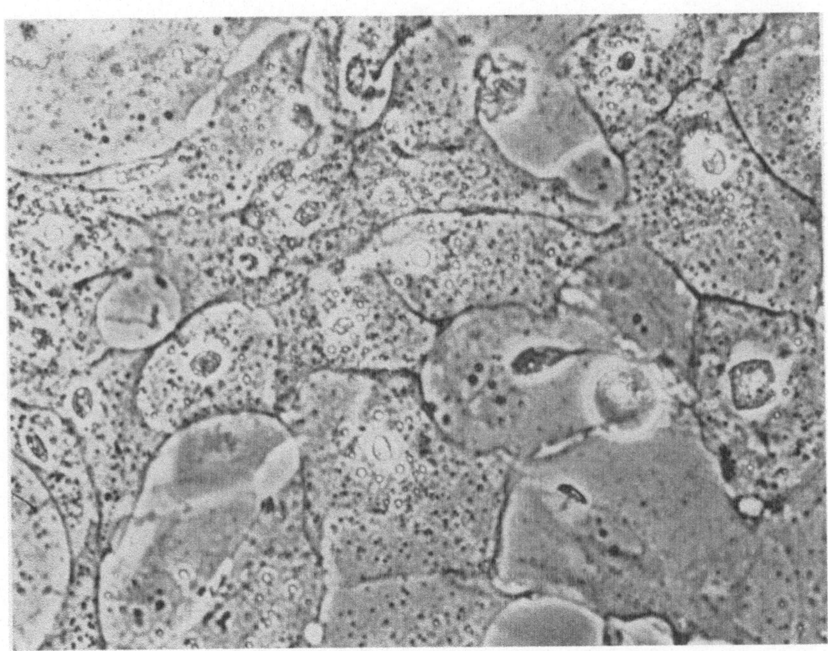

Abb. 8. 12 Tage alte Epidermis-Kultur. Die oberste Zellage weist Kernpyknose, Plasma-Granulierung und stark verdickte Zellmembranen auf (Phasen-Kontrast; × 350)

In 10–14 Tage alten Kulturen tritt eine starke Schrumpfung der oberen Schichten ein, was meist zur Zerreißung aller Zellschichten führt. Die Haftung der Zellagen aneinander ist offenbar stärker als die der Zellen an der Plastikoberfläche. Die Hornschicht löst sich ab. Die übrigbleibenden, geschrumpften Zellinseln degenerieren in wenigen Tagen. Unterkulturen konnten bisher nur wenige Tage am Leben erhalten werden, da sie nur geringe Wachstumstendenz zeigen.

Fassen wir zusammen:

1. Es ist uns – soweit uns nach sorgfältiger Prüfung der Literatur bekannt ist – zum ersten Mal gelungen, ausgehend von Zellsuspensionen der embryonalen Mäusehaut, rein epidermale Zellkulturen zu erhalten.

Außer mit morphologischen ist auch mit immunologischen Methoden [*8*] der epidermale Charakter der Kulturen nachgewiesen.

2. Neben einer guten Proliferationsaktivität über 8–10 Tage weisen diese Kulturen zellmorphologische Veränderungen auf, die im Sinne einer Differenzierung zu interpretieren sind.

Literatur

1. Berwald, Y., Sachs, L.: In vitro cell transformation with chemical carcinogens. Nature **200**, 1182 (1963).
2. Briggaman, R. A., Abele, D. C., Harris, S. R., Wheeler, C. E.: Preparation and characterization of a viable suspension of postembryonic human epidermal cells. J. Invest. Dermat. **48**, 159 (1967).
3. Giovanella, B. C., Heidelberger, C.: Mouse epidermal cells and carcinogenesis I. Isolation of skin constituents. Cancer Res. **25**, 161 (1965).
4. Hecker, E.: Cocarcinogenic principles from seed oil of croton tiglium and from other euphorbiaceae. Cancer Res. **28**, 2338 (1969).
5. Perry, V. P., Evans, V. J., Earl, W. R., Wyatt, G. W., Bedell, W. C.: Long-term tissue culture of human skin. Amer. J. Hyg. **63**, 52 (1956).
6. Reaven, E. P., Cox, A. J.: Organ culture of human skin. J. Invest. Dermat. **44**, 151 (1965).
7. Sanford, K. K., Hoemann, R. E.: Neoplastic transformation of mouse and hamster cell in vitro with and without polyoma virus. J. nat. Cancer Inst. **39**, 691 (1967).
8. Worst, P., Fusenig, N. E.: In Vorbereitung.

Über die Proteinbindung carcinogener Kohlenwasserstoffe und cocarcinogener Phorbolester

Von

M. Traut, G. Kreibich und E. Hecker

Den vorliegenden Experimenten liegt die Auffassung zugrunde, daß Substanzen, die eine so tiefgreifende und über die Zellteilung hinaus bleibende Wirkung auf Zellen ausüben wie Carcinogene und Cocarcinogene, in irgendeiner Weise mit den Molekülen in Wechselwirkung treten müssen, die die Information der Zellen tragen. Diese informationstragenden Moleküle sind die Nucleinsäuren und die Proteine. Im folgenden soll über die Bindung von carcinogenen Kohlenwasserstoffen und cocarcinogenen Phorbolestern an die Proteine der Mäusehaut berichtet werden.

Weibliche NMRI-Mäuse wurden geschoren; sie erhielten eine acetonische Lösung der mit Tritium markierten Testsubstanz auf die Rückenhaut und wurden nach bestimmten Zeitintervallen getötet. Die Rückenhaut wurde abgezogen, Fett- und Bindegewebe abgekratzt und die zurückbleibende Epidermis unter flüssigem Stickstoff im Mörser pulverisiert. Aus dem Hautpulver wurde das lösliche Protein mit isotonischer KCl-Lösung 3mal extrahiert; die vereinigten Extrakte wurden zur Entfernung von allen Partikeln bei 105000 g zentrifugiert. In dieser Lösung wurde die an Protein gebundene Radioaktivität nach der Plättchen-Methode von Novelli [*3*] in der Modifikation von Volm u. Süss [*4*] gemessen: Ein Aliquot wird auf ein Filterplättchen pipettiert, dieses wird getrocknet und anschließend nacheinander für je eine Stunde in 10%-ige TCA-Lösung und zweimal in 5%-ige TCA-Lösung getaucht. Hierbei wird das Protein auf dem Filterplättchen fixiert und die in Lösung befindliche Aktivität ausgewaschen; durch nachfolgende Extraktion mit Äther/Alkohol, Äther, Benzol, Dioxan und Aceton wird adsorptiv gebundene Aktivität entfernt.

Abb. 1 zeigt den zeitlichen Verlauf der Proteinbindung. Der Vergleich der mit der Plättchen-Methode gefundenen Werte für 1.2.3.4-DBA mit den von Heidelberger u. Moldenhauer [*2*] nach einer anderen Methode erhaltenen Werte zeigt gute Übereinstimmung. Vergleicht man die Bindung von Kohlenwasserstoff und Phorbolderivaten, so fällt als erstes auf, daß der Kohlenwasserstoff um etwa zwei Größenordnungen stärker gebunden wird als die Phorbolderivate. Weiter ist die hohe Nullpunktbindung der Phorbolester bemerkenswert. Allerdings stellen diese Werte Artefakte dar, denn die Nullpunktbindung ist deutlich niedriger, wenn man die Aktivität, die nur an der Hautoberfläche klebt, vor der Homogenisierung mit in Aceton getränkten Kleenex-Tüchern abwischt. Ein solches Abwischen beeinflußt dagegen den Wert der Nullpunktbindung des Kohlenwasserstoffes nicht.

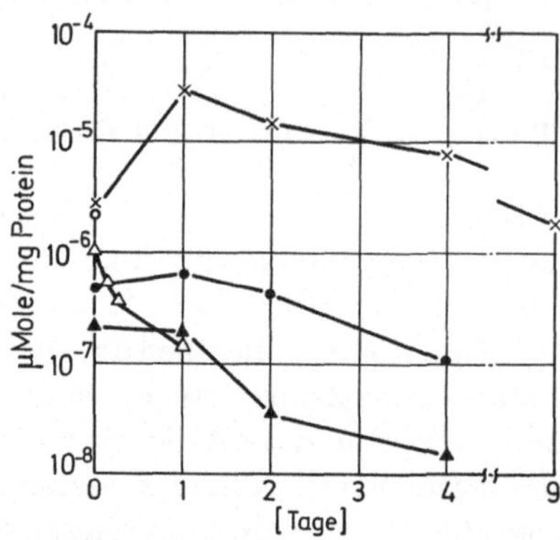

Abb. 1. Bindung von 1.2.3.4.-DBA-^{3}H, TPA-20-^{3}H und 4α-PDD-20-^{3}H an die löslichen Proteine der Mäusehaut, bestimmt nach der Plättchen-Methode. 1.2.3.4.-DBA-^{3}H (x); TPA-20-^{3}H mit (▲) und ohne (△) Entfernung der oberflächlich abgelagerten Substanz; 4α-PDD-^{3}H mit (●) und ohne (○) Entfernung der oberflächlich abgelagerten Substanz

Weiter sollte geprüft werden, ob die Bindung der Phorbolderivate an die löslichen Proteine der Mäusehaut irgendeine Spezifität zeigt und wie sie im Vergleich zur Bindung der kondensierten aromatischen Kohlenwasserstoffe aussieht. Hierzu wurde wiederum der geschorene Mäuserücken mit radioaktivem Material (TPA als cocarcinogenem, 4α-PDD als nicht cocarcinogenem Phorbolester, 1.2.3.4-DBA als nichtcarcinogenem KW und DMBA als carcinogenem KW) behandelt. Das lösliche Protein wurde, wie oben beschrieben, extrahiert; die Proteinlösung wurde dialysiert und lyophilisiert. Der Rückstand wurde dann in einer kleinen Menge isotonischer KCl-Lösung aufgenommen und an Sephadex-G100 chromatographiert. Abb. 2 zeigt die Elutionskurven von löslichem Protein aus der Mäusehaut von Tieren, die zuvor mit markiertem DMBA bzw. 1.2.3.4-DBA behandelt worden waren. Die durchgezogene Linie gibt Proteingehalt (Folin) an; sie ist gut reproduzierbar. Das Elutionsmuster der löslichen Proteine mit und ohne Gabe von Kohlenwasserstoff ist identisch.

Im Falle von DBA oder DMBA ist die Radioaktivitätsverteilung unterschiedlich. Zunächst fällt auf, daß eine beachtliche Portion des DBA am Ende der Chromatographie – lange nach der Elution der hochmolekularen Substanzen – in einem recht scharfen Peak aus der Säule läuft. Ein solcher Endpeak fehlt beim DMBA, Daß dies nicht auf die Abwesenheit freien, ungebundenen Kohlenwasserstoffs zurückzuführen ist, erkennt man beim *In-vitro*-Versuch; auch dort kommt das ungebundene

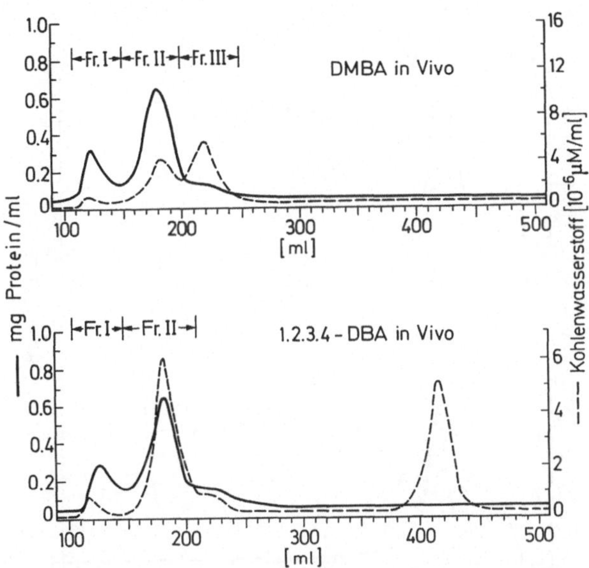

Abb. 2. Chromatographie der löslichen Proteine der Mäusehaut, die jeweils 12 Std. nach Gabe des aromatischen Kohlenwasserstoffs *in vivo* isoliert wurden, auf Sephadex G-100

DMBA über viele Fraktionen verteilt, ohne einen ausgeprägten Peak zu bilden. Hinzuweisen ist ferner auf den relativ hohen Aktivitätspeak bei den niedermolekularen Proteinen; ob es sich hierbei um eine spezifische Bindung handelt, konnten wir nicht nachweisen. Wir haben jedoch unsere Zweifel, wenn wir die Abb. 3 betrachten. Hier wurden die löslichen Proteine der Mäusehaut durch Extraktion, Dialyse und Lyophilisation isoliert. Unmittelbar bevor die Proteinlösung auf die Säule gegeben wurde, mischten wir eine gewisse Menge radioaktiven Kohlenwasserstoffs zu; die Chromatographie erfolgte wie beim *In-vivo*-Versuch. Auch hier sehen wir einen ganz massiven Endpeak beim DBA, beim DMBA jedoch nur die Andeutung eines Endpeaks. Was jedoch im Gegensatz zu den *In-vivo*-Versuchen auffällt, ist einmal das Fehlen eines Aktivitätspeaks unter der Proteinfraktion III im Falle von DMBA; wir sehen zwei gleich hohe Aktivitätsgipfel unter den Fraktionen I und II (beim *In-vivo*-Versuch war in Fraktion I nur sehr wenig Aktivität zu finden, während ein beachtlicher Berg unter Fraktion III lag). Gerade umgekehrt sieht es beim DBA aus. Ähnlich wie beim *In-vivo*-Experiment haben wir hohe Aktivität im Endpeak und unter Proteinfraktion II, aber nur wenig Aktivität unter Fraktion I. Im Gegensatz zum *In-vivo*-Versuch finden wir *in vitro* jedoch beachtliche Aktivität in Fraktion III.

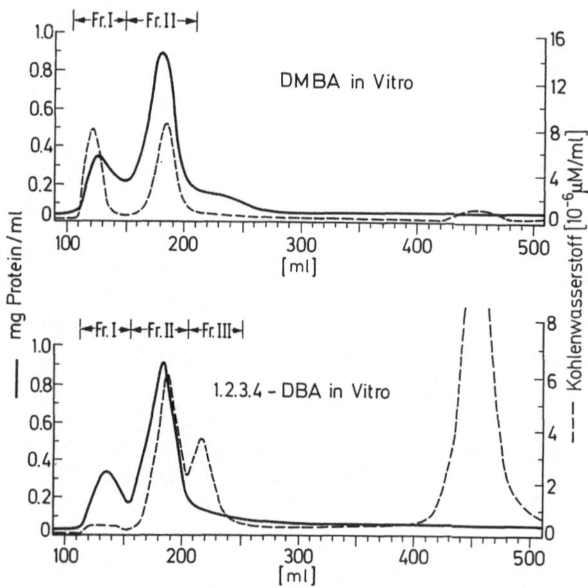

Abb. 3. Chromatographie der löslichen Proteine der Mäusehaut, nach Inkubation mit dem aromatischen Kohlenwasserstoff *in vitro*, auf Sephadex G-100

Nun zu den Phorbolestern: Abb. 4 zeigt die Elutionsprofile von löslichem Protein aus der Haut von Mäusen, die 12 Std zuvor mit PDD bzw. 4α-PDD behandelt worden waren. Überraschend ist die Veränderung des Elutionsmusters des Proteins nach Behandlung mit dem inaktiven 4α-PDD. Die Proteinfraktion I wird nicht mehr sauber von II getrennt; beide gehen ineinander über. Worauf dies zurückzuführen ist, bleibt unklar. Übereinstimmend kommt der Großteil der Radioaktivität sowohl beim aktiven PDD als auch beim inaktiven 4α-PDD zusammen mit den hochmolekularen Proteinen von der Säule. Unter Fraktion II wird nur noch wenig gefunden; auch der Endpeak ist nur verhältnismäßig schwach ausgebildet.

In Abb. 5 sehen wir das Ergebnis des *In-vitro*-Versuchs. Fast die gesamte Aktivität kommt mit der hochmolekularen Fraktion I; in Fraktion

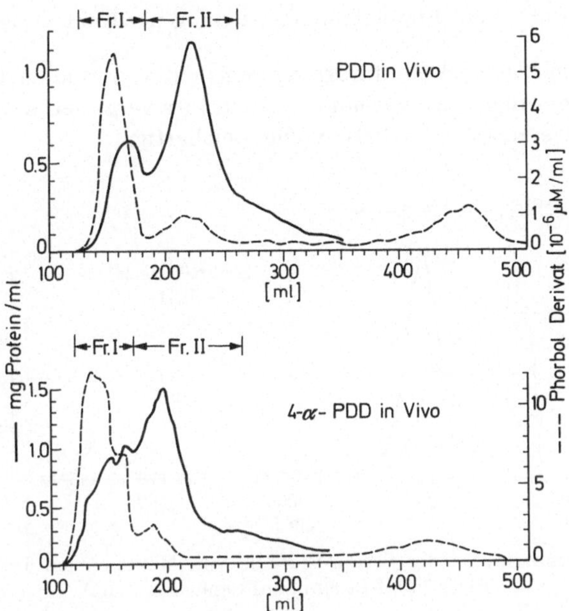

Abb. 4. Chromatographie der löslichen Proteine der Mäusehaut, die 12 Std. nach Gaben von PDD-20-^{3}H bzw. 4α-PDD-20-$_3$H *in vivo* isoliert wurden, auf Sephadex G-100

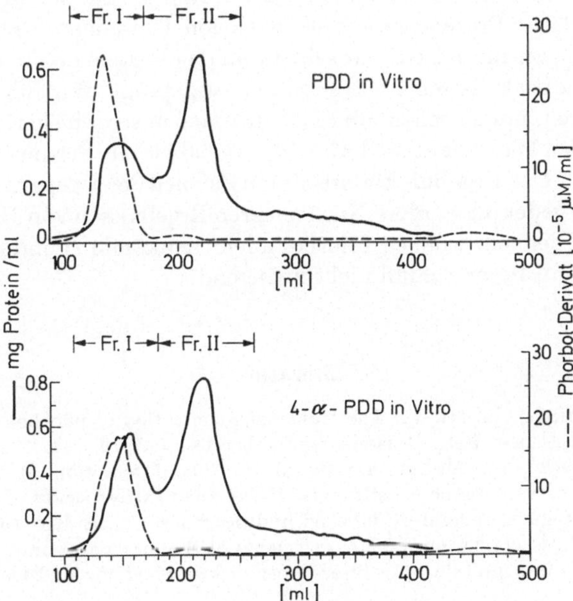

Abb. 5. Chromatographie der löslichen Proteine der Mäusehaut, jeweils nach Inkubation mit PDD-20-^{3}H bzw. 4α-PDD-20-$_3$H *in vitro*, auf Sephadex G-100

II ist nur ein kleiner Aktivitätsgipfel angedeutet, und auch der Endpeak ist nur andeutungsweise vorhanden. Auch hier verhalten sich das aktive PDD und das inaktive 4α-PDD völlig gleichartig.

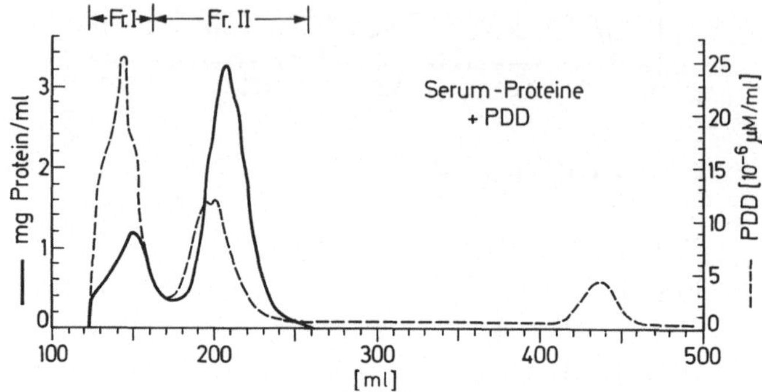

Abb. 6. Chromatographie der Serum-Proteine von Mäusen nach Inkubation mit PDD-20-^{3}H *in vitro*, auf Sephadex G-100

Abb. 6 zeigt das Ergebnis einer Sephadex-G100-Chromatographie von Mäuseserum, das zuvor mit PDD *in vitro* inkubiert worden war. Auch hier finden wir den höchsten Aktivitätspeak bei der Fraktion der hochmolekularen Proteine, während Fraktion II weniger Aktivität enthält. Fast die gesamte Aktivität scheint an das Protein gebunden zu sein, denn der Endpeak ist nur noch schwach ausgeprägt. Wir führten diesen Versuch durch, um zu sehen, ob PDD, das nach unserer bisherigen Kenntnis nur in der Mäusehaut wirksam ist, irgendwie an Serumproteine gebunden wird. Das Ergebnis könnte als ein Zeichen der Unspezität der Proteinbindung gedeutet werden. Nach neueren Ergebnissen von Berenblum u. Lonai [*1*] jedoch, wonach Phorbol allein Leukämie zu induzieren vermag, erscheint dieser Schluß nicht zwingend.

Literatur

1. Berenblum, H., Lonai, V.: The leukaemogenic action of phorbol. 1. Congress Europ. Ass. Cancer Res., Brussels, September 14–17, 1970.
2. Heidelberger, C., Moldenhauer, M. G.: The interaction of carcinogenic hydrocarbons with tissue constituents. IV. A quantitative study of the binding to skin proteins of several ^{14}C-labelled hydrocarbons. Cancer Res. **16**, 442 (1956).
3. Mans, R. J., Novelli, G. D.: Measurements of the incorporation of radioactive amino acids into protein by a filter-paper disk method. Arch. Biochem. **94**, 48 (1961).
4. Süss, R., Volm, M.: Rapid screening of macromolecular synthesis in single cell cultures. Naturwissenschaften **55**, 134 (1968).

Über ein neues Cocarcinogen aus Euphorbia ingens

Von

H. J. Opferkuch und E. Hecker

Zusammenfassung

Aus dem Latex von Euphorbia ingens, einer in Südafrika wachsenden Species der Familie der Wolfsmilchgewächse, konnten die entzündlich und cocarcinogen wirkenden Inhaltsstoffe isoliert und charakterisiert werden. Die Struktur des den Wirkstoffen zugrunde liegenden neuen Diterpens Ingenol wurde durch Röntgenstrukturanalyse ermittelt. Einer der Wirkstoffe – das Ingenol-3-hexadekanoat ($C_{36}H_{58}O_6$) – ist entzündlich und cocarcinogen etwas weniger wirksam als der Phorbolester A1. Entzündlich wesentlich wirksamer als Ingenol-3-hexadekanoat sind die Inhaltsstoffe Ingenol-3-dekatrienoat ($C_{30}H_{40}O_6$) und Dekatrienoyl-16-hydroxyingenol-tigliat, ein Diester des in Position 16 hydroxylierten Ingenols.

Ausführliche Darstellung in Zechmeister, K., Brandl, F., Hoppe, W., Hecker, E., Opferkuch, H. J., Adolf, W.: Tetrahedron Letters No. 47, pp. 4075 (1970) und Opferkuch, H. J.: Dissertation Universität Heidelberg 1971.

Untersuchungen über die Beziehungen zwischen Struktur und Wirkung von Phorbolestern

Von

R. Schmidt und E. Hecker

Die aus Crotonöl isolierten natürlichen Cocarcinogene sind Ester von Phorbol (Abb. 1) mit jeweils einer lang- und einer kurzkettigen Fettsäure an den Positionen 12 und 13 [*4*]. Sie besitzen mehrere funktionelle Gruppen, über deren Beitrag zur biologischen Wirksamkeit im Berenblum-Experiment [4] man durch gewisse chemische Veränderungen des Moleküls Aussagen machen kann.

Als Bezugssubstanz für solche Untersuchungen über die Struktur-Wirkungs-Beziehungen wird das partialsynthetisch leicht zugängliche Phorbol-12.13-didekanoat „PDD" verwendet, das praktisch dieselbe entzündliche und cocarcinogene Wirkung wie der Crotonöl-Faktor Al („TPA") besitzt [*10, 11*].

Da schon die Veränderung einzelner funktioneller Gruppen im PDD zu partiellem oder vollständigem Verlust der biologischen Aktivität führen kann [*10, 11*], erscheint es zweckmäßig, jeweils nur eine funktionelle Gruppe in möglichst systematischer Weise zu variieren.

Veränderungen des Moleküls durch Angriff an den Hydroxylgruppen

Frühere Versuche haben gezeigt, daß die chemische Veränderung der Hydroxylgruppe an C-20 durch Veresterung, Verätherung, Substitution durch Chlor bzw. partielle Oxydation zu einem starken und teilweise zu vollständigem Wirkungsverlust führt [*10, 11*]. Zur Darstellung des Derivates mit vollständig oxydierter primärer Hydroxylgruppe geht man von Phorbol-12.13-didekanoat (1) aus (Abb. 2). Der durch Behandlung mit Braunstein als Zwischenprodukt erhaltene Aldehyd (2) wird mit Selendioxid/Wasserstoffperoxid zur entsprechenden Säure (3) weiteroxydiert.

Die Substitution der Hydroxylgruppe an C-20 durch Wasserstoff ist auf folgendem Wege möglich: man tauscht in dem in Abb. 2 mit (4) bezeichneten Phorbol-12.13-diacetat die primäre Hydroxylgruppe durch Reaktion mit Methansulfonsäurechlorid in Pyridin gegen Chlor aus und erhält als Zwischenprodukt die Verbindung (5). Das Halogen ersetzt man

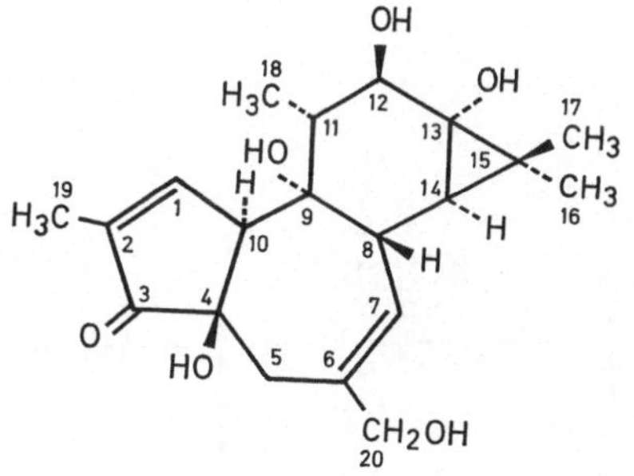

Abb. 1. Phorbol

reduktiv durch Wasserstoff und reinigt auf der Stufe des nicht abgebildeten 20-Desoxyphorbol-12.13-diacetats. Aus diesem erhält man nach Verseifung mit Natriummethylat/Methanol und anschließender Veresterung mit Dekanoylchlorid in Pyridin das 20-Desoxy-phorbol-12.13-didekanoat (6). Diese Verbindung wurde auf anderem Wege schon früher dargestellt [1].

12.13-Di-O-dekanoyl-
-phorbol-säure-(20)

20-Desoxy-phorbol-
-12.13-didekanoat

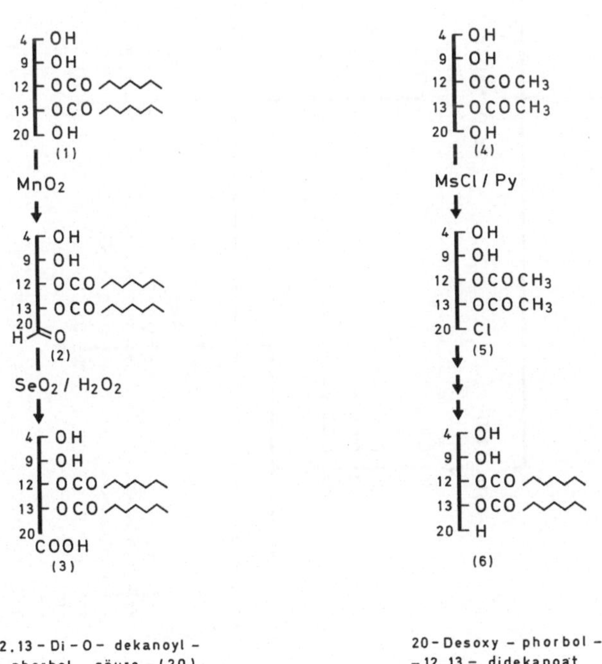

Abb. 2. Darstellung von Phorbol-12.13-didekanoaten mit veränderter Hydroxymethylgruppe (schematisch)

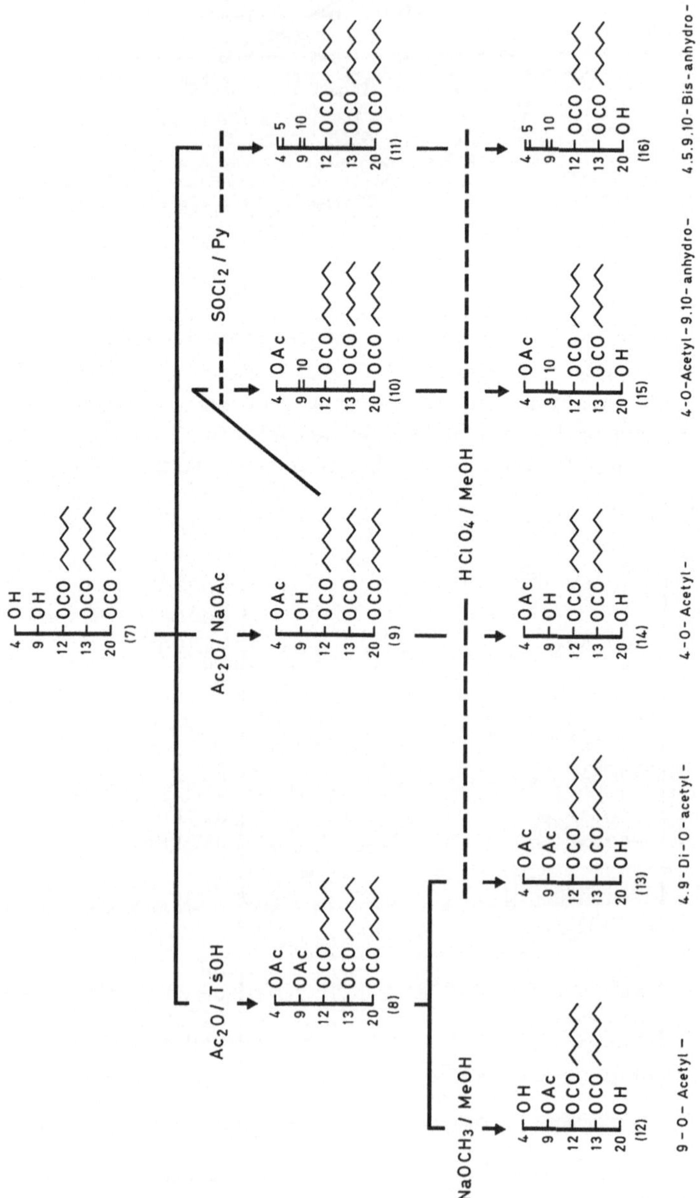

Abb. 3. Darstellung von Phorbol-12.13-didekanoaten mit veränderten Hydroxylgruppen 4 und 9 (schematisch)

Die Hydroxylgruppen 4 bzw. 9 konnten bis jetzt noch nicht gegen Wasserstoff ausgetauscht werden. Um dennoch Hinweise für die Bedeutung dieser funktionellen Gruppen zu erhalten, wurden Versuche unternommen, sie selektiv zu verestern bzw. abzuspalten (Abb. 3).

Im Phorbol-12.13.20-tridekanoat (7) lassen sich mit Acetanhydrid durch basische Katalyse in der Hitze die tertiäre Ketol-Hydroxylgruppe an C-4 bzw. durch saure Katalyse [*6*] die Hydroxylgruppen 4 und 9 acetylieren. Auf diese Weise werden die Zwischenprodukte (8) und (9) erhalten. Aus (9) – dem 4-O-Acetyl-phorbol-12.13.20-tridekanoat – wird durch Behandlung mit Thionylchlorid in Pyridin die OH-Gruppe an C-9 formal als Wasser abgespalten und somit eine Doppelbindung von C-9 nach C-10 eingeführt. Man erhält das Zwischenprodukt (10).

Die gleiche Reaktion auf das Phorbol-12.13.20-tridekanoat (7) selbst angewandt, führt zum Zwischenprodukt (11) mit zwei Doppelbindungen von C-4 nach C-5 und von C-9 nach C-10.

Aus den Zwischenprodukten (8–11) setzt man die für die biologische Wirkung bereits als wesentlich erkannte [*10*, *11*] Hydroxylgruppe an C-20 durch sauer katalysierte Umesterung [*2*] frei.

Aus (8) – dem 4.9-Di-O-acetyl-phorbol-12.13.20-tridekanoat – wird bei basisch katalysierter Umesterung zusätzlich die Hydroxylgruppe an C-4 freigesetzt.

Auf diese Weise werden Derivate des Phorbol-12.13-didekanoats erhalten, die entweder zwei zusätzliche Acetylgruppen in 4- und 9-Stellung im Derivat (13) bzw. eine zusätzliche Acetylgruppe in 4- oder 9-Stellung in den Derivaten (12) und (14) tragen. Im Derivat (15) ist bei acetylierter 4-Stellung die Hydroxylgruppe an C-9 entfernt und im Derivat (16) sind beide Hydroxylgruppen 4 und 9 abgespalten.

Veränderungen des Moleküls durch Angriff an den Doppelbindungen

Von dem an der Doppelbindung $\Delta 6$ epoxydierten Derivat des Phorbol-12.13-didekanoats ist bereits bekannt, daß es nur geringe biologische Wirksamkeit besitzt [*10*, *11*]. Es sollte daher versucht werden, auch das Derivat mit durch Wasserstoff gesättigten Doppelbindungen darzustellen (siehe Abb. 4).

Bei der direkten Hydrierung von Phorbolderivaten wird neben der Absättigung der Doppelbindungen stets auch die Hydroxylgruppe 20 aus der Hydroxymethylgruppe des Phorbols reduktiv entfernt [*6*]. So würde man z. B. bei der Hydrierung von Phorbol-12.13-didekanoat (1) das Tetrahydro-20-desoxy-phorbol-12.13-didekanoat (17) erhalten. Daher muß zur Darstellung eines Derivates mit hydrierten Doppelbindungen allein ein Umweg beschritten werden. Man geht dazu von dem durch Oxydation von (1) mit Braunstein zugänglichen Aldehyd (2) aus (Abb. 4).

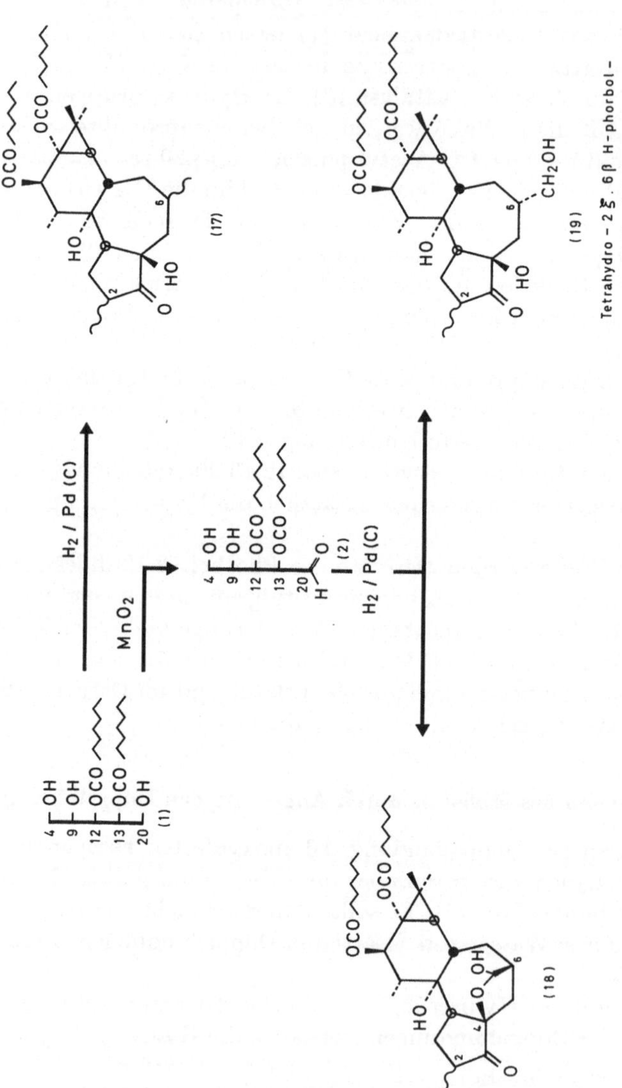

Abb. 4. Darstellung von Tetrahydro-phorbol-12.13-didekanoat

Bei dessen katalytischer Hydrierung entsteht zunächst durch Absättigung der beiden Doppelbindungen ein Gemisch von Epimeren sowohl bezüglich C-2 als auch bezüglich C-6. Das eine der beiden Epimeren an C-6, bei dem die Aldehydfunktion β-ständig ist, also über der Ebene des Moleküls liegt, bildet unter Beteiligung der ebenfalls β-ständigen Hydroxylgruppe an C-4 spontan ein inneres Halbacetal (18), das nicht weiter bearbeitet wird.

Das andere Epimere bezüglich C-6 enthält eine α-ständige, d.h. unter die Ebene des Moleküls gerichtete Aldehydfunktion; diese wird unter den Bedingungen der Hydrierung zur Hydroxymethylgruppe reduziert. Das so erhaltene Tetrahydro-phorbol-12.13-didekanoat (19) ist noch ein Epimerengemisch bezüglich C-2.

Veränderungen des Moleküls durch Isomerisierungen

Die Behandlung von Phorbol (20) mit Natriummethylat/Methanol (Abb. 5) ergibt nach Acetylierung des Gemisches neben Phorbol-12.13. 20-triacetat (22), das aus nicht umgesetztem Phorbol entsteht [*6*], das bekannte Epimere 4α-Phorbol-12.13.20-triacetat (21) [*7*], sowie das bisher unbekannte 10β-Phorbol-12.13.20-triacetat (23) und das mit (22) isomere Δ1-Iso-phorbol-12.13.20-triacetat (24).

Durch sauer katalysierte Umesterung erhält man aus (23) und (24) die entsprechenden 12.13-Diacetate (25) und (26).

Biologische Wirksamkeit der dargestellten Verbindungen

Die biologische Wirksamkeit der neuen Phorbolderivate wurde mit derjenigen von PDD bzw. Phorbol-12.13-diacetat verglichen.

Als Maß für die entzündliche Wirkung dienen die Entzündungseinheit (EE) bzw. die entzündliche Dosis 50 (ED_{50}), gemessen am Mäuseohr [*3,5*]. Die cocarcinogene Wirkung wurde im standardisierten Berenblum-Experiment [4] jeweils mit 0,1 μM DMBA als Initiator und 2mal wöchentlicher Applikation der in den Tabellen 1 und 2 aufgeführten Einzeldosen des Promotors über 12 Wochen gemessen. Die Tumorrate der überlebenden Tiere wird in Prozent, die mittlere Tumorausbeute in Tumoren pro überlebende Maus angegeben. Die ED_{50} des Phorbol-12.13-didekanoats (PDD) liegt bei 0,01μM/Ohr. Im Tumorpromotionstest tragen bei der Standarddosierung nach 12 Wochen 82% der überlebenden Tiere Tumoren und zwar im Mittel 3,6 Tumoren/Überlebende (Tab. 1).

Wenn, wie im 4-O-Acetyl-PDD, die OH-Gruppe 4 zusätzlich verestert ist, dann steigt die ED_{50} etwa um den Faktor 2×10^2; im Tumorpromotionstest erhält man auch mit dem Dreifachen der Standarddosierung

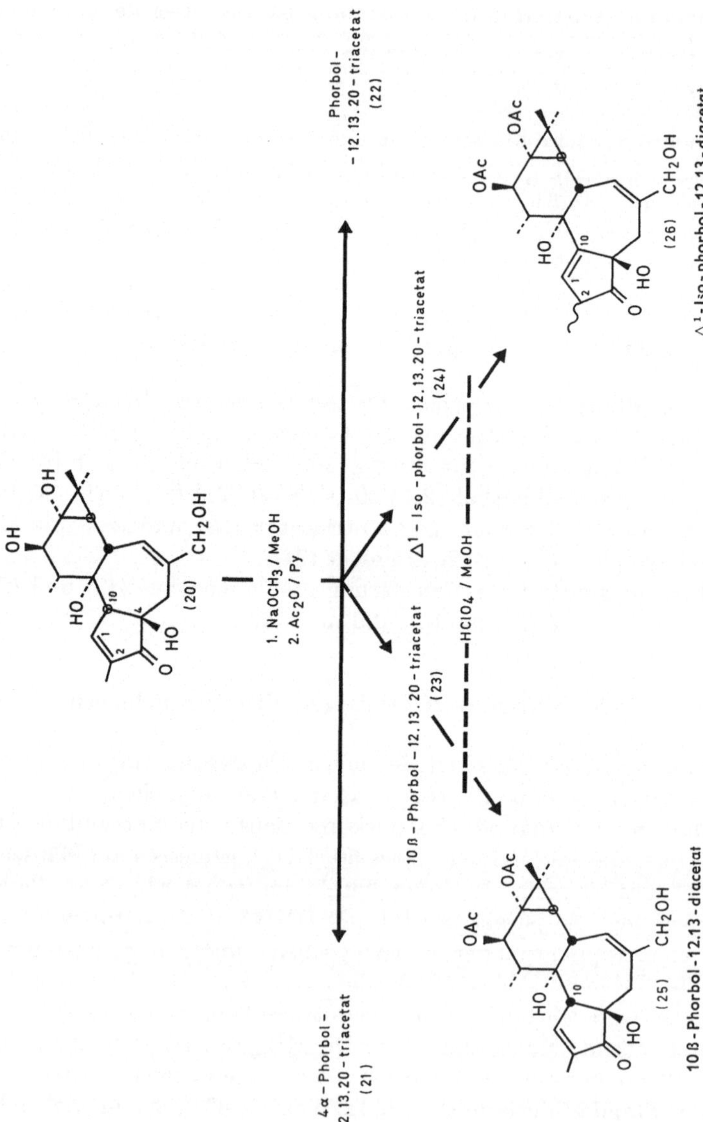

Abb. 5. Darstellung von Δ^1-Iso-phorbol- und 10β-Phorbol-12.13-diacetat

keine Tumoren. Die an Hydroxylgruppe 9 zusätzlich acetylierte Verbindung 9-O-Acetyl-PDD zeigt eine nur um den Faktor 30 erhöhte ED_{50}. Im Cocarcinogentest wird nach 12 Wochen 1 Tumorträger (entsprechend 4%) mit 1 Tumor gezählt (Tab. 1).

Tabelle 1. *Biologische Aktivität der dargestellten Phorbol-Derivate I*

Substanz	Entzündliche[a] Wirksamkeit		Cocarcinogene[c] Wirksamkeit		
	EE	ED_{50}[b]	Einzeldosis p	Tumorrate[d]	mittl. Tumorausbeute[d]
	[mμM/Ohr]	[mμM/Ohr]	[μM]	[%]	[Tumoren/Überl.]
Phorbol-12.13-didekanoat (PDD)	0,1	0,01	0,02	82	3,6
4-0-Acetyl-PDD	21,0	1,9	0,06	—	—
9-0-Acetyl-PDD	1,1	0,28	0,02	4	0,04
4.9-Di-0-acetyl-PDD	> 100,0	—	0,02	—	—
4-0-Acetyl-9.10-anhydro-PDD	> 100,0	—	0,12	—	—
4.5.9.10-Bis-anhydro-PDD	> 100,0	—	0,02	—	—

[a] Standard-Methode, Mäuseohr (Hecker, 1963; Hecker et al., 1966).
[b] Einfache Standardabweichung σ:1,3; Signifikanzniveau $\alpha = 0,05$.
[c] Standard-Methode, NMRI-Mäuse (Hecker, 1971); Initiator: 0,1 μM 7.12-Dimethyl-benz(a)anthracen.
[d] nach 12 Wochen = 24 Applikationen.

Die Verbindungen 4.9-Di-O-Acetyl-PDD, 4-O-Acetyl-9.10-anhydro-PDD und 4.5,9.10-Bis-anhydro-PDD, in denen die Hydroxylgruppen 4 und 9 beide acetyliert bzw. bei acetylierter Hydroxylgruppe 4 die Hydroxylgruppe 9 oder die beiden freien Hydroxylgruppen 4 und 9 abgespalten wurden, sind in beiden Tests mit den applizierten Dosen unwirksam.

Derivate des Phorbol-12.13-didekanoats, in denen die Hydroxymethylgruppe an C-20 zur Säure oxydiert bzw. zur Methylgruppe reduziert ist, sind in den applizierten Dosen ebenfalls wirkungslos. Sind die Doppelbindungen hydriert, wie im Tetrahydro-PDD, so erhöht sich die ED_{50} um den Faktor 10^2; bei der angegebenen Dosierung treten im Tumorpromotiontest keine Tumoren auf (siehe Tab. 2).

Δ^1-Iso-phorbol-12.13-diacetat und 10β-Phorbol-12.13-diacetat sind bei einer Dosis von 45 mμM bzw. 100 mμM entzündlich nicht wirksam, während Phorbol-12.13-diacetat eine ED_{50} von 1,5 mμM/Ohr aufweist (Tab. 2).

Tabelle 2. *Biologische Aktivität der dargestellten Phorbol-Derivate II*

Substanz	Entzündliche[a] Wirksamkeit		Cocarcinogene[c] Wirksamkeit		
	EE [mμM/Ohr]	ED_{50}[b] [mμM/Ohr]	Einzeldosis p [μM]	Tumor-[d] rate [%]	mittl. Tumor-[d] ausbeute [Tumoren/Überl.]
PDD-Säure-(20)	> 100,0	—	0,02	—	—
20-Desoxy-PDD	> 100,0	—	0,02	—	—
Tetrahydro-PDD	4,6	1,0	0,02	—	—
Phorbol-12.13-diacetat	17,0	1,5	4,0	—	—
Δ^1-Iso-phorbol-12.13-diacetat	> 45,0	—	nicht untersucht		
10β-Phorbol-12.13-diacetat	> 100,0	—	nicht untersucht		

[a] Standard-Methode, Mäuseohr (Hecker, 1963; Hecker et al., 1966).
[b] Einfache Standardabweichung σ: 1,3; Signifikanzniveau $\alpha = 0{,}05$.
[c] Standard-Methode, NMRI-Mäuse (Hecker, 1971); Initiator: 0,1 μM 7.12-Dimethyl-benz(a)anthracen.
[d] nach 12 Wochen = 24 Applikationen.

Die biologischen Daten der jeweiligen Phorbol-Derivate können mit den chemischen und demzufolge sterischen Veränderungen an Hand von räumlichen Molekülmodellen in Zusammenhang gebracht werden (Abb. 6).

So erkennt man z. B. am Modell des Phorbol-12.13-didekanoats, daß der starke Wirkungsverlust bei den Derivaten mit acetylierten Hydroxylgruppen 4 und/oder 9 zwei Gründe haben kann: entweder wird durch Einführung der Acetylgruppen die Raumerfüllung des gesamten Moleküls zu stark verändert oder die freien Hydroxylgruppen sind essentiell für die Wirkung (so könnte die mit spektroskopischen Methoden nachgewiesene [*9*] intramolekulare Wasserstoffbrücke von OH-9 zum Carbonyl der Estergruppierung an C-13 von wesentlicher Bedeutung dafür sein, daß Verbindungen vom Typ der Phorbolester cocarcinogen wirksam sind). Ein Hinweis dafür, daß die Hydroxylgruppe an C-4, wenn sie schon vorhanden ist, frei sein muß, ist die Tatsache, daß auch der 4-O-Methyläther des PDD nur sehr geringe biologische Wirksamkeit besitzt [*8*].

Einen Beitrag zur Bedeutung der freien Hydroxylgruppen 4 und 9 sollte das Derivat mit abgespaltenen OH-Funktionen liefern. Allerdings läßt die Tatsache, daß auch diese Substanz biologisch unwirksam ist, keine Entscheidung zu, da gleichzeitig mit der Einführung der beiden Doppelbindungen eine Änderung der Konformation des 6-Ringes eingetreten ist: der Ester-Rest an C-12 ragt nach dem Raummodell – verglichen mit dem des Phorbol-12.13-didekanoats – mehr aus der Ebene des Sechsringes heraus, da die veresterte Hydroxylgruppe 12 jetzt axiale Stellung einnimmt (siehe Abb. 6).

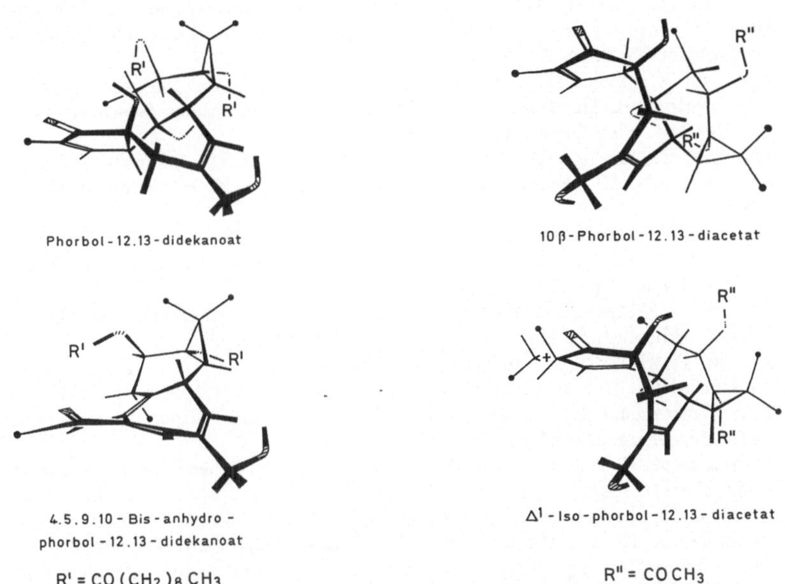

Abb. 6. Räumliche Darstellung von einigen Phorbolderivaten

Für die geringe Wirksamkeit des Tetrahydro-PDD ist möglicherweise nicht allein die Absättigung der Doppelbindungen, sondern auch die gleichzeitig damit eintretende Konformationsänderung des Siebenringes entscheidend; ähnlich läßt sich die Unwirksamkeit des $\triangle^1$-Iso-phorbol- bzw. 10β-Phorbol-12.13-diacetats durch die infolge der Isomerisierung der Doppelbindung von C-1 nach C-2 bzw. auf Grund der cis-Verknüpfung des 5-Ringes mit dem 7-Ring eintretende Konformationsänderung im Siebenring erklären (siehe Abb. 6): in diesen Verbindungen nimmt die Hydroxymethylgruppe, verglichen mit PDD und bezogen auf die Ebene des 5-Ringes, eine völlig veränderte Lage ein.

Offenbar ist für die entzündliche und cocarcinogene Wirksamkeit von Phorbol-12.13-diestern und deren Derivaten neben der freien Hydroxylgruppe an C-9 und möglicherweise der freien Hydroxylgruppe an C-4 nicht nur wichtig, daß an C-20 eine unveresterte Hydroxylgruppe steht, sondern auch, daß diese eine bestimmte Lage in Bezug auf die anderen funktionellen Gruppen einnimmt.

Literatur

1. Borchert, P.: Über Desoxyphorbole. Diplomarbeit Univ. Heidelberg 1968.
2. Bresch, H., Kreibich, G., Kubinyi, H., Schairer, H. U., Thielmann, H. W., Hecker, E.: Über die Wirkstoffe des Crotonöls, IX. Partialsynthese von Wirkstoffen des Crotonöls. Z. Naturforsch. **23 b**, 538 (1968).
3. Hecker, E.: Über die Wirkstoffe des Crotonöls, I. Biologische Teste zur quantitativen Messung der entzündlichen, cocarcinogenen und toxischen Wirkung. Z. Krebsforsch. **65**, 325 (1963).
4. Hecker, E.: Isolation and characterization of the cocarcinogenic principles from croton oil. In Busch, H. (Edit.): Methods in Cancer Research Vol. 6, pp. 439–484. New York: Academic Press 1971.
5. Hecker, E., Immich, H., Bresch, H., Schairer, H. U.: Über die Wirkstoffe des Crotonöls, VI. Entzündungsteste am Mäuseohr. Z. Krebsforsch. **68**, 366 (1966).
6. Hecker, E., Szczepanski, Ch. v., Kubinyi, H., Bresch, H., Härle, E., Schairer, H. U., Bartsch, H.: Über die Wirkstoffe des Crotonöls, VII. Phorbol. Z. Naturforsch. **21 b**, 1204 (1966).
7. Jacobi, P., Härle, E., Schairer, H. U., Hecker, E.: Zur Chemie des Phorbols, XVI. 4α-Phorbol. Liebigs Ann. Chem. **741**, 13 (1970).
8. Jacobi, P., Hecker, E.: unveröffentlichte Versuche.
9. Kreibich, G.: Zur Struktur des polyfunktionellen Diterpens Phorbol, sowie zum Wirkungsmechanismus seiner entzündlichen und tumorpromovierenden Derivate. Dissertation Univ. Heidelberg 1968.
10. Thielmann, H. W., Hecker, E.: Beziehungen zwischen der Struktur von Phorbolestern und ihren entzündlichen sowie tumorpromovierenden Eigenschaften. Hoppe-Seylers Z. physiol. Chem. **349**, 17 (1968).
11. Thielmann, H. W., Hecker, E.: Beziehungen zwischen der Struktur von Phorbolderivaten und ihren entzündlichen und tumorpromovierenden Eigenschaften. In C. G. Schmidt u. O. Wetter (Hrsg.): Fortschritte der Krebsforschung – Molekularbiologie, Wachstum, Klinik, S. 171–179. Stuttgart-New York: Schattauer 1969.

Wirkung von biologisch aktiven Phorbolestern auf Hela-Zellen

Von

R. SÜSS, V. KINZEL und G. KREIBICH

Heute morgen noch einmal Phorbolformeln zu projizieren, bedeutet eigentlich, Eulen nach Athen zu tragen; trotzdem: es erleichtert die Verständigung (Abb. 1) [*1*, *3*].

Mit folgenden 3 Verbindungen haben wir zunächst gearbeitet:

1. Mit dem natürlichen Crotonölfaktor, der am Phorbolgerüst einmal einen Tetradecanoylrest und einmal einen Acetatrest an den Positionen 12 und 13 trägt. Tetradecanoylphorbolacetat ist daher die Abkürzung; früher hieß es A1.

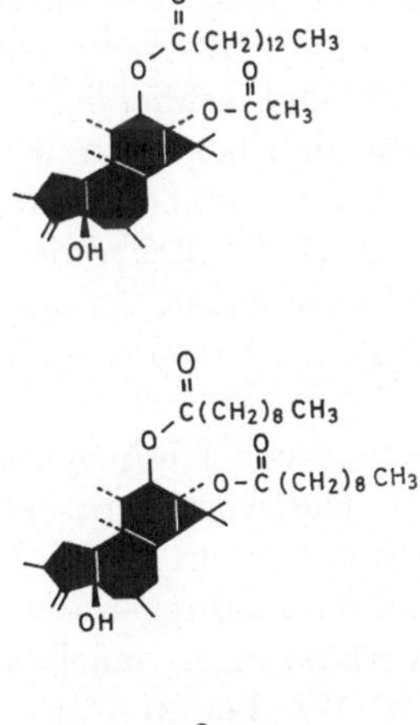

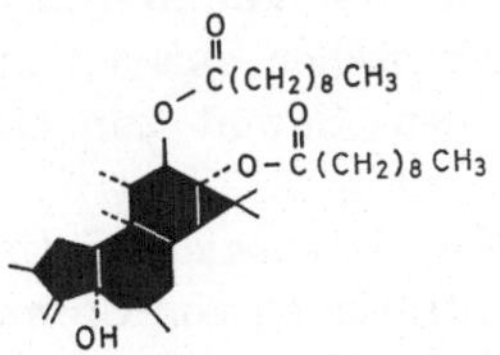

Abb. 1. Schematische Darstellung dreier Phorbolderivate (TPA — 12-O-Tetradecanoyl-phorbol-13-acetat [natürlicher Crotonölfaktor A1]; PDD = Phorbol-12,13-di-decanoat und 4α-PDD = 4α-Phorbol-12,13-di-decanoat [biologisch inaktiv])

2. Mit einem synthetischen Faktor der an den Positionen 12 und 13 jeweils eine Fettsäure mit 10 C-Atomen trägt; daher die Abkürzung PDD (Phorbol-Di-Decanoat).

3. Schließlich noch mit einer biologisch inaktiven Verbindung: 4α-PDD. Diese Verbindung ist ein Stereoisomeres zu PDD; sie unterscheidet sich „lediglich" in der räumlichen Anordnung am C-Atom 4: einmal steht die Hydroxylgruppe hier nach oben und einmal nach unten.

Als leicht zu messende biochemische Parameter für Wirkungen in der Gewebekultur wählten wir den Einbau radioaktiven Cholins und Thymidins, mit dem Hintergedanken, dabei etwas über DNA-Snythese und Membranstoffwechsel zu erfahren. Die Aufarbeitung war sehr einfach: Die Zellen wurden mit den Wirkstoffen inkubiert und erhielten dann für 1 Std Cholin bzw. Thymidin; der Einbau wurde mit SDS gestoppt, und dabei lysierten die Zellen. Das Lysat wurde dann auf Papierfilter aufgebracht, extrahiert und die verbleibende Radioaktivität direkt in einem Szintillationszähler gemessen [5].

Abb. 2 zeigt einen Versuch, in dem steigende Mengen Crotonölfaktor für 6 Std auf HeLa-Zellen einwirkten und danach der *Thymidineinbau* gemessen wurde: Bei sehr niedrigen Konzentrationen kein Unterschied gegenüber der Kontrolle, dann Absinken auf eine mittlere Terrasse zwischen 10^{-8} und 10^{-6} M und schließlich Rückgang auf Null. Im Mikroskop kann man sehen, daß bei hohen Konzentrationen die Zellen lysiert, also tot sind. Im Terrassenbereich dagegen bleiben die Zellen intakt. Es lassen sich demnach 2 Effekte des Crotonölfaktors auf den Thymidineinbau in HeLa-Zellen konstatieren:

1. Einfache Lyse; tote Zellen bauen dann auch kein Thymidin mehr ein und
2. Nicht-lytische Blockade der DNA-Synthese bei niedrigen Wirkstoffkonzentrationen. Die Konzentrationen sind in der Tat sehr niedrig: 10^{-8} M TPA entspricht 0.006 γ/ml.

Wir haben nun die drei Verbindungen der Abb. 1 miteinander verglichen: Beide aktiven Verbindungen machen die Thymidin-Terrasse, die inaktive dagegen nicht. Wir könnten also den vorsichtigen Schluß ziehen, daß HeLa-Zellen zwischen aktiven und inaktiven Phorbolderivaten unterscheiden können. Soweit zunächst einmal die Thymidin-Experimente.

Nun zu unseren *Cholin-Einbaustudien.* Im Gegensatz zu Thymidin wird bei niedrigen Konzentrationen von Crotonölfaktor TPA der Cholineinbau dramatisch gesteigert [7]. Cholin wird in Lecithin, Lecithin in Lipide, Lipide in Membranen eingebaut. Daher könnte die Steigerung des Cholineinbaues bedeuten, daß der Crotonölfaktor die Membransynthese stimuliert. Diese Steigerung bei niedrigen Konzentrationen ist wiederum auf aktive Verbindungen beschränkt: TPA und PDD steigern,

4α-PDD – also das inaktive Isomere – steigert dagegen nicht. Die Steigerung findet bei den gleichen Konzentrationen statt, bei denen auch die Thymidinterrasse eingestellt wird. Wir wurden nun schon etwas kühner und postulierten, daß aktive Phorbolderivate bei niedrigen Konzentrationen Thymidinterrasse und Cholinsteigerung machen, wenn man HeLa-Zellen als Testsystem verwendet.

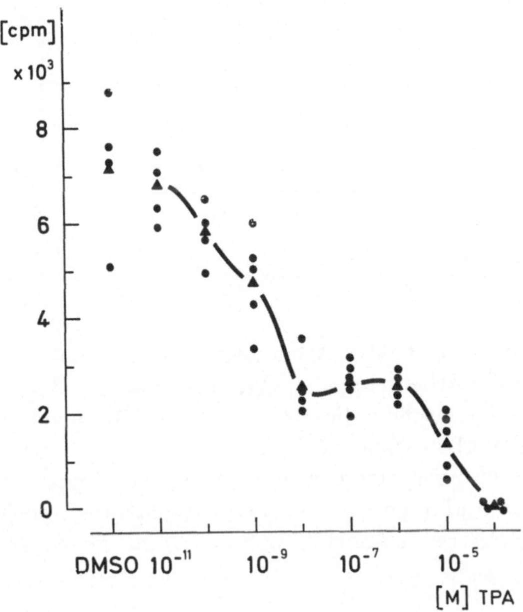

Abb. 2. Einbau ^{3}H-markierten Thymidins in HeLa-Zellen, die für sechs Stunden mit steigenden Konzentrationen Crotonölfaktor (TPA) inkubiert wurden

Tabelle 1 zeigt einige Verbindungen, die wir nun getestet haben: Die Kreuze stehen für entzündliche Aktivität, für tumorpromovierende Aktivität bei der Maus und für Thymidindepression und Cholinsteigerung bei HeLa-Zellen. Ein flüchtiger Blick zeigt: Aktive Verbindungen sind überall aktiv, inaktive überall inaktiv.

Deutlich zeigt sich auch die Korrelation bei Phorbolestern mit verschiedener Kettenlänge (DiC_2 und DiC_{14} sind keine Cocarcinogene und auch bei unserem Test negativ). Auf dieser Tabelle sind zwei isomere Äther aufgeführt (12-O-Äthyl-phorbol-13-tetradecanoat = EPT und 12-O-Tetradecanoyl-phorbol-13-äthyläther = TPE): der eine ist bei der Maus cocarcinogen, der andere nicht [*4*].

Tabelle 1. *In-vitro- und In-vivo-Aktivitäten von Phorbolestern. (Vgl. Text)*

	Mäusehaut		Hela-Zellen	
	Entzündung	Tumorpromotion	Thy >	Chol <
TPA	+	+	+	+
PDD (DiC_{10})	+	+	+	+
4α-PDD (ISO)	—	—	—	—
P-DiC_2	—	—	—	—
P-DiC_4	+	+	+	+
P-DiC_6	+	+	+	+
P-DiC_8	+	+	+	+
P-DiC_{10}	+	+	+	+
P-DiC_{14}	—	—	—	—
EPT	+	+	+	+
TPE	—	—	—	—

Die Formeln dieser beiden Äther zeigen nur „minimale" Verschiedenheiten: einmal die Äthergruppe an C_{12}, einmal an C_{13}. Trotzdem kann die Maus sehr wohl zwischen diesen beiden Verbindungen unterscheiden und HeLa-Zellen eben auch.

Tabelle 2 gibt noch einige weitere Beispiele: Ingenol-5-palmitat ist biologisch aktiv und auch in unserem *In-vitro*-System positiv. Mezerein, eine Substanz aus Schildknechts Laboratorium, ist cocarcinogen aktiv

Tabelle 2. *Cocarcinogene und nicht-cocarcinogene Substanzen in vivo und in vitro. (vgl. Text)*

	Mäusehaut		HeLa-Zellen	
	Entzündung	Tumorpromotion	Thy >	Chol <
Ingenol-5-palmitate	+	+	+	+
Mezerein (Schildknecht)	+	+	+	+
P-Di-C_{10}-4-9 diacetate	—	—	—	—
P-13-monoacetate	—	—	—	—
Phorbol	—	—	—	—
Anthralin	+	+	—	—
Tween 80	+	+	—	—
Cantharidine	+	+	—	—
Triton X-100	?	—	—	—

und auch bei uns +. Inaktiv ist beispielsweise der Grundkörper Phorbol, ebenso ein diacetyliertes Derivat von PDD, über das Herr SCHMIDT gerade berichtet hat.

Anthralin ist bei uns negativ, und damit kommen wir zur ersten Ausnahme. Anthralin ist etabliertes Cocarcinogen, allerdings – und dies könnte der Grund für die Ausnahme sein – braucht man sehr viel mehr Substanz (ca. Faktor 100!), um Tumoren zu erzeugen, als bei den Phorbolestern, und es ist eigentlich nicht anzunehmen, daß Substanzen, die so verschieden dosiert werden müssen, über den gleichen Mechanismus wirken. Ähnliches gilt auch für Tween und Cantharidin; Triton X-100 dagegen ist eindeutig kein Cocarcinogen und zeigt auch *in vitro* keine Wirksamkeit.

Zum Abschluß sei noch einmal auf die Thymidinterrasse verwiesen. Wenn man die Terrasse nach verschiedenen Zeiten mißt, sieht man, wie sie im Laufe der Zeit immer mehr absackt. Werden Cholineinbau und Thymidineinbau gleichzeitig gemessen, so kommt folgende Kinetik heraus: Die Cholinsteigerung schwingt wieder zurück, der Thymidineinbau dagegen nimmt annähernd linear ab. Eine mögliche Interpretation ist folgende: Der Crotonölfaktor könnte im Zellcyclus ein Tor vor der S-Phase schließen. Keine Zelle könnte neu in die S-Phase gehen; alle in der S-Phase befindlichen Zellen könnten noch herauslaufen. Wir würden also schließen, daß *der Crotonölfaktor die S-Phase blockiert, ohne die DNA-Synthese zu beeinflussen* [*6*].

Dieses Modell hat eine einfache Konsequenz: Wenn das Tor zur S-Phase durch den Crotonölfaktor geschlossen wird, dann müßten im Laufe der Zeit immer mehr Zellen vor diesem Tor auflaufen, es müßte ein Stau entstehen. Würde dann das Tor wieder geöffnet, dann sollten mehr Zellen durch die S-Phase laufen als normalerweise. Genau dies zeigt nun das Experiment [*2*]:

Wir haben HeLa-Zellen mit Crotonölfaktor behandelt, ihnen nach 24 Std frisches Medium gegeben und den Thymidineinbau nach verschiedenen Zeiten gemessen. Dabei zeigte es sich deutlich, daß Thymidin überschießend eingebaut wird. Ob dieses Modell einer Hyperplasie durch Partialsynchronisierung auch für die Hyperplasie *in vivo* relevant ist, darüber geben diese Kurven allerdings keine Auskunft.

Literatur

1. BRESCH, H., KREIBICH, G., KUBINYI, H., SCHAIRER, H.-U., THIELMANN, H. W., HECKER, E.: Über die Wirkstoffe des Crotonöls, IX. Partialsynthese von Wirkstoffen des Crotonöls. Z. Naturforsch. **23b**, 538 (1968).
2. FREIENSTEIN, C., FREIENSTEIN, S., KREIBICH, G., KINZEL, V., SÜSS, R.: Thymidine Incorporation into HeLa-Cells Increased by Tumorpromoting Crotonoilfactor TPA. Naturwissenschaften **57**, 675 (1970).

3. Hecker, E., Bresch, H.: Über die Wirkstoffe des Crotonöls. III. Reindarstellung und Charakterisierung eines toxisch, entzündlich und cocarcinogen hochaktiven Wirkstoffes. Z. Naturforsch. **20b**, 216 (1965).
4. Kreibich, G., Hecker, E.: Zur Chemie des Phorbols, V. Über einige Äther des Phorbols. Z. Naturfosch. **23b**, 1444 (1968).
5. Mans, R. J., Novelli, G. D.: Measurement of the incorporation of radioactive amino acids into protein by a filter-paper disk method. Arch. Biochem. **94**, 48 (1961).
6. Mueller, G. C., Kajiwara, K.: Regulatory steps in the replication of mammalian cell nuclei. In: Developmental and metabolic control mechanisms and neoplasia. 19th Annual Symposium on Fundamental Cancer Research, 1965, p. 452–474. Baltimore: Williams and Wilkins 1965.
7. Süss, R., Kinzel, V., Kreibich, G.: Cocarcinogenic croton oil factor A1 stimulates lipid synthesis in cell cultures. Experientia **27**, 46 (1971).

Morphologische Untersuchungen zur hyperplaseogenen Wirkung eines biologisch aktiven Phorbolesters

Von

H. BACH und KL. GOERTTLER

Zusammenfassung

Mittels kombinierter histologischer, histometrischer und cytophotometrischer Methoden wurde die zeitabhängige Wirkung einer einmaligen Pinselung der Mäuseepidermis mit einer Lösung des Phorbolesters A1 zwischen 0 und 240 Std untersucht. Morphologische, histometrische und cytophotometrische Veränderungen zeigen dabei einen parallelen Verlauf. Die ersten erfaßbaren Wirkungen bestehen in einer Volumenvergrößerung der Zellkerne nach 8 Std, der eine epidermale Hyperplasie mit einem Maximum nach 32 Std folgt. Erste Anzeichen entzündlicher Reaktionen werden nach ca. 16 Std beobachtet. Alle Effekte klingen zwischen 72 und 240 Std nach Applikation allmählich bis zur Norm ab. Aus der zeitlichen Verschiebung zwischen Kernschwellung und DNS-Synthese wird auf eine direkte Stimulation infolge Einwirkung auf die Kernmembran durch den Phorbolester A1 geschlossen. Die cocarcinogene Wirkung wird auf eine Permeabilitätsänderung der Kernmembran bezogen.

Erschienen in Virchows Arch. Abt. B. – cell pathology · Zellpathologie – **8**, 196–205 (1971).

Reliefautoradiographie in der Mäusehaut

Von

M. KARATSCHAI

Zusammenfassung

Es wird über eine Methode berichtet, mit deren Hilfe man die Populationskinetik in der Epidermis der Mäusehaut in allen drei Dimensionen verfolgen kann. Unter Zuhilfenahme der Autoradiographie erlaubt unsere Methode auch eine Aussage über den horizontalen und vertikalen Zellnachschub. Durch Arretierung der Mitosen mit Colcemid konnte das Zellteilungsmuster der Basalzellen im Stratum basale erfaßt werden. Dabei ließ sich eine enge Beziehung der Zellteilungsvorgänge besonders zu den Kanten der überlagernden Hornzellen bzw. Hornschuppen nachweisen.

Der Vortrag ist einbezogen in eine von KARATSCHAI, M., KINZEL, V., GOERTTLER, Kl. und SÜSS, R. verfaßte Studie über „Geography of Mitoses and Cell Divisions in the Basal Cell Layer of Mouse Epidermis".

Erschienen in Z. Krebsforsch. **76**, 59–64 (1971).

Cytophotometrische Untersuchungen an Zellkernen von experimentell erzeugten Neoplasmen

Von

KL. GOERTTLER, D. HAAG und C. TASCA

Zusammenfassung

Durch cytophotometrische Messungen an 8000 Zellkernen von normalen, initiierten bzw. promovierten und auch tumorös umgewandelten, hypo- und hyperchromen Zellkernen wird gezeigt, daß während der experimentellen Carcinogenese zunächst keine meßbaren Änderungen des DNS-Gehaltes auftreten. Während bei der Carcinogenese der Epidermis durch 3,4-Benzpyren erst in den ausgeprägteren Erscheinungsformen mit zunehmender Malignitätsstufe auch eine zunehmende Aneuploidie der Zellkerne beobachtet wird, bleibt der durchschnittliche DNS-Gehalt in Zellkernen von experimentell durch Diäthylnitrosamin erzeugten Hepatomen gegenüber Normalwerten unverändert. Dagegen ist die Korrelation zwischen DNS-Gehalt und Zellkernvolumen vermindert, die sich durch stochastische Funktionen der Form

DNS-Gehalt = mittlere DNS-Dichte mal Kernvolumen + Konst.

beschreiben läßt. Dies wurde bei allen bisher untersuchten Fällen von neoplastischem Wachstum im Vergleich zu Normalwerten beobachtet. Die Verminderung ist bereits an carcinogen-beeinflußten (initiierten) jedoch histologisch noch unauffälligen Gewebspartien zu beobachten. Durch den cocarcinogenen (promovierenden) hyperplasiogenen Phorbolester A1 wird die Korrelation im Gegensatz zu Carcinogenen nicht beeinflußt. Die Verminderung der Kernvolumen-DNS-Korrelation kann somit als erster meßbarer Indikator einer geänderten Zellfunktion gelten und wird als irreversible Schädigung des Zellkernstoffwechsels infolge Veränderungen der Kernmembranen durch Carcinogene gedeutet.

Erscheint in Z. Krebsforsch.

Granulocytic Chalone and Leukaemia

By

T. Rytömaa

Summary

Granulocytic chalone was extracted from granulocytes of men, cattle and rats as well as from subcutaneous chloromas of rats and leukaemic human cells (chronic myeloic leukaemia) and concentrated by ultrafiltration. The chalone inhibits DNS-synthesis in normal and leukaemic granulocytes in a tissue- but not species-specific form. Generalized leukaemia (chloroleukaemia of the rat) can be completely and permanently cured by repeated injections of chalone. In all animals thus treated it was possible to distinctly extend the survival time; with 9 out of 40 rats the leukaemia was made to disappear permanently. Possibilities of application for the treatment of human leukaemia are discussed.

The substance of the lecture is fully covered by the following two articles:

1. Rytömaa, T., Kiviniemi, K.: Chloroma regression induced by the granulocytic chalone. Nature (Lond.) **222**, 995–996 (1969).

2. Rytömaa, T., Kiviniemi, K.: Regression of generalized leukaemia in rat induced by the granulocytic chalone. Europ. J. Cancer **6**, 401–410 (1970).

Einfluß des Tumorwachstums auf den Kupfer- und Mangan-Spiegel in Organen des Wirtstieres

(Untersuchungen mit Hilfe der Neutronenaktivierungsanalyse)

Von

J. Zimmerer, M. Volm, K. Wayss und H. Wesch

In zahlreichen Untersuchungen wurden verschiedenste Wirkungen der Tumoren auf den Wirts-Stoffwechsel festgestellt. Jedoch fehlen bisher systematische Untersuchungen über einen Einfluß der Tumoren auf den Spurenelementhaushalt der Tumorträger. Ziel unserer Untersuchungen war es daher, an experimentellen Tumoren der Ratte Änderungen des Spurenelementspiegels zum Tumorwachstum in Beziehung zu setzen.

In ersten Experimenten konnten beim Vergleich zwischen Tumor- und Kontrolltieren Unterschiede der Kupfer- und vor allem der Mangankonzentration einiger Organe nachgewiesen werden (Tabelle).

Für die Kupfer- und insbesondere die Mangananalysen der untersuchten Organproben bietet sich die Neutronenaktivierungsanalyse als optimales Verfahren an. Bei einem Neutronenfluß von 2×10^{12} n s^{-1} cm^{-2} (TRIGA Mark I-Reaktor des DKFZ) liegt die Nachweisgrenze für die Bestimmung von Kupfer bei 10^{-4} μg, für Mangan sogar bei 10^{-5} μg. Daher genügen schon einige mg biologischen Materials für eine Analyse. Im Unterschied zur konventionellen chemischen Analyse kann bei dieser Methode das Ergebnis nicht durch nach der Bestrahlung eingeschleppte Verunreinigungen verfälscht werden. Der Fehler des Verfahrens ist $\leqslant 5\%$.

Die DNS-Synthese der Tumoren wurde mit Hilfe von radioaktiven Vorläufern und des Flüssigkeitsscintillationsspektrometers bestimmt. Einzelheiten der Methoden werden an anderer Stelle ausführlich beschrieben [*1*, *2*, *3*].

Die bisher durchgeführten Untersuchungen mit dem Yoshida-Sarkom und dem Walker-256-Carcinosarkom der Ratte umfassen den Zeitraum zwischen dem 1. und 16. Tag nach Transplantation der Tumorzellen. Dabei wurden täglich mindestens 4 Tumortiere und etwa jeden 2. Tag ebensoviele Kontrolltiere getötet. Neben den Spurenelementkonzentrationen wurde die Aktivität der Leberkatalase bestimmt, da andere Experimente Hinweise auf eine mögliche Beziehung zwischen der Erniedrigung der Mangan- und der Katalasewerte der Leber während des Tumorwachstums gegeben hatten [*4*]. Ferner wurde neben den Tumorgewichten (Abb. 1) der ³H-Thymidineinbau in die Tumor-DNS bestimmt (Abb. 2).

Tabelle *Kupfer- und Mangankonzentrationen (Mittelwerte und Standardfehler) in Organen von Ratten (SD, ♂, Gewicht 200–300* g, *Standarddiät Altromin-R). Die Konzentrationen sind auf Feuchtgewicht bezogen. K = Kontrolltiere, T = Tumortiere (Y = Yoshida-Sarkom; W = Walker-256-Carcinosarkom). Die Tumortiere wurden am 11. Tag (W) bzw. zwischen dem 5. und 12. Tag (Y) nach Transplantation getötet*

Organ	Gruppe	Cu (μg/g)	Mn (μg/g)
Plasma	K	1,15 ± 0,05	—
	T (W)	> 2	—
Leber	K	3,18 ± 0,12	1,92 ± 0,10
	T (Y)	3,03 ± 0,05	1,27 ± 0,09
Niere	K	6,29 ± 0,88	0,61 ± 0,06
	T (W)	4,56 ± 0,26	0,50 ± 0,03
Nebenniere	K	1,62 ± 0,09	3,25 ± 0,38
	T (W)	1,73 ± 0,18	1,51 ± 0,24
Milz	K	1,84 ± 0,18	0,25 ± 0,01
	T (Y)	1,80 ± 0,09	0,18 ± 0,02
Thymus	K	1,52 ± 0,15	0,13 ± 0,01
	T (Y)	1,67 ± 0,08	0,13 ± 0,01
Herz	K	6,06 ± 0,13	0,36 ± 0,01
	T (W)	6,43 ± 0,35	0,39 ± 0,01
Muskel	K	1,16 ± 0,02	0,08 ± 0,01
	T (W)	1,36 ± 0,12	0,12 ± 0,02

Die Tumorgewichte steigen bis etwa zum 8. Tag rasch an, um dann im Mittel annähernd konstant zu bleiben. Dem entspricht der Anstieg der DNS-Syntheserate zu maximalen Werten zwischen dem 6. und 10. Tag, gefolgt von einem Abfall gerade in dem Zeitraum, in dem sich die mittleren Tumorgewichte nur wenig ändern.

Da der ³H-Thymidineinbau, das Tumorgewicht sowie die Spurenelementkonzentrationen der Organe für jedes Tier einzeln bestimmt wurden, ist die Möglichkeit gegeben, durch Kovarianzanalysen Beziehungen zwischen diesen Größen zu prüfen. Insbesondere kann getestet werden, ob zeitliche Änderungen der Spurenelementwerte (abhängige Variable) nach Elimination des Faktors Zeit allein durch die Änderung der Tumorgewichte oder der Tumorwachstumsrate (unabhängige Variable) beschrieben werden können, oder ob zusätzliche zeitabhängige Effekte (z. B. immunologischer Art) angenommen werden müssen. Für die statistischen Tests wurden die Originaldaten logarithmiert, um wenigstens angenähert die geforderte Normalverteilung der Werte zu erreichen.

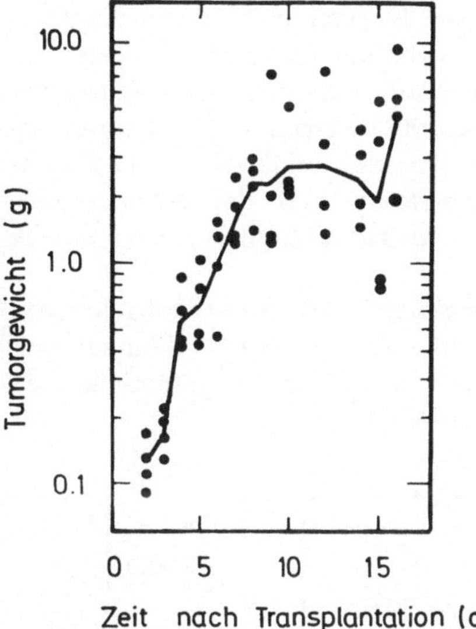

Abb. 1. Tumorgewichte (Yoshida-Sarkom)

In Abb. 3 erkennt man den ähnlichen zeitlichen Verlauf der Kupferkonzentration im Plasma, der Mangankonzentration in Leber und Niere sowie der Katalaseaktivität der Leber. Maximale Abweichungen von den Kontrollen treten zwischen dem 6. und 10. Tag nach Transplantation des Tumors auf, also genau in dem Zeitraum, in dem die DNS-Syntheserate der Tumoren am größten ist (siehe Abb. 2).

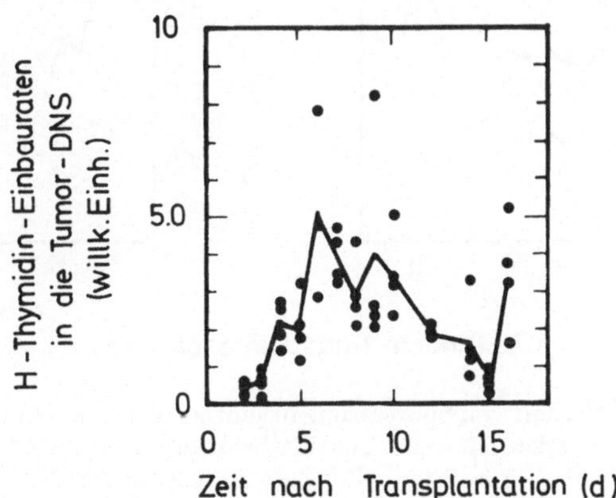

Abb. 2. DNS-Syntheserate der Tumoren (Yoshida-Sarkom)

Die eingezeichneten Kurven sind aus den ^{3}H-Thymidineinbauwerten berechnet. Dieser Berechnung liegen die linearen Regressionen zwischen (log) ^{3}H-Thymidineinbau und (log) der Spurenelementkonzentration bzw. der Katalaseaktivität zugrunde. Die Regressionen sind durch Kovarianzanalysen gesichert. Mit anderen Worten, der zeitliche Verlauf der Spurenelementkonzentration und der Katalaseaktivität kann allein durch Änderung der ^{3}H-Thymidinmarkierung des Tumors beschrieben werden.

Damit ist erstens gezeigt, daß für die beobachteten Effekte die Tumorgröße nicht entscheidend ist, zweitens können auch Abbauprodukte nekrotischen Materials nicht für die gefundenen Änderungen verantwortlich gemacht werden.

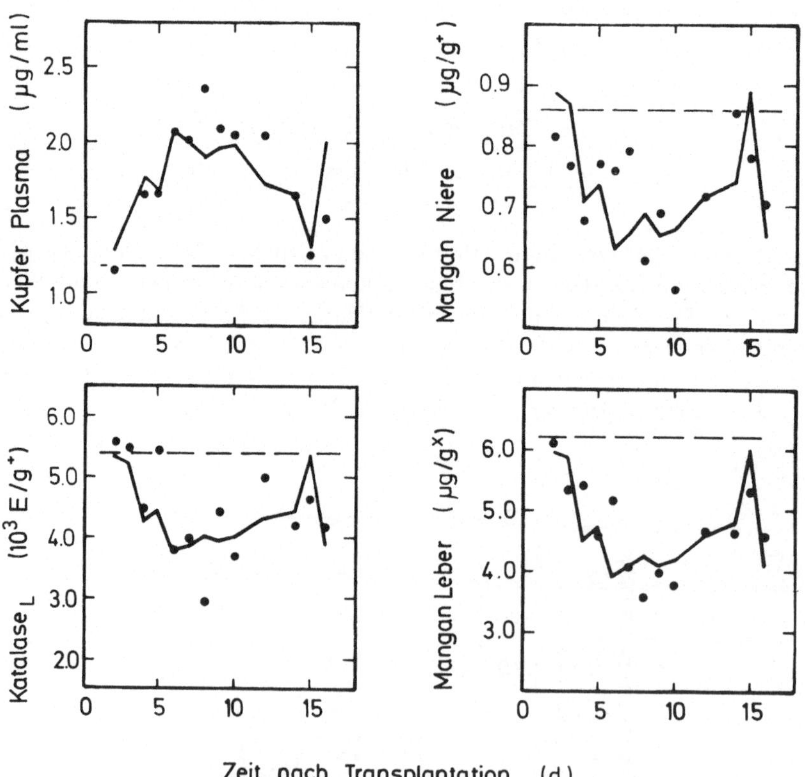

Abb. 3. Zeitlicher Verlauf von Spurenelementkonzentrationen und Katalaseaktivität in Organen der Tumortiere (Ratten) (Yoshida-Sarkom). (Werte auf Frischgewicht (+) oder Trockengewicht (×) bezogen). Punkte: (logarithmische) Mittel aus 3 Einzelwerten; gestrichelte Linien: Mittelwert aller Kontrollen (SD < 15%). Die Kurven sind aus der DNS-Syntheserate der Tumoren über die linearen Regressionen berechnet

Offen bleibt, ob die beobachteten Veränderungen tatsächlich nur von proliferierenden Tumorzellen verursacht werden. Die Korrelation zwischen der DNS-Synthese und den anderen Größen könnte beim Yoshida-Sarkom dadurch vorgetäuscht sein, daß alle nicht-nekrotischen Zellen zugleich proliferationsaktiv sind.

Literatur

1. Lück, H.: Katalase. In Bergmeyer, H. U. (Hrsg.): Methoden der enzymatischen Analyse, S. 885ff. Weinheim: Verlag Chemie 1962.
2. Volm, M., Spielhoff, R., Süss, R.: Schnellbestimmung der DNS-Synthese mit ^{3}H-Thymidin. Naturwissenschaften **55**, 390 (1968).
3. Wesch, H., Zimmerer, J., Schuhmacher, J.: Simultaneous determination of copper, manganese and zinc in biological materials by means of neutron activation analysis and chelate extraction. Int. J. appl. Radiat. **21**, 431 (1970).
4. Zimmerer, J., Wesch, H., Dogan, E. B.: Zeitlicher Verlauf der Konzentration von Mn, Cu und Zn in Leber, Milz und Thymus von Ratten mit Yoshida-Ascites-sarkom. Z. Krebsforsch. **74**, 15 (1970).

C.

3. Wissenschaftliche Sitzung am Donnerstag, den 24. 9. 1970

Vorsitz: H. Lettré

The Role of Exogenous RNA in Cell Function

By

M. C. Niu

Summary

The function of exogenous RNA has been studied in a variety of living systems. Available data can readily be grouped into three categories showing (a) it enters into the recipient cells without apparent degradation, (b) the effect on living system is shown by the change of its structural and/or physiological (biosynthetic) properties and the type of changes is related to the property of RNA donor tissue, and (c) it is capable of regulating the nuclear (DNA) function. As to the mechanism, we are working with the assumption that exogenous RNA derepresses the DNA function through indirect association with the chromosomal protein.

For further details see C. M. Niu in Tritsch, G. L. (Ed.): Axenic Mammalian Cell Reactions, pp. 155-180. New York – London: Marcel Dekker 1969.

Elektronenmikroskopische Untersuchungen an Unterlinien des Ehrlich'schen Mäuse-Ascites-Tumors

Von

N. PAWELETZ

Zusammenfassung

Fünf Unterlinien des Ehrlich'schen Mäuse-Ascites-Tumors wurden elektronenmikroskopisch untersucht. Dabei konnten starke morphologische Unterschiede zwischen den einzelnen Unterlinien beobachtet werden. Eine besonders gravierende Veränderung gegenüber dem Originalstamm zeigte eine Unterlinie, die inzwischen als G+-Unterlinie bezeichnet wird: Ihre Zellen sind in der Lage, große Mengen Glykogen im Kern zu speichern, während bei allen anderen Linien keine Glykogenspeicherung festgestellt werden konnte.

Ein Vergleich der Untersuchungen des Originalstammes im Jahre 1956 durch SELBY et al. [Ann. N. Y. Acad. Sci. 63 (1956)] mit den Ergebnissen der Beobachtungen am Originalstamm von 1969/70 in unserem Institut zeigt, daß sich im Laufe der Zeit starke morphologische Veränderungen manifestieren können.

Erscheint in Cytobiologie.

Unterschiedliches Verhalten des Leberglykogens der Maus beim Wachstum einer glykogenhaltigen und einer glykogenfreien Linie des Ehrlich-Lettré-Ascitestumors

Von

C. Granzow und P. Beheim

Zusammenfassung

Mit histochemischen und biochemischen Verfahren wurden die Entwicklung einer glykogenhaltigen Tumorlinie und die Veränderungen des Leberglykogenbestandes der Tumortiere beim Wachstum einer glykogenfreien und einer glykogenhaltigen Linie des Ehrlich-Lettré-Ascitestumors untersucht.

Das Wachstum des glykogenhaltigen Ascitestumors ist von einer intranucleären Thesaurierung von Glykogen begleitet, die sich an einen initialen Abfall des Glykogengehaltes der Tumorzellen anschließt und gegenüber dem Beginn des Tumorwachstums um 3 Tage verzögert einsetzt.

Im Zuge der Entwicklung des glykogenfreien Tumors sinkt das Leberglykogen der Mäuse innerhalb von 10 Tagen anfangs rasch, später langsamer und gleichmäßig bis auf 10% der Norm ab. Beim glykogenhaltigen Ascitestumor führt ein initialer Steilabfall zu nahezu vollständigem Schwund des Leberglykogens, dem nach relativer Sättigung des Tumors mit Glykogen ein Wiederanstieg folgt.

Erscheint in European Journal of Cancer.

Über den Stand der experimentellen Chemotherapie in der Krebsforschung

Von

E. GRUNDMANN

Das Thema, über das ich zu referieren habe, fasse ich am einfachsten in 3 Fragen zusammen:

1. Welchen Wert hat die Chemotherapie heute in der Krebsforschung?
2. Welche Ziele hat die experimentelle Chemotherapie in der Krebsforschung?
3. Welche neuen Wege lassen sich heute zur Erreichung dieser Ziele erkennen?

Damit ist der Rahmen abgesteckt. Er schließt ausdrücklich die klinische Beurteilung mit ein, denn das Ziel jedes Zweiges der Krebsforschung ist es, die bösartigen Geschwülste des Menschen – einschließlich der Hämoblastosen – durch neue Erkenntnisse auf prophylaktischem oder therapeutischem Wege besser in den Griff zu bekommen, d. h., sie entweder zu verhüten oder zu heilen.

Der mit diesen drei Fragen gegebene Rahmen schließt andererseits alle Bemühungen aus, durch Anregung körpereigener Mechanismen das genannte Ziel zu erreichen. Vielleicht sind solche körpereigenen Mechanismen sogar wichtiger als die Chemotherapie. (Ich erinnere nur an die mehr und mehr Konturen gewinnende Immuntherapie oder an die Ausführungen von Herrn RYTÖMAA vom heutigen Vormittag über die Stellung der Chalone in der Leukämiebehandlung.) Die Beschränkung auf das obengenannte Thema beruht allein darauf, daß unsere Arbeitsgruppe in der Chemotherapie mehr Erfahrung besitzt als in den anderen Wegen der medikamentösen Krebsbehandlung.

Der Platz der Chemotherapie in der Krebsforschung

Der Wert der Chemotherapie in der Krebsforschung ist noch immer umstritten. Während heute Erkrankungen durch Bakterien, Pilze oder Parasiten durch chemotherapeutische Maßnahmen in der Mehrzahl der Fälle geheilt werden können, sind chemotherapeutische Heilungen maligner Tumoren noch immer Seltenheiten. Vielleicht ist es kein Zufall, daß wir in der Behandlung der Virusinfektionen heute noch vor dem gleichen unbefriedigenden Resultat stehen. Man muß freilich berücksichtigen, daß die gezielte Suche nach Krebschemotherapeutica erst vor ca. 25 Jahren begann. Erst nach dem Ende des zweiten Weltkrieges wurde die Möglichkeit ausgebaut, mit den 30 Jahre vorher zur Menschenvernichtung entwickelten Senfgasen maligne Wucherungen zu bremsen. Die nach 1945 entwickelten Verbindungen mit der N-Lost-Gruppe werden noch heute in weitem Maße angewandt, und ihre therapeutischen Möglichkeiten erscheinen noch immer nicht ausgeschöpft. Nachdem man festgestellt hatte, daß die antineoplastische Wirkung mit der alkylierenden Eigenschaft dieser Verbindungen zusammenhängt, wurden andere Alkylantien geprüft, und auch sie fanden Eingang in die Klinik. Ich nenne als Beispiel die Äthylenimine oder die Methansulfonsäureester. Eine neue Stoffklasse, die sowohl alkylierend als auch über eine Peroxydbildung wirkt, sind die Methylhydrazine. Hauptangriffsorte aller dieser Verbindungen sind die Nucleinsäuren, und an den gleichen Molekülen greifen auch bevorzugt die tumorhemmenden Antibiotica an. Unmittelbar im Nucleinsäurestoffwechsel wirken auch die Purin- und Pyrimidin-Analoga und die sogenannten Folsäureantagonisten.

Alle diese hiermit bei weitem nicht vollständig aufgezählten tumorhemmenden Verbindungsklassen haben eines gemeinsam: sie stören oder verhindern die mitotische Zellteilung, und zwar aller Zellteilungen innerhalb und außerhalb des Organismus. Ihre Wirkung ist also ubiquitär. Bei der Anwendung an experimentellen und dann an menschlichen Tumoren ging man – grob gesprochen – von der Vorstellung aus, daß die bösartig wachsenden Gewebe eine besonders hohe Proliferationsrate haben und deshalb empfindlicher sind als normale Gewebe. Wir wissen heute, daß das durchaus nicht immer der Fall ist. Freilich ist die Variation der Ergebnisse beim Studium der Proliferationsgeschwindigkeit von normalen oder malignen Geweben beträchtlich. Das liegt einmal an den verschiedenen biologischen Abhängigkeiten, denen die Gewebe unterworfen sind (wie z. B. Alter, Hormone, Tagesrhythmen, Polyploidie usw.), zum anderen an der Schwierigkeit aller Zähl- und Meßmethoden in diesem Bereich.

Am gesichertsten erscheint mir noch die Bestimmung der Verdoppelungszeit der Tumorzellen durch ^{3}H-Thymidin [*2*]. Einige der damit gewonnenen Werte sind in der Tabelle zusammengestellt. Sie variieren zwischen 22,6 Std (Portiocarcinom) bis zu 3 Monaten (Mammacarcinom). Die Verdoppelungszeit menschlicher Normoblasten beträgt dagegen 15–18 Std, die menschlicher Dickdarmzellen z. B. 10–30 Std [*17*]. Bei aller Vorsicht, die schon aus methodischen Gründen diesen Zahlen gegenüber geboten ist, ergibt sich doch eindeutig, daß die meisten Tumorzellen des Menschen wesentlich langsamer proliferieren als die

Zellen der menschlichen Wechselgewebe. Tierische Impftumoren verhalten sich anders, können aber hier nicht als Vergleich herangezogen werden. Jeder Krebstherapeut weiß, daß manche Tumoren langsamer, manche schneller wachsen, daß das Wachstum von Primär- oder Tochtergeschwülsten oft lange Zeit sistieren und dann sich plötzlich stark beschleunigen kann.

Tabelle. *Generationszeiten normaler menschlicher Gewebe und menschlicher Tumoren nach autoradiographischen Untersuchungen (zusammengestellt aus* Bond *et al.* [*2*], Lipkin [*17*] *und* Oehlert [*18*]*)*

Normoblasten	15–18 Std
Dickdarmzellen	10–30 Std
Portio uteri-Ca	22,6 Std
Rectum-Ca	35 Std
Corpus uteri-Ca	62,5 Std
Magen-Ca	66 Std
Leber-Ca	10 Tage
Ovarial-Ca	1,5 Mon
Mamma-Ca	3,0 Mon

Bei diesen biologischen Eigenschaften des Tumorgewebes ist es nicht verwunderlich, daß diejenigen chemischen Substanzen, die etwa über eine alkylierende Eigenschaft oder als sog. Antimetaboliten in den Nucleinsäurestoffwechsel eingreifen, in der Behandlung der soliden bösartigen Tumoren bislang keinen durchschlagenden Erfolg gebracht haben. Leider ist die Kenntnis von der relativ langen Verdoppelungsdauer der meisten Carcinomzellen noch jung und nicht weit genug verbreitet.

Freilich ist diese Antwort wieder grob vereinfachend: die Verhältnisse sind komplizierter, und das heutige Gesamtbild über den Wert der Chemotherapie der Tumoren mit den genannten cytostatischen Substanzen ist bei differenzierter Betrachtung erheblich positiver. Es gibt nämlich Tumorarten, bei denen mit den Cytostatica der herkömmlichen Form echte Erfolge zu verzeichnen sind. Hier ist an erster Stelle das Chorionepitheliom der Frau zu nennen, ein bislang besonders gefürchteter Tumor, der meist in wenigen Monaten durch diffuse Metastasierung zum Tode führte. Heute gelingt es, mit Amethopterin nicht nur Remissionen, sondern Heilungen zu erzielen. Als Beleg hierfür sei eine Studie des National Cancer Institute in Bethesda erwähnt (Hammond et al. [*11*]): von 58 Patientinnen mit Chorionepitheliom lebten nach 7 Jahren noch 54, also 93%. Im Roswell Park Memorial Institute, Buffalo, wurden von Holland *et al.* [*12*] kontrollierte Studien an 27 Kliniken in verschiedenen Ländern überwacht. 144 Patientinnen wurden mit Amethopterin in ausreichenden Dosen behandelt. Die Überlebensrate nach 18 Monaten lag unter Einbezug auch der bereits metastasierten Chorionepitheliome bei 85%. Vorherige Radikaloperation verschlechterte die chemotherapeutischen Ergebnisse; die Operation ist also kontraindiziert. Patientinnen, die mit Amethopterin von ihrem Chorionepitheliom geheilt worden waren, können gesunde Kinder gebären.

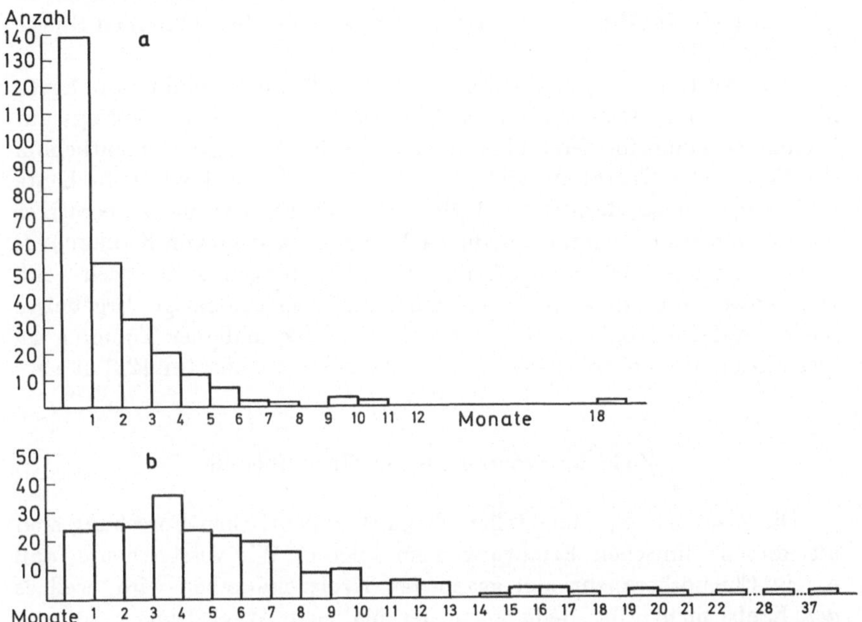

Abb. 1a u. b. Überlebensdauer (nach Krankenhauseinweisung) von Patienten mit akuter Leukämie a) ohne Chemotherapie, b) mit Chemotherapie. (Aus Iversen [*13*])

Wenn bei diesem Tumor die *Chemotherapie heute die Behandlung der Wahl* ist, so liegt das an seiner besonderen Eigenart: er ist eine Art menschlicher Impftumor, da er von fetalen Zellen ausgeht, also letztlich körperfremd ist. Immerhin sollten solche Ergebnisse allen prinzipiellen Skeptikern der Chemotherapie zu denken geben.

Solche Beobachtungen stehen auch keineswegs isoliert. Langdauernde Remissionen, möglicherweise sogar Heilungen, lassen sich bei dem meist foudroyant verlaufenden afrikanischen Lymphom – dem sog. Burkitt-Tumor – mit Alkylantien erzielen (Ziegler et al. [*31*]). Das in Japan entwickelte Antibioticum Bleomycin scheint bei Hautcarcinomen zu Remissionen, in einigen Fällen zu Heilungen zu führen. Weitere chemotherapeutisch mit Erfolg behandelte Tumoren sind das Ewing-Sarkom, der Wilms-Tumor und maligne Teratome und Seminome.

Die Behandlung der Hämoblastosen ist heute ohne die Chemotherapie nicht mehr vorstellbar. Bei den Leukämien werden meist verschiedene Medikamente kombiniert, um zwischen der Effektivität und der Toxicität das Optimum zu finden. Die mittlere Lebenserwartung der akuten Lymphoblasten-Leukämien ist in den 20 Jahren von 1946–1966 von 4 auf 37 Monate angestiegen, hat sich also fast verzehnfacht. Einzeldaten gibt beispielhaft Abb. 1 aus einer zusammenfassenden dänischen Studie (Iversen [*13*]).

Der Wert der Chemotherapie maligner Tumoren kann also heute nicht mehr bestritten werden. Er beschränkt sich bisher allerdings auf bestimmte Tumorformen und ist in einem Fall – beim Chorionepitheliom der Frau – der Operation eindeutig überlegen. Hinzu kommt die heute breit angewandte Rezidiv- und Metastasenprophylaxe nach operativer Entfernung des Primärtumors, die nach Beobachtungen von Karrer [*14*] beim Bronchuscarcinom, nach anderen Mitteilungen z. B. auch beim Ovarialcarcinom günstige, wenn auch nicht so eindeutige Ergebnisse liefert. Auf die Möglichkeiten der Lokaltherapie maligner Tumoren sei hier nur ergänzend hingewiesen (Grundmann [*9*], Schmähl [*23*] u. a.).

Ziele der experimentellen Chemotherapie

Die Ziele der experimentellen chemotherapeutischen Forschung sind aus diesen klinischen Erfahrungen zu folgern. Wir wissen heute, daß es *ein* Chemotherapeuticum gegen *den* Krebs nie geben wird, weil es *den* Krebs nicht gibt. Jede Form des malignen Wachstums zeigt eine andere Sensibilität gegen die heute verfügbaren Medikamente. Diese Sensibilität hat sich bisher in keinem Fall durch Tierexperimente voraussagen lassen. Sie ist jeweils erst in langen, mehrjährigen, klinischen Studien herausgearbeitet worden. Dazu waren Beobachtungen an Tausenden von Patienten nötig. Jeder Experimentator, der an der Krebschemotherapie arbeitet, sollte das vor Augen haben. Die Situation ist also vom experimentellen Standpunkt aus recht unbefriedigend. *Wie kann man sie bessern?* Naheliegend ist die Folgerung, daß wir ja noch immer ungenügend über die Vorgänge unterrichtet sind, welche zur malignen Entartung führen, und daß wir im Grunde noch immer zu wenig über die prinzipiellen Unterschiede zwischen den normalen Somazellen und den Tumorzellen wissen. Zweifellos liegt hier ein wesentlicher Ansatzpunkt für die weiteren Arbeiten. Vielleicht ergeben sich aus der besseren Kenntnis der Carcinogenesemechanismen in der cellulären und molekularbiologischen Ebene Hinweise auf die Prophylaxe und die Therapie. Allerdings ist hier Skepsis am Platze. Die Entdeckung des Tuberkelbacteriums durch ROBERT KOCH hatte keineswegs die erfolgreiche Therapie der Tuberkulose zur Folge. Strenggenommen wären zwar nicht die hygienischen, aber die modernen chemotherapeutischen Methoden der Tuberkulosebekämpfung auch ohne die Pioniertat ROBERT KOCHS möglich gewesen. Wer den Ablauf der experimentellen Forschungen, die zur Entwicklung der Antituberkulotica geführt haben, kritisch-historisch verfolgt, muß zu diesem Schluß kommen. In der gesamten Arzneimittelforschung gilt die Regel, daß erst die Wirkung einer neuen Substanz und dann der Wirkungsmechanismus entdeckt werden – denken Sie an die Sulfonamide oder die Penicilline. Es gibt nur ganz wenige Ausnahmen von dieser Regel. Die bekanntesten sind die Insulinbehandlung des Diabetes und die Vitamin B_{12}-Behandlung der perniziösen Anämie – beides übrigens reine Substitutionsbehandlungen. Die malignen Tumoren scheinen jedenfalls nicht zu diesen Ausnahmen zu gehören.

Wenn wir uns auf das Phänomen der selektiven Tumorwirksamkeit konzentrieren, tritt sofort die Aufgabe in den Vordergrund, diese Selektivität besser und rascher zu erkennen. Nach der allgemeinen Grundlagenforschung ist also das zweite Ziel der experimentellen Chemotherapie die Suche nach Methoden, die Empfindlichkeit der Tumoren *vor* der unmittelbaren Anwendung am Menschen zu erkennen. Welche Wege da heute gegeben erscheinen, soll weiter unten aufgezeigt werden.

Das dritte und meines Erachtens wichtigste Ziel der experimentellen Chemotherapie ist aber *der kliniknahe Tierversuch*. Man vergegenwärtige sich, daß bis heute schätzungsweise 1,2 Millionen verschiedene chemische Substanzen, Pflanzenextrakte usw. auf Tumorwirksamkeit im Tierexperiment geprüft worden sind, und daß alle diese Bemühungen eine nur sehr schmale Basis für die Anwendung beim Menschen gebracht haben. In jedem Fall konnten erst langjährige klinische Erfahrungen das Wirkungsspektrum der relativ wenigen wirksamen Medikamente aufzeigen. Gerade bei der Suche nach den speziellen Wirkungsspektren hat die experimentelle Forschung weitgehend versagt. Das läßt nur eine harte Folgerung zu: die Parameter, an denen bisher tierexperimentell geprüft worden ist, sind ungenügend, wenn nicht gar falsch. Alle Laboratorien, die sich mit der experimentellen Krebstherapie befassen, sind sich darin einig, daß wir neue Beurteilungskriterien brauchen, daß in mühsamer experimenteller Arbeit neue Methoden gefunden werden müssen, die den Verhältnissen beim Menschen besser entsprechen als die bisherigen Verfahren. Niemand kann die Möglichkeit leugnen, daß unter den obengenannten 1,2 Millionen Extrakten und Substanzen sich auch solche befinden, die gegen bestimmte menschliche Tumoren wirksam sind. Nur weil ihre Wirksamkeit im Tierexperiment nicht feststellbar war, ist eine Prüfung am krebskranken Patienten bisher nicht erfolgt.

Neue Wege der experimentellen Chemotherapie

Die Frage nach neuen experimentellen Wegen ist nur von der Eigenart und von der Ätiologie der bösartigen Tumoren her zu beantworten. Da die Krebszellen sich in der Regel weniger oft teilen als die Zellen der normalen Wechselgewebe, verlieren - grob gesprochen - alle Substanzen an Bedeutung, die allein auf die Zellvermehrung wirken. Proliferationsgifte sind also vergleichsweise uninteressant. Das Analoge gilt für Testmethoden in der Gewebekultur, wenn sie allein die Hemmung bzw. Störung des Zellteilungsmechanismus als Parameter heranziehen. Damit ist nichts gegen die Untersuchungen an Gewebekulturen gesagt; diese können sehr wertvoll sein. Es geht hier allein um die Prüfkriterien.

Ein gutes Beispiel für einen neuen experimentellen Weg sind Untersuchungen mit dem ersten Chemotherapeuticum, das an einer Stoffwechselanomalie von bösartig wachsenden Zellen ansetzt, der L-Asparaginase. Die Wirkung dieses Enzyms auf bestimmte Mäuse-Leukämien wurde von Kidd [*15*] und Broome [*3*] entdeckt. De Barros et al. [*4*], Dolowy et al. [*5*] und in breiterem Rahmen Oettgen et al. [*19*] sowie Schmidt u. Gallmeier [*25*] haben festgestellt, daß *eine* bestimmte Leukämieform, nämlich die akute lymphatische Leukämie, und einige Lymphosarkome durch L-Asparaginase in komplette Remissionen gebracht werden können. Die normalen Wechselgewebe werden dabei nur sehr wenig beeinflußt. Dem Ziel einer selektiven Tumorzellschädigung bzw. -zerstörung ist man hier also erstmals sehr nahe gekommen. Das Wirkprinzip ist relativ einfach: die normalen Zellen können die Aminosäure L-Asparagin selbst produzieren; die Leukämiezellen beziehen diese Aminosäure aus dem umgebenden Blut bzw. aus der Gewebslymphe. L-Asparaginase zerstört das L-Asparagin im Blut und in der Gewebslymphe. Die gegen Entzug dieser Aminosäure empfindlichen Leukämiezellen sterben am Mangel einer für sie essentiellen Aminosäure (Abb. 2). Die klinische Anwendbarkeit dieses Prinzips ist inzwischen in mehreren internationalen Studien belegt worden.

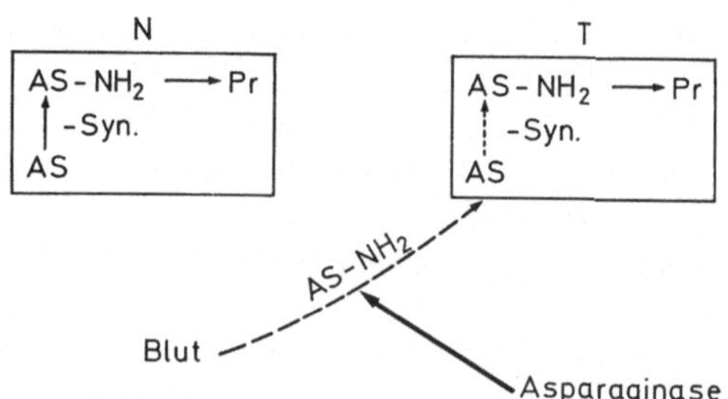

Abb. 2. Schematische Darstellung des Wirkungsmechanismus der L-Asparaginase

Für den Experimentator ist besonders von Interesse, daß von 134 geprüften lymphatischen Leukämien und Lymphosarkomen der Maus nur 32 gegen den Asparaginentzug empfindlich sind. Nach den heutigen klinischen Erfahrungen sind unter allen Formen der menschlichen Leukämie bevorzugt die akute lymphatische Leukämie, und von dieser wiederum nur etwa 50% mit L-Asparaginase zu beeinflussen. Sensible Tierleukämien sind z. B. das Gardner-Lymphom oder die $EARAD_1$-Leukämie, bei denen nach Untersuchungen von BIERLING [*1*] in unserem Arbeitskreis durch L-Asparaginase in wenigen Tagen Vollremissionen, in vielen Fällen auch Heilungen zu erzielen sind. Histologisch sieht man schon nach einer einzigen Injektion des Enzyms Nekrosen einzelner, nach mehreren Injektionen nahezu aller Leukämiezellen. In der elektronenmikroskopischen Dimension reagieren sehr früh die mit der Proteinsynthese befaßten Zellorganellen, also bevorzugt die Ribosomen, die sich nach Untersuchungen von VOIGT [*30*] in unserer Gruppe zuerst kompensatorisch vermehren, später zugrunde gehen.

Wir haben hier also Tiermodelle, die unmittelbar auf die Verhältnisse beim Menschen zu übertragen sind. Hier war der Rückschluß vom Tier auf den Menschen unmittelbar möglich: bestimmte Mäuse-Leukämien sprachen auf die Enzymbehandlung an, also mußten die analogen menschlichen Leukämien gefunden werden. Heute kennen wir sie.

Wenn man die an der L-Asparaginase gewonnenen positiven Erfahrungen auf das hier zu behandelnde Thema überträgt, dann ergeben sich 2 Folgerungen:

1. Ist experimentell die Wirkung eines neuen Stoffes festgestellt worden, muß der Kliniker versuchen, den oder die mit den Tiermodellen korrelierenden menschlichen Tumorkrankheiten zu finden. Es kann natürlich sein, daß es diese gar nicht gibt, aber sie müssen gesucht werden. Ein neuer Stoff ist dann von besonderem Interesse, wenn er kein ubiquitäres Proliferationsgift ist. PETERSEN et al. [*20*] und wir (GRUNDMANN et al. [*10*]) haben über eine solche Stoffklasse kürzlich berichtet. Es handelt sich um bestimmte Derivate des 2-Amino-1,4-naphthochinons, die selektiv bestimmte Formen des soliden Ehrlich-Carcinoms, des Sarkoms 180 und des C3H-Mamma-Carcinoms zu heilen vermögen, und zwar ohne Depression des granulopoetischen Systems und ohne Immunsuppression. Es gibt also prinzipiell tumorselektiv wirkende Substanzen auch außerhalb der Aminosäure-Enzyme. Ob damit Krebskranken geholfen werden kann, ist freilich noch offen. Es geht mir hier nur um den experimentellen Ansatz.

2. Wenn eine selektive Tumorwirkung klinisch untersucht werden soll, muß nach Wegen zur prätherapeutischen Sensibilitätstestung gesucht werden. Auch hier haben die L-Asparaginase-Forschungen erste Erfolge gebracht. Von OETTGEN et al. [*19*], in Deutschland vor allem von SCHMIDT

u. Gallmeier [*6*, *25*], wurde ein solcher „Predictiv-Test“ entwickelt, der vor der Therapie die Empfindlichkeit der Leukämiezellen zu prüfen erlaubt. Gemessen wird der Einbau von radioaktiv markierten Aminosäuren, z. B. Valin, in die Leukämiezellen mit und ohne L-Asparaginase-Einwirkung, wiederum ein einfaches Prinzip. Technisch hat es allerdings seine Schwierigkeiten, und leider ist die Vorhersage nicht in jedem Falle sicher.

Dieses Prinzip kann aber auch auf andere Tumorzellen und auf andere Substanzklassen angewendet werden. Seit mehreren Jahren beschäftigen sich einige Arbeitsgruppen mit diesen Methoden der prätherapeutischen Sensibilitätsprüfung von Cytostatica. Ich nenne als Beispiele Garattini et al. [*7*], Limburg u. Krahe [*16*] und Tanneberger [*27*]. Die zuletzt genannte Gruppe hat in einer kürzlich erschienenen Arbeit (Tanneberger u. Bacigalupo [*28*]) festgestellt, daß die Vorhersage „sensibel“ oder „wenig sensibel“ in 60% der Fälle durch das Ergebnis der Krebschemotherapie klinisch bestätigt wurde.

Methodisch kann man verschieden vorgehen: man kann – wie die zuletzt genannten Autoren – Primärkulturen der Tumorzellen als Testobjekte verwenden. Man kann solche Kulturen in Behältern mit semipermeablen Membranen anderen Tieren implantieren, um auch indirekte Wirkungen zu erfassen. Man kann an ganzen Tumorstückchen prüfen. Das hat in unserer Arbeitsgruppe Seidel [*26*] versucht. Im Mittelpunkt stand hier die Frage, ob experimentell eine Beziehung zwischen der Beeinflussung des Nucleinsäurestoffwechsels durch Cytostatica *in vitro* und dem Ansprechen des analogen Tumors *in vivo* gefunden werden kann. Seidel benutzte dabei verschiedene Systeme, u. a. den GW 77-Tumor, ein in der Hamsterbackentasche wachsendes menschliches Dickdarm-Carcinom (Goldenberg et al. [*8*]). Vereinfacht brachten die Untersuchungen folgende Ergebnisse: Actinomycin C hemmt den Einbau von ^{3}H-Thymidin und von ^{3}H-Cytidin *in vitro* signifikant und hemmt das Wachstum des Tumors *in vivo*. Triaziquon (Trenimon) hemmt den Einbau von ^{3}H-Cytidin *in vitro* und auch das Wachstum des Tumors *in vivo*. Rubidomycin (Ondena) hemmt bevorzugt den ^{3}H-Thymidin-Einbau *in vitro*, aber nicht das Wachstum des Tumors *in vivo*. Der Hydroxyharnstoff, der *in vitro* eine starke ^{3}H-Thymidin-Hemmung bewirkt, verhindert das Tumorwachstum nur während der Therapie. Nach Absetzen der Behandlung wächst der Tumor um so rascher, was ja leider in der Klinik nach Cytostatica-Behandlung nicht selten beobachtet wird.

Hydroxyharnstoff wirkt nach Pfeiffer u. Tolmach [*21*] über eine Blockade der S-Phase, also über die gegen viele Cytostatica besonders sensible DNS-Synthesephase im Mitosecyclus. Das reicht für die Therapie normalerweise also nicht aus. Hier kann aber ein sich logisch ergebender Kunstgriff weiterhelfen: Wenn es nämlich gelingt, die Masse der Tumorzellpopulation in ihrer Mitosefolge zu synchronisieren und dann ein solches Cytostaticum zu geben, werden wesentlich mehr Zellen getroffen, je nach dem erreichten Synchronisierungsgrad. Das ist das Prinzip des sogenannten „Timings“, das in der Tat klinisch zu eindrucksvollen Ergebnissen führen kann. Freilich werden dabei ebenfalls – wenn auch nur vereinfacht – alle sich teilenden Zellen eines Organismus erfaßt. Die Methode der Synchronisation verspricht also eine bessere Anwendung des herkömmlichen cytostatischen Prinzips. Wenn man sie aber mit dem Prinzip der Tumorzell-Selektivität kombinieren kann, wäre der Effekt mit Sicherheit besser, und so bleibt für den Experimentator diese Frage weiter im Vordergrund.

Ein Weg zur Prüfung dieser Sensibilität ist die Untersuchung von menschlichen Geschwülsten, die im Tier als Impftumor wachsen. Der schon erwähnte GW 77-Tumor, den GOLDENBERG et al. [*8*] auf die Hamsterbackentasche übertragen haben, wächst in unserem Laboratorium jetzt bereits in mehr als 150 Passagen und ist histologisch noch immer ein typisches Gallert-Carcinom mit sogenannten Siegelringzellen (TROSSMANN [*29*]). Das schließt freilich nicht aus, daß er sich trotzdem an den Hamster adaptiert hat, worauf vielleicht Chromosomenveränderungen hinweisen. Immerhin haben wir hier ein dem Menschen nahestehendes Tiermodell.

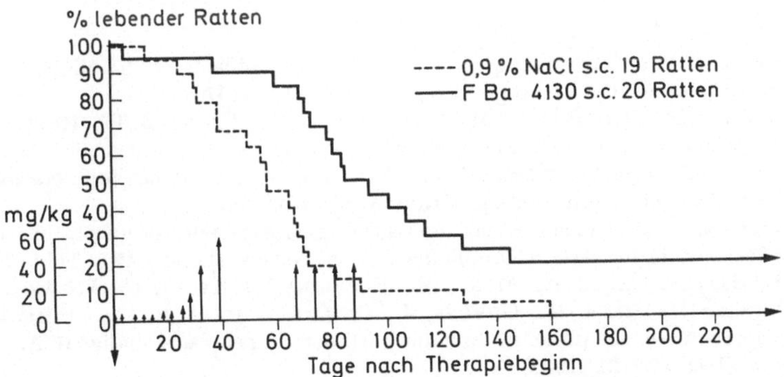

Abb. 3. Beispiel eines Tierexperiments mit einem autochthonen Tumor: Behandlung des durch Diäthylnitrosamin induzierten Lebercarcinoms der Ratte durch ein Prüfpräparat

Pathogenetisch-ätiologisch entstehen die meisten menschlichen Tumoren nach heutiger Kenntnis durch cancerogene Substanzen oder Strahlen. Es liegt also nahe, die Prüfmodelle auf diese Erkenntnis abzustimmen und z. B. an chemisch induzierten Tumoren die Wirksamkeit von potentiell krebstherapeutisch anwendbaren Substanzen zu testen, wie das kürzlich auch SCHMÄHL [23, 24] betont hat. Hier bietet sich wesentlich sicherer die Möglichkeit, mit den menschlichen Geschwülsten analogen Tiermodellen zu arbeiten. Herr STEINHOFF konnte in unserer Arbeitsgruppe in den letzten Jahren ausführliche Studien, z. B. an dem durch Diäthylnitrosamin induzierten Leberkrebs der Ratte, vornehmen und dabei Verbindungen finden, die diesen Tumor signifikant beeinflussen (Abb. 3). SCHMÄHL [22] hatte **1963** gezeigt, daß das Wachstum dieses chemisch induzierten Tumors durch die herkömmlichen Cytostatica nicht beeinflußt werden kann; wir konnten dies bestätigen. Die Prüfung an chemisch induzierten Tumoren ist naturgemäß um ein Vielfaches aufwendiger als die an den herkömmlichen Impftumoren. Sie wird aber inzwischen in mehreren Laboratorien angewandt.

Niemand wird behaupten, daß damit ein sicherer Weg zum Erfolg offensteht. Sicher aber ist, daß die experimentelle Krebsforschung ihr Hauptaugenmerk auf die Übertragbarkeit ihrer Befunde auf die Verhältnisse beim Menschen richten muß. Sie kann also nicht isoliert stehen, sondern bedarf der engen Zusammenarbeit mit der Klinik. Die Klinik ist das entscheidende Prüffeld für alle medizinischen Theorien. Auch hier kann nur die Verbindung zwischen theoretischer Erkenntnis und klinischer Praxis erfolgreich sein.

Literatur

1. BIERLING, R.: Experimental investigations on problems of the clinical use of l-asparaginase. Recent Progr. Cancer Res. **33**, 114 (1970).
2. BOND, V. P., FLIEDNER, T. M., CRONKITE, E. P., RUBINI, J. R., ROBERTSON, J. S.: Cell turnover in blood and blood-forming tissues studied with tritiated thymidine. In F. STOHLMAN (Ed.): The kinetics of cellular proliferation, p. 188ff. New York and London: Grune & Stratton 1959.
3. BROOME, J. D.: Evidence that the l-asparaginase activity of guinea pig serum is responsible for its antilymphoma effects. Nature (Lond.) **191**, 1114 (1961).
4. DE BARROS, T., CUNHA FILHO, M., FERREIRA DE SANTA, C., VALENCA, M., PEREIRA DA SILVA, M., GUEDES, J., DE CARVALHO, A. R. L.: Utilizacao da l-asparaginase em paciente humano portador de neoplasia maligna. An. Fac. Med. Recife **25**, 21 (1965).
5. DOLOWY, W. C., HENSON, D., CORNET, J., SELLIN, H.: Toxic and antineoplastic effects of l-asparaginase. Study of mice with lymphome and normal monkeys and report on a child with leukemia. Cancer (Philad.) **19**, 1813 (1966).
6. GALLMEIER, W. M., SCHMIDT, C. G.: Stoffwechseluntersuchungen als Kriterien der Enzymtherapie. In SCHMIDT, C. G. und WETTE, O. (Hrsg.): Fortschritte der Krebsforschung–Molekularbiologie, Wachstum, Klinik. Stuttgart-New York: Schattauer 1969.
7. GARATTINI, G., GUAITANI, A., NANNI, E., PALMA, V.: Studies on the selectivity of antitumor agents. Cancer Res. **27**, 1309 (1967).
8. GOLDENBERG, D. M., MÜLLER, E., WITTE, S.: *In vivo* proliferation of heterotransplanted human cancer cells. Europ. J. Cancer **3**, 315 (1967).

9. GRUNDMANN, E.: Die Möglichkeiten cytostatischer Lokaltherapie. HNO-Wegweiser **14**, 129 (1966).
10. — JÜHLING, L., PÜTTER, J., SEIDEL, H. J.: Carcinostase durch hetero-cyclische Derivate des 2-Amino-1,4-naphthochinons bei Transplantations-Tumoren. Z. Krebsforsch. **72**, 185 (1969).
11. HAMMOND, C. B., HERTZ, R., ROSS, G. T., LIPSETT, M. B., ODELL, W. D.: Primary chemotherapy for nonmetastatic gestational trophoblastic neoplasms. Amer. J. Obstet. Gynec. **98**, 71 (1967).
12. HOLLAND, J. F., HRESHCHYSHYN, M. M., GLIDEWELL, O.: Controlled clinical trials of methotrexate in treatment and prophylaxis of trophoblastic neoplasia. 10. Internat. Cancer Congr. Houston **1970**, Abstr. S. 461.
13. IVERSEN, T.: Leukaemia in infancy and childhood. Copenhagen: Munksgaard 1966.
14. KARRER, K.: Kombinierte chirurgische und zytostatische Therapie des Bronchialkarzinoms. Münch. med. Wschr. **109**, 1320 und 1609 (1967).
15. KIDD, J. G.: Regression of transplanted lymphomas induced in vivo by means of normal guinea pig serum. J. exp. Med. **98**, 565, 583 (1953).
16. LIMBURG, H., KRAHE, M.: Die Züchtung von menschlichem Krebsgewebe in der Gewebekultur und seine Sensibilitätstestung gegen neuere Zytostatika. Dtsch. med. Wschr. **89**, 1938 (1968).
17. LIPKIN, M.: Cell proliferation in the gastrointestinal tract of man. Fed. Proc. **24**, 10 (1965).
18. OEHLERT, W.: Charakterisierung menschlicher Tumoren durch autoradiographische Untersuchung von Biopsiematerial. Europ. J. Cancer **3**, 457 (1968).
19. OETTGEN, H. F., OLD, L. J., BOYSE, E. A., CAMPBELL, H. A., PHILIPS, F. S., CLARKSON, B. D., TALLAL, L., LEEPER, R. D., SCHWARTZ, M. K., KIM, J. H.: Inhibition of leukemias in man by l-asparaginase. Cancer Res. **27**, 2619 (1967).
20. PETERSEN, S., GAUSS, W., KIEHNE, H., JÜHLING, L.: Derivate des 2-Amino-1,4-naphthochinons als Carcinostatica. Z. Krebsforsch. **72**, 162 (1969).
21. PFEIFFER, S. E., TOLMACH, L. J.: Inhibition of DNA synthesis in HeLa cells by hydroxyurea. Cancer Res. **27**, 124 (1967).
22. SCHMÄHL, D.: Wert und Gefahr der Krebs-Chemotherapie. Dtsch. med. Wschr. **88**, 1463 (1963).
23. —: Entstehung, Wachstum und Chemotherapie maligner Tumoren, 2. Aufl. Aulendorf: Editio Cantor 1970.
24. —: Autochthone Tiertumoren als Testmodelle für Krebs-Chemotherapeutika. Mitt. dtsch. pharm. Ges. **40**, 173 (1970).
25. SCHMIDT, C. G., GALLMEIER, W. M.: Zur Enzymtherapie der Leukämien. (In-vitro-Vortest und Klinik). In SCHMIDT C. G. und WETTER O. (Hrsg.): Fortschritte der Krebsforschung, S. 67–97. Stuttgart: Schattauer 1969.
26. SEIDEL, H. J.: Zur Sensibilitätsbestimmung von Tumoren in vitro. II. Testungen am soliden Ehrlich-Carcinom der Maus und an einem menschlichen Colon-Carcinom nach Heterotransplantation (GW 77). Z. Krebsforsch. **74**, 131 (1970).
27. TANNEBERGER, St.: Gewebekultur und Krebschemotherapie. Arch. Geschwulstforsch. **31**, 387 (1968).
28. — BACIGALUPO, G.: Klinische Vorhersage der Krebschemotherapie durch in-vitro-Studien. Arch. Geschwulstforsch. **35**, 44 (1970).
29. TROSSMANN, G.: Wachstumsverhalten eines menschlichen Dickdarm-Carcinoms nach mehrfacher Transplantation im Hamster (unveröffentlicht).
30. VOIGT, W.-H.: unveröffentlichte Ergebnisse.
31. ZIEGLER, J. L., MORROW, R. H., FASS, L., KYALWAZI, S. K., CARBONE, P. P.: Treatment of Burkitt's lymphoma with cyclophosphamide. 10. Internat. Cancer Congr. Houston **1970**, Abstr. S. 485.

Potenzierung der chemotherapeutischen Cyclophosphamid-Wirkung durch Thymidin

Von

H. Osswald

Zusammenfassung

Beim Ehrlich-Ascites-Tumor bewirkte die vorhergehende Thymidingabe eine überadditive Wirkung von Endoxan (Cyclophosphamid), wenn die Thymidin-Vorbehandlung 6 Std vor der Endoxan-Injektion erfolgte. Verlängerung oder Verkürzung des Zeitintervalls verringerte die chemotherapeutische Wirksamkeit der Kombination. Der mögliche Wirkungsmechanismus wird diskutiert.

Erschienen in Z. Krebsforsch. **74**, 376 (1970).

Neue Colchicin-Derivate

Von

H. Lettré und K. H. Dönges

Von Lettré sind in früheren Jahren eingehende Untersuchungen über die Beziehungen zwischen der Konstitution und der mitosehemmenden Wirksamkeit des Colchicins durchgeführt worden [*1*]. Diese Arbeiten wurden im Jahre 1966 durch einen amerikanischen Chemiker, Th. Fitzgerald, im hiesigen Institut wieder aufgenommen [*2*].

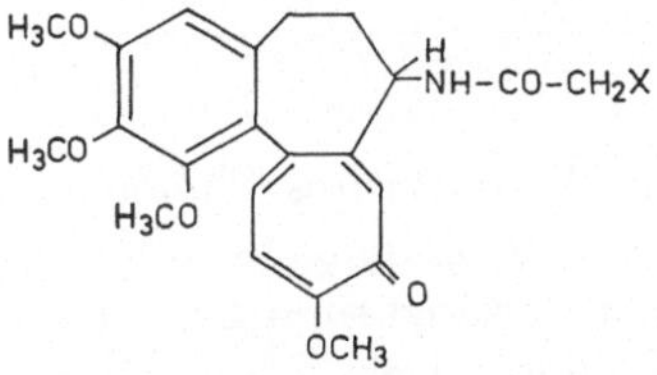

X = H	$C_{22}H_{25}O_6N$	400
X = F	$C_{22}H_{24}O_6NF$	418
X = Cl	$C_{22}H_{24}O_6NCl$	434,5
X = Br	$C_{22}H_{24}O_6NBr$	479
X = J	$C_{22}H_{24}O_6NJ$	526

Abb. 1. Halogen-Acyl-Derivate des Colchicins

In Abb. 1 sind einige Derivate des Colchicins aufgeführt, die Fitzgerald seinerzeit hergestellt hat. Die bis dahin noch nicht durchgeführte Variation am Molekül bestand darin, daß die im Naturprodukt enthaltene Acetylgruppe durch Halogen-acyl-Gruppen ersetzt wurde. Die ganze Reihe der Halogen-Derivate, Fluor, Chlor, Brom und Jod, wurde dargestellt. In der letzten Spalte der Abbildung sind die Molekulargewichte wiedergegeben, ansteigend entsprechend den Atomgewichten der verwendeten Halogene.

In Tabelle 1 sind die Grenzwerte der Wirksamkeit von Colchicin und dieser Halogen-Derivate vergleichend gegenübergestellt, wie sie sich in unserem Routinesystem an Hühnerfibroblasten in der Gewebekultur ergaben. Es zeigt sich einmal, daß das Fluor-colchicin – auf Gewichtsbasis bezogen – eine dreimal so starke Wirksamkeit besitzt wie das Colchicin, die des Chlorcolchicins der des Colchicins entspricht und deren Wirksamkeit bei den anderen Derivaten abfällt. Wegen der veränderten Molekulargewichte werden diese Grenzkonzentrationen der Wirksamkeit auch noch auf molarer Basis gegenübergestellt.

Tabelle 1. *Wirksamkeit von Colchicin und seiner Halogenderivate an Hühnerfibroblasten in der Gewebekultur*

	Wirksamkeit an Hühner-Fibroblasten	
	γ/ml	molar
Colchicin	0,01	$2,5 \cdot 10^{-8}$
Fluor-colchicin	0,003	$0,7 \cdot 10^{-8}$
Chlor-colchicin	0,01	$2,3 \cdot 10^{-8}$
Brom-colchicin	0,05	$10,0 \cdot 10^{-8}$
Jod-colchicin	0,08	$15,0 \cdot 10^{-8}$

Im Testsystem des Mäuse-Ascites-Tumors (Abb. 2) zeigte nun das Chlor-Acetyl-Derivat eine besonders starke Wirksamkeit: während mit Colchicin bei allgemeiner Verlangsamung des Tumorwachstums nur 10% der Tiere eine echte Heilung zeigen, gelang es mit geeigneter Injektionsfolge von Chlorcolchicin eine Überlebenschance von über 50% zu erhalten. Diese gute Wirksamkeit des Chlor-Derivates gab Anlaß, die Verbindung auch an äußerlich zugänglichen menschlichen Tumoren in der Klinik zu erproben.

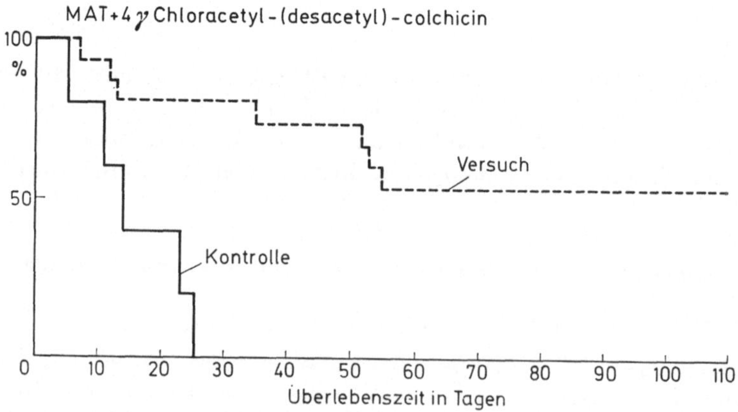

Abb. 2. Wirksamkeit von Chlorcolchicin im Testsystem des Mäuse-Ascites-Tumors

Abb. 3 zeigt ein Basaliom, das Herr Oberarzt Dr. JUNG in der hiesigen Hautklinik als 1. Fall lokal mit einer Chlorcolchicin-Salbe behandelt hat. Der linke Teil zeigt den Zustand vor Therapiebeginn (am 29. November 1967), der rechte Teil den Zustand nach 5 Wochen. Histologisch ergab eine spätere Untersuchung des behandelten Falles keine Anzeichen für das Persistieren von Tumorzellen.

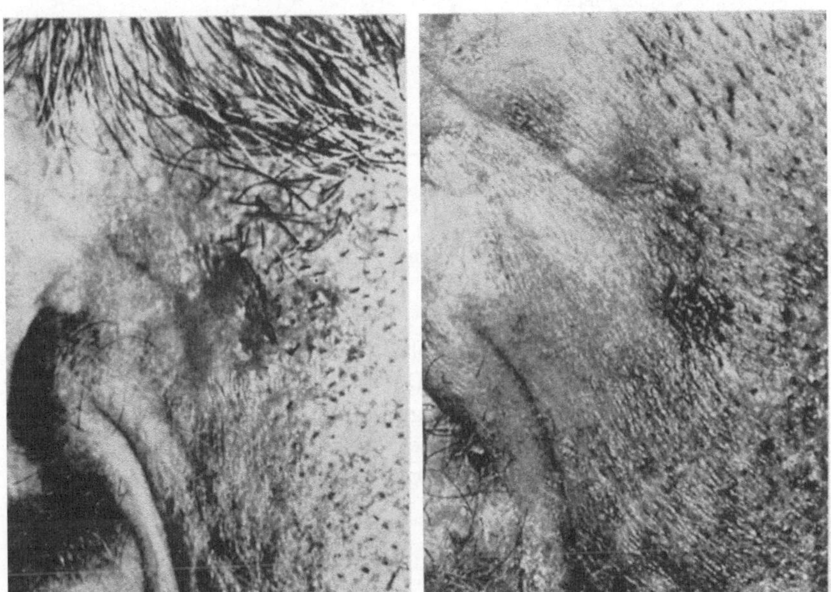

Abb. 3. Behandlung eines Hautcarcinoms (Basaliom) mit Chlorcolchicin. a vor Therapie, 29. 11. 1967; b nach 5 Wochen, 8. 1. 1968

Eine andere Qualität des Chlorcolchicins wurde wiederum experimentell festgestellt, und zwar an einer colchicinresistenten Unterlinie des Ascites-Tumors, die im hiesigen Institut schon lange gezüchtet wird (Abb. 4). Während dabei das Colchicin keine mitosearretierende Wirkung erkennen läßt, bewirkt das Chlorcolchicin eine starke Arretierung der Metaphasen.

In den folgenden Jahren haben wir nun weitere Variationen am Colchicinmolekül durchgeführt. Herr Dr. K. BARTHOLD hat die OCH_3-Gruppe im Ring C durch die $N(CH_3)_2$-Gruppe ersetzt und auch von dieser Ausgangsverbindung die Reihe der Halogen-Acyl-Verbindungen hergestellt, die aber hinsichtlich ihrer Wirksamkeit keine Besonderheiten boten.

Unsere Aufgabe bestand nun darin, die analogen Verbindungen herzustellen, die eine Thio-methyl-Gruppe enthalten. In Abb. 5 ist die Me-

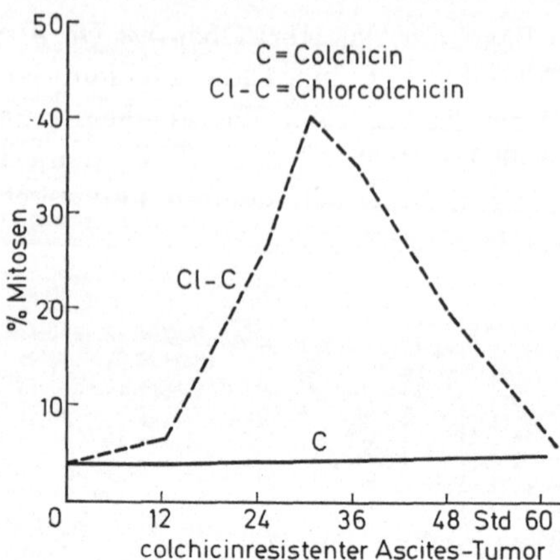

Abb. 4. Wirkung von Chlorcolchicin auf eine colchicinresistente Ascites-Tumor-Linie

thode dargestellt, nach der wir vorgingen. Colchicin wird mit Methylmercaptan in Gegenwart von p-Toluolsulfonsäure umgesetzt, wodurch ein Austausch der Gruppen erfolgt. Durch Hydrolyse mit methanolischer Salzsäure wird die Acetylgruppe abgespalten und dann durch eine Reacylierung der gewünschte Rest eingeführt. Auf diese Weise wurde auch hier die vollständige Reihe der Halogen-acyl-Derivate erhalten.

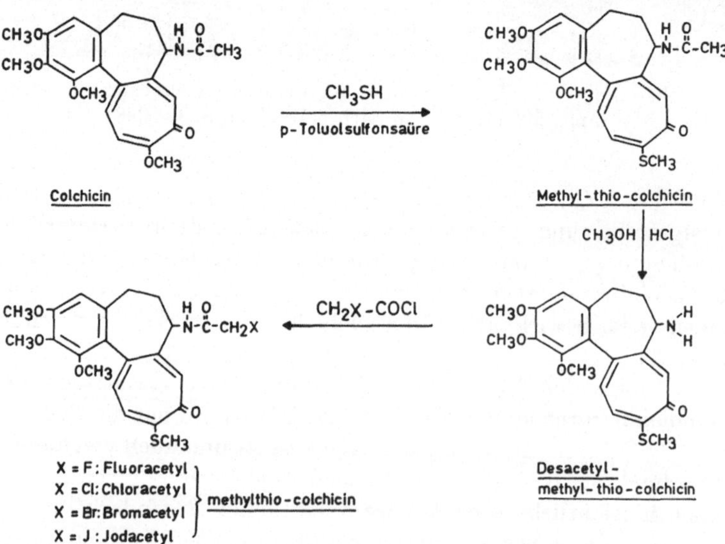

Abb. 5. Darstellung von Halogenderivaten des Thiocolchicins

Durch Untersuchungen französischer Autoren [4, 5] war bekannt, daß die Thio-methyl-Verbindung gegenüber dem Colchicin eine verstärkte Wirksamkeit zeigt, was wir durch unsere Untersuchungen bestätigen konnten. Die Wirksamkeit ist etwa 5mal größer (Tabelle 2).

Tabelle 2. *Vergleich der Wirksamkeit von Colchicin, einiger Thiocolchicin-Derivate und Vincaleukoblastin an Hühnerfibroblasten in der Gewebekultur*

	Molgew.	Wirksamkeit an Hühner-Fibroblasten	
		γ/ml	molar
Colchicin	400	0,01	$2,5 \cdot 10^{-8}$
Thio-colchicin	416	0,002	$0,5 \cdot 10^{-8}$
Fluor-thio-colchicin	434	0,001	$0,23 \cdot 10^{-8}$
Chlor-thio-colchicin	450,5	0,004	$0,9 \cdot 10^{-8}$
Vincaleukoblastin	810	0,002	$0,24 \cdot 10^{-8}$

In dem von uns dargestellten Fluorderivat zeigte sich nun eine nochmalige Steigerung der Wirksamkeit, während die Chlorverbindung etwas geringere Wirkung zeigte. Im Gesamtgebiet der Untersuchungen mitosehemmender Verbindungen ist es von Interesse, daß wir in dem Fluor-thio-Colchicin zum ersten Mal eine Verbindung erhalten haben, die in ihrer Wirksamkeit mit der des Vincaleukoblastins (eines Alkaloids aus Vinca rosea, einer Immergrünart) zu vergleichen ist. Die bisherige Lücke, die zwischen Colchicin und Vincaleukoblastin in der quantitativen Wirksamkeit bestand, wurde nun durch diese Derivate kontinuierlich ausgefüllt. Auch alle diese Verbindungen sind im Tierversuch und in geringerem Umfange auch im klinischen Versuch erprobt worden. Sie zeigen – ähnlich wie das Chlorcolchicin – positive Ergebnisse. Die Darstellung weiterer Derivate aus dieser Gruppe von Colchicin-Verbindungen wird im hiesigen Institut fortgesetzt.

Unsere gegenwärtigen Untersuchungen beschäftigen sich mit dem Versuch, den Wirkungsmechanismus und die Besonderheiten der dargestellten Colchicin-Derivate zu analysieren.

Shelanski und Taylor [3] haben nachgewiesen, daß in sich teilenden Zellen ein Protein enthalten ist, das Colchicin zu binden vermag. Die Wirksamkeit eines Mitosegiftes läßt sich auf biochemischer Basis wahrscheinlich als Ausdruck der Bindungsfestigkeit des betreffenden Stoffes an dieses Protein auffassen. Wir versuchen nun zu klären, wie dieses Protein im colchicinempfindlichen und im colchicinresistenten Ascites vorliegt und wie sich weiterhin das Colchicin und die hier beschriebenen Halogen-acyl-Verbindungen in ihrem Verhalten gegenüber diesem Protein unterscheiden.

Literatur

1. LETTRÉ, H.: Über Mitosegifte. Ergebn. Physiol. **46**, 379 (1950).
2. LETTRÉ, H., FITZGERALD, Th.: Konstitution und Wirkung von Mitosegiften. In LETTRÉ, H. u. WAGNER, G. (Hrsg.): Aktuelle Probleme aus dem Gebiet der Cancerologie II, S. 200–205. Heidelberg: Springer 1968.
3. SHELANSKI, M. L., TAYLOR, E. W.: Isolation of a protein subunit from microtubules. J. Cell Biol. **34**, 549 (1957).
4. VELLUZ, L., MULLER, G.: La thiocolchicine. Bull. Soc. Chim. **1954**, 755.
5. VELLUZ, L., MULLER, G.: La thiocolchicine II. – Produits d'hydrolyse, de réduction et d'oxydation, avec exemples de soufre asymétrique. Bull. Soc. Chim. **1954**, 1072.

Hemmung von Zellsynthesen durch cytotoxische Substanzen

Von

D. Werner

Jede cytotoxische Substanz hemmt zumindest eine, meist jedoch mehrere celluläre Synthesen. Die Messung von Zellsynthesen unter Substanzeinfluß ist deshalb eine Standardmethode bei der Aufklärung der Wirkungsmechanismen cytotoxischer Verbindungen. Im Idealfall gelingt es, den oder die Stoffwechselschritte aufzufinden, die von der cytotoxischen Substanz spezifisch gehemmt werden. Diese spezifische Hemmung kann dann als biochemisches Äquivalent für die morphologisch erkennbare Wirkung betrachtet werden.

Bei der Messung von Synthesen *in vitro* werden Zellen unter gleichen Bedingungen mit dem radioaktiv markierten Vorläufer einer Synthese (z. B. Aminosäure für Proteinsynthese) einmal ohne Hemmsubstanz (Kontrollen) und einmal mit Hemmsubstanz (Versuchsproben) inkubiert. Die Differenz zwischen der Einbaurate in Kontrollen und Versuchsproben gilt als Maß für die Hemmung der Synthese.

Wir haben nun untersucht, ob es möglich ist, aufgrund des zeitlichen Einbaus eines markierten Vorläufers in Zellen mehr Information über den Wirkungsmechanismus eines Hemmstoffes zu erhalten. Es ist bekannt, daß Zellen bei Inkubation mit markiertem Vorläufer auch bei langer Inkubationszeit nicht die gesamte dem Medium zugesetzte Aktivität einbauen. Nach einer bestimmten Zeit erreicht die Einbaukurve ein Plateau (Abb. 1). Mit Hemmstoff wird dieses Plateau nicht einfach nur später erreicht (einfache Verzögerung), sondern die Einbaukurve biegt früher ab, d.h. das Plateau liegt bei niedrigeren Einbauwerten. Die Differenz der Plateaus entspricht der bereits beschriebenen „Hemmung“. Die Form der Kurven enthält aber einen weiteren Informationswert, der nicht sofort ersichtlich ist, der aber eine Analyse lohnend erscheinen läßt. Zunächst wurde untersucht, wie die in Abb. 1 dargestellten Einbaukurven theoretisch zustande kommen.

A priori ist anzunehmen, daß die in Zellen eingebaute Aktivität (M^+) während einer Zeit (t) proportional der dem Medium zugesetzten

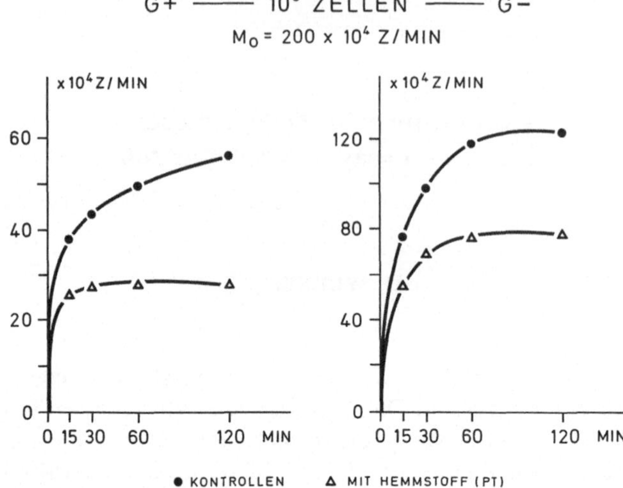

Abb. 1. Einbau von L-Lysin-^{14}C in Ascites-Tumor-Zellen *in vitro*. Für jede Inkubationszeit wurden pro Zellinie sechs unabhängige Proben angesetzt, und zwar für Kontrollen und Versuchsproben: 0,5–1 · 10^8 Zellen, 5 ml „Hanks balanced salt solution" vom pH 7,4, 1 μCi L-Lysin-^{14}C (13,45 mCi/mM) (Mo), bei Proben mit Hemmstoff 100 μg/ml Puryl-6-tryptamin (PT) (Abb. 2). Inkubationsstop durch Eingießen in 1 ml 30%ige Trichloressigsäure (4°). Der hochmolekulare Niederschlag wurde in 3 ml Protosol (NEN-Chemicals) gelöst und mit 10 ml Scintillationsflüssigkeit auf Toluolbasis in einem Tri-Carb-Scintillationsspektrometer (Packard 3380) gemessen. Einbauwerte wurden gemittelt und auf 10^8 Zellen pro Ansatz umgerechnet

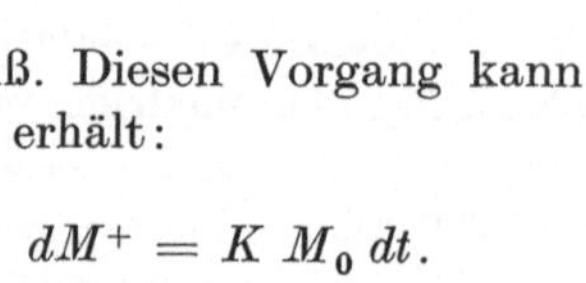

Abb. 2. Puryl-6-tryptamin (PT)

Aktivität (M_0) sein muß. Diesen Vorgang kann man als Differentialgleichung schreiben und erhält:

$$\text{Zelle} \leftarrow\text{-------}\quad dM^+ = K\,M_0\,dt. \tag{1}$$

Würde nur dieser Prozeß ablaufen, so müßte die Aktivität in der Zelle zunächst rasch ansteigen, mit der Verarmung des Mediums an Aktivität müßte die Einbaukurve abflachen, jedoch würde bei genügend langer Inkubationszeit die gesamte Aktivität in die Zelle eingebaut werden. Es ist jedoch experimentell nachweisbar, daß markierte Zellen auch Aktivität bei der Inkubation an das Medium abgeben (Abbaureaktionen). Ganz analog zum Einbau ist deshalb anzunehmen, daß die an das Medium während einer Zeit (t) abgegebene Aktivität (M) proportional der bereits in die Zelle eingebauten Aktivität (M^+) sein muß. Auch dieser Vorgang kann als Differentialgleichung geschrieben werden:

$$dM = K^+ M^+ dt \dashrightarrow \text{Medium}. \tag{2}$$

Der Einbau des markierten Vorläufers der Synthese stellt sich demnach als ein Austauschprozeß dar, der auf dem Plateau seinen Gleichgewichtszustand erreicht. Die Koppelung der Differentialgleichungen (1) und (2) ergibt die den Gesamtvorgang beschreibende Funktion:

$$M^+ = \frac{K M_0}{K - K^+} (1 - e^{(K^+ - K)t}). \tag{3}$$

Während der Inkubationszeit kann ein Teil des markierten Vorläufers noch in andere Metaboliten umgewandelt werden. Die hierbei entstehenden Produkte unterliegen dann sicher nicht mehr dem Austauschprozeß (3). Bei meßbarer Metabolisierungsrate während der Inkubationszeit wird also in der Zelle noch etwas mehr Aktivität eingebaut als Gl. (3) angibt. Damit der Gesamtprozeß auch für diesen Fall beschrieben ist, muß an die Gl. (3) noch ein Korrekturglied angefügt werden. Die Metabolisierungsrate wird sicher in erster Näherung proportional der Zeit sein. Weiter wird sie proportional der verfügbaren markierten Moleküle sein, d. h. der Startkonzentration M_0. Die Gleichung, die also die gesamten Vorgänge beschreiben kann, hat dann folgendes Aussehen:

$$M^+ = \frac{K M_0}{K - K^+} (1 - e^{(K^+ - K)t}) + K^{++} M_0 t. \tag{4}$$

Wir haben somit eine Funktion gefunden, die den Einbau eines radioaktiv markierten Vorläufers einer cellulären Synthese *in vitro* voll beschreiben sollte. Es muß darauf hingewiesen werden, daß wir nicht eine Kurvengleichung gesucht haben, die möglichst gut auf die gemessenen Einbaukurven „paßt", sondern wir haben aus rein theoretischen Überlegungen heraus eine Funktion gefunden, die alle Eigenschaften hat, um *ganz allgemein* Einbauvorgänge der beschriebenen Art darzustellen. Die Anpassung an das spezielle System (Zellart, Inkubationsbedingungen usw.) muß durch Einsetzen geeigneter Konstanten K, K^+ und K^{++} erfolgen. Vor der Ermittlung dieser Konstanten für ein spezielles Beispiel muß nochmals kurz ihre Bedeutung herausgestellt werden:

Aus Gl. (1) folgt, daß K ein Maß für die Einbauprozesse ist, denen der markierte Vorläufer unterliegt. Da die Zellen nach der Inkubation mit

Trichloressigsäure denaturiert werden und die Aktivität nur im hochmolekularen Niederschlag bestimmt wird, steht K nur für die Einbauprozesse, nicht aber für die Membranpermeation und auch nicht für die Anreicherung des Vorläufers in ungebundener Form in der Zelle. Aus Gl. (2) folgt, daß K^+ für die umgekehrten Vorgänge steht, d.h. Abbau von hochmolekularem Material. K^{++} ist nach Gl. (4) ein Maß für die während der Inkubationszeit metabolisierte Menge des Vorläufers.

In Abb. 1 ist der zeitliche Einbau von L-Lysin-^{14}C in Zellen zweier verschiedener Ascites-Tumor-Stämme dargestellt. Die Inkubationszeiten wurden so gelegt, daß die starke Krümmung der Einbaukurve und das Plateau mit erfaßt wurden. Aus je drei Meßpunkten lassen sich für jede der Kurven die entsprechenden K-, K^+- und K^{++}-Werte errechnen. Da eine exakte Übereinstimmung zwischen Funktionswerten und gemessenen Werten nicht erwartet werden kann, variieren die Werte für die einzelnen Konstanten geringfügig, je nachdem, welche Kombination der vier Meßpunkte zur Errechnung verwendet wird. Als vorläufig beste Lösungen haben sich folgende Konstanten ergeben:

G+ STAMM

Kontrolle: $K = 2{,}09$ $K^+ = -\ 8{,}51$ $K^{++} = 0{,}0425$
Hemmstoff: $K = 2{,}25$ $K^+ = -\ 14{,}74$ $K^{++} = 0{,}0025$

G− STAMM

Kontrolle: $K = 2{,}37$ $K^+ = -\ 1{,}63$ $K^{++} = 0$
Hemmstoff: $K = 3{,}60$ $K^+ = -\ 5{,}90$ $K^{++} = 0$

Werden diese Konstanten in Gl. (4) eingesetzt, ergeben sich folgende Funktionswerte im Vergleich mit den gemessenen Werten (Zähler/min $\times$ 10^{-4}):

	G+ Kontrolle		*G+ Hemmstoff*	
t	gefunden/	berechnet	gefunden/	berechnet
15′	38,9	38,8	26,0	26,2
30′	43,5	43,5	26,7	26,7
60′	49,5	47,9	27,7	27,0
120′	56,3	56,4	27,9	27,4

	G− Kontrolle		*G− Hemmstoff*	
t	gefunden/	berechnet	gefunden/	berechnet
15′	78,5	74,9	65,0	68,7
30′	98,5	102,5	69,5	75,1
60′	118,3	116,3	76,1	75,8
120′	122,0	118,5	76,6	75,8

Es wird deutlich, daß die Gl. (4) durch Einsetzen geeigneter Konstanten an die gemessenen Einbaukurven angepaßt werden kann. Der Informationsgehalt der Kurvenform wurde also in eine Kombination von jeweils drei Konstanten übersetzt. Da die Bedeutung der einzelnen Konstanten bekannt ist, läßt sich die gewonnene Information in Zusammenhang mit unserem Problem diskutieren.

Der klassische Informationsgehalt der Experimente von Abb. 1 wären die Hemmungsprozente gewesen. Man hätte erfahren, daß der Hemmstoff (PT) die Proteinsynthese des $G+$ Stammes zu etwa 43% und die Proteinsynthese des G— Stammes zu etwa 31% hemmt. Betrachtet man die Konstanten, erhält man weitere Informationen:

1. K^{++} zeigt, daß bei den Kontrollen des G+ Stammes ein Teil des markierten Vorläufers metabolisiert wird. Diese Umwandlung des Vorläufers wird durch den Hemmstoff zu über 90% gehemmt.

2. Im Falle des $G-$ Stammes ist K^{++} sowohl für die Kontrollen als auch für die Versuche mit Hemmstoff gleich 0. Diese Zellinie metabolisiert während der Inkubationszeit keinen Vorläufer. L-Lysin-^{14}C unterliegt hier nur den Austauschprozessen. Es gilt Gl. (3).

3. K ist bei $G+$ Stamm und $G-$ Stamm in der gleichen Größenordnung. Beide Stämme bauen also in der gleichen Zeit ungefähr gleich viel Lysin ein. K^+ ist jedoch bei $G+$ Stamm größer (5mal), so daß hier pro Zeiteinheit mehr Lysin ans Medium abgegeben wird. In der Bilanz resultiert ein geringerer Einbau pro Zelle.

4. K ändert sich beim Zusatz von „Hemmstoff" bei beiden Stämmen wenig. K^+ wird dagegen absolut größer. Das besagt, daß der sogenannte Hemmstoff die anabolischen Prozesse nicht hemmt, sondern die katabolischen Prozesse aktiviert. PT ist demnach kein „Hemmstoff" für den Lysin-Einbau, sondern es aktiviert besonders den Proteinabbau.

5. Zieht man von der Einbauhemmung beim $G+$ Stamm den auf die Hemmung der Metabolisierung entfallenden Anteil ab, wird der reine Lysin-Einbau bei beiden Stämmen zu gleichen Raten gehemmt.

Wird im Zusammenhang mit cellulären Synthesen von einer Hemmung gesprochen, so bedeutet das nicht unbedingt verminderten Einbau oder verminderte Synthese. Es bedeutet nur, daß die Bilanz von Einbauprozessen und Ausbauprozessen niedriger ist als bei Kontrollen. Hemmung einer Synthese *kann* auf verminderte Synthese zurückgeführt werden, ebensogut können aber auch die Abbauprozesse aktiviert sein. Für das Puryl-6-tryptamin haben wir an dem Beispiel nachgewiesen, daß hier eine Aktivierung des Abbaus vorliegt. Die Analyse der Vorgänge am mathematischen Modell hat also zu wichtigen Hinweisen für den Wirkungsmechanismus der Substanz geführt. Wir glauben, daß dieses Modell auch für die Analyse weiterer Probleme geeignet ist. Insbesondere denken wir an die Charakterisierung von verschiedenen Zellinien durch Konstanten. Bei Beibehaltung des Systems müssen bei Wiederholung der Versuche immer wieder die gleichen zellspezifischen Konstanten gefunden werden. Verändern sich die Konstanten mit der Zeit, verändern sich auch die Eigenschaften der Zellinie.

Wir haben Frau G. Bosold (Institut für Dokumentation, Information und Statistik am Deutschen Krebsforschungszentrum) sowie den Herren W. Wendel und W. Müller (Institut für physikalische Chemie der Universität Heidelberg) für Beratung und Diskussion sehr herzlich zu danken.

D.

Round-Table-Diskussion über „Konzeptionshemmer und Krebsentstehung“

Leitung: KL. GOERTTLER

Diskussionsteilnehmer:

F. DALLENBACH, H. G. HILLEMANNS, H. KRAUTKRÄMER, H. J. STAEMMLER, L. WANZEK

Das Rundtischgespräch wurde unter dem Titel „Wissenschaft in der Entscheidung: Fördert die Pille die Krebsentstehung?“ am 10. Oktober 1970 im Süddeutschen Rundfunk gesendet.

Beziehungen zwischen Östrogen und Carcinogenese

Von

F. D. Dallenbach

Zusammenfassung

Seit ca. 70 Jahren haben Wissenschaftler aus aller Welt immer wieder und bei vielen Tierarten über das Auftreten von gut- und bösartigen Tumoren (insbesondere in Uterus, Ovar, Mamma, Hypophyse und Niere) nach langdauernder Zufuhr von Östrogen in kleinen Dosen berichtet. Neuerdings mehren sich die tierexperimentellen Hinweise darauf, daß es nach Einnahme von Ovulationshemmern ebenfalls zum Auftreten von Tumoren kommen kann, insbesondere dann, wenn in diesen Präparaten die Östrogenkomponente überwiegt.

Nach heutiger Vorstellung besitzen bestimmte Zellen der sog. Targetorgane die Fähigkeit, mit Östrogen einen Eiweißkomplex zu bilden, der im Zellkern als Derepressor eines Genoms die DNS aktiviert, worauf eine RNS-Vermehrung mit Eiweißproduktion und Steigerung der Proliferationsvorgänge folgt. Östrogen verkürzt somit die Dauer der Zellgeneration und löst eine Mitosewelle aus. Dieser Vorgang dürfte beim Menschen in gleicher Weise ablaufen wie bei den bisher untersuchten Säugetierarten.

Nach zahlreichen Beobachtungen induziert Östrogen die Proliferation des Endometriums nach der Menstruation; Längerdauernde Östrogenstimulierung verursacht eine glandulär-cystische Hyperplasie des Endometriums, die über die adenomatöse Hyperplasie und das Adenocarcinom *in situ* zur Entwicklung eines Adenocarcinoms führen kann. Bei östrogenbehandelten Männern ist das Auftreten von Mammacarcinomen kasuistisch beschrieben worden.

Epidemiologische Untersuchungen der letzten Zeit haben gezeigt, daß die zur Entwicklung des Mammacarcinoms führenden hormonellen Abwegigkeiten bereits in den ersten Jahren nach der Pubertät einsetzen. Danach erscheint die Annahme naheliegend, daß die chronische Einnahme von Ovulationshemmern mit ihrer Hemmwirkung auf den Hypothalamus und die Hypophyse das hormonelle Gleichgewicht solcher junger Frauen zu der für die Entstehung des Mammacarcinoms gefährlichsten Zeit stört.

Erschienen in Fortschr. Med. **89**, 626–631 (1971).

Hormonale Kontrazeptiva und Krebsentstehung

Von

H. G. Hillemanns

Hormone und Krebs

1889, 7 Jahre vor dem englischen Chirurgen Beatson, empfahl der Freiburger Professor Albert S. Schinzinger, ein vorwiegend praktischer Chirurg, die prophylaktische Oophorektomie bei Prämenopause-Patientinnen mit Brustkrebs vor operativer Entfernung der erkrankten Brust. Schinzinger hatte damit als erster die Frage der hormonellen Induktion des Krebses aufgeworfen (Simmer [*29*]).

Bald nachdem Butenandt [*2*] 1929 das Östrogen dargestellt hatte, wurde die enge chemische Beziehung zwischen den Steroiden und den krebserzeugenden aromatischen Kohlenwasserstoffen erkannt. Damit stellte sich die Frage: Ist die Entstehung von Tumoren auf die Bildung carcinogener Stoffe aus endogenen oder exogenen Steroiden zurückzuführen? (Machen doch nach Dannenberg [*5*] die enzymatischen Reaktionen der Steroide *in vivo* die Umwandlung in carcinogene Verbindungen im Sinne eines fehlgeleiteten Steroidstoffwechsels möglich.)

Die Beobachtung von Brustkrebs beim Mann nach langdauernder Östrogen-Therapie wegen Prostata-Carcinoms – die erste Mitteilung kam wieder aus Freiburg durch den Pathologen Liebegott [*20–22*] – stimulierte nachdrücklich und erneut das Problem Östrogen und Krebsinduktion.

Heute besteht weithin die Meinung, daß Sexualhormone zu Krebs von Brust und Uterus führen können. Diese Ansicht scheint berechtigt, nachdem die Industrie 1969 das Präparat „Neonovum“ und 1970 alle Präparate, die Chlormadinon enthalten, aus dem Handel zog. Besteht diese Gefahr, müssen wir unsere Patienten schützen; besteht sie aber nicht, so müssen wir durch klare Information und Stellungnahme diese wertvollen Medikamente – die Östrogene und die „Pille“ – vor Diskriminierung bewahren.

Die Voranstellung folgender Grundtatsachen erscheint wichtig: Die Frage „Pille und Krebs“ ist nur unter dem Gesamtaspekt „Hormone und Krebs“ zu besprechen, so daß nicht nur die im Vordergrund stehenden Östrogene als Proliferationsaktivatoren diskutiert werden dürfen.

Die Grundwirkung der Östrogene ist die Proliferation, d.h. die Aktivierung der Nucleinsäuren (Abb. 1).

Zellwachstum, Zellbewegung – gleich durch welche Ursache – ist unspezifische Vorbedingung einer Sensibilität gegenüber Carcinogenen. Die Grundwirkung der Gestagene ist der Proliferationsstop, die Umschal-

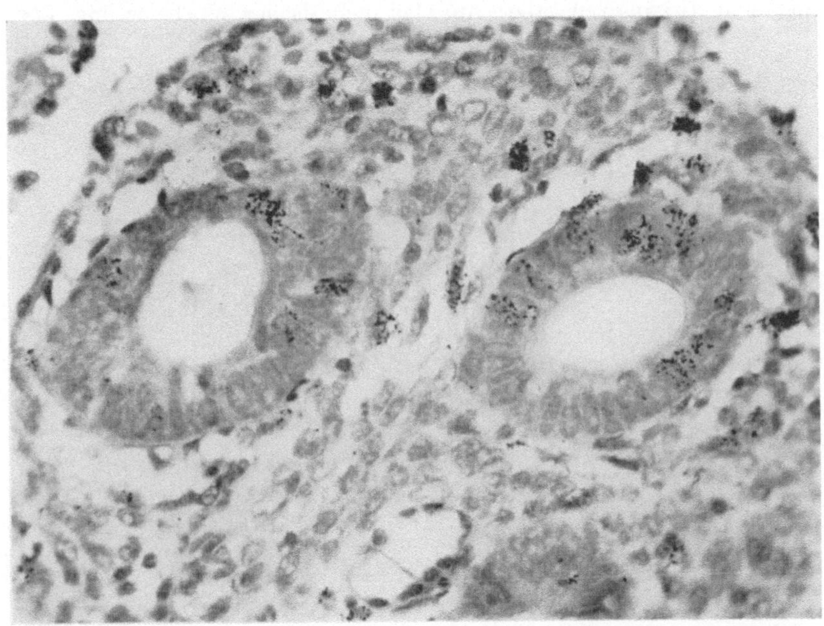

Abb. 1. Endometrium am 10. Cyclustag unter voller östrogener Stimulation. Starke mitotische Aktivität von Drüsenepithel und Stroma (Markierung: ^{3}H-Thymidin + G5 Emulsion. Vergr. 160mal. Doz. Dr. O. Fettig, Univ.-Frauenklinik Freiburg)

tung auf Differenzierung (Abb. 2), mit Dauer der Einwirkung die Rückbildung, die Atrophie. Das aber bedeutet weitgehende Immunität gegenüber Carcinogenen. Hormonale Konzeptionshemmer haben nicht östrogene, sondern gestagene, d.h. antiöstrogene Wirkung an Zelle und Gewebe.

Brustkrebs

Tierversuch. Was besagt der Grundversuch von Leo Loeb [*23*]: Nach Oophorektomie bei sehr jungen weiblichen Mäusen eines Stammes mit hoher spontaner Brustkrebsrate entwickelt sich später kein Brustkrebs. Das heißt: Ohne östrogen-bedingte Organentwicklung entsteht kein Organkrebs.

Der zweite Grundversuch von LACASSAGNE [*18*]: Induktion von Brustkrebs bei *männlichen* Mäusen nach extremen Dauerdosen von Östrogenen über lange Zeit bei krebssensiblen Stämmen, nicht bei Stämmen mit seltenem spontanem Brustkrebs. Das heißt: Die durch maximale Östrogendosen auch bei männlichen Individuen mögliche Brustentwicklung kann Ort für Organkrebs werden, ganz analog der Beobachtung von LIEBEGOTT, aber nur bei genetischer Vorbelastung [*18*].

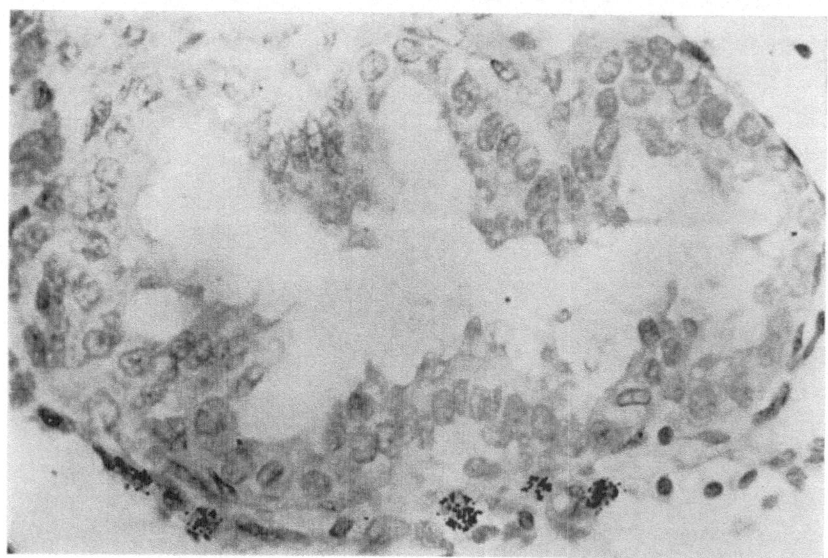

Abb. 2. Endometrium am 21. Cyclustag unter östrogener und gestagener Stimulation. Keine mitotische Aktivität am sekretorisch transformierten Drüsenepithel (keine Markierung), nur vereinzelt Stromazellen in Teilung (markiert). Durch Gestageneinwirkung resultiert Wachstumshemmung am Drüsenepithel, sowohl physiologisch wie unter hormonaler Ovulationshemmung. (^{3}H-Thymidin + G5 Emulsion. Vergr. 160mal. Doz. Dr. O. FETTIG, Univ.-Frauenklinik Freiburg)

GARDNER [*6*] gab Östrogene den weiblichen Nachkommen von hybriden Mäusen aus einem krebssensiblen und aus einem krebsresistenten Stamm. Brustkrebs entwickelte sich nur bei Mäusen, deren Mütter zum krebssensiblen Stamm gehörten.

In Bestätigung dieser Befunde bezeichneten 1943 BUTENANDT, DANNENBERG u. FRIEDRICH-FREKSA [*3*] diesen unspezifischen Einfluß des Follikelhormons auf die Tumorentstehung als „bedingt“ krebsauslösenden Co-Faktor. Östrogene sind selbst an der Brust kein Carcinogen, sondern entwickeln nur das hormonabhängige Organ, das dann Angriffspunkt für Carcinogene werden kann.

Bis vor kurzem wurden das Progesteron und die Gruppe der Gestagene (Hauptbestandteile der Pille) kaum ernstlich in Beziehung zur Krebsinduktion gebracht. POEL [*27*, *28*] fand, daß Progesteron die Carcinogenität des Brusttumorvirus (MTV) und auch des Methylcholanthren verstärkt. Fehlt das MTV-Virus, so entwickeln sich keine Brusttumoren. Diese Untersuchungen demonstrierten, daß Gestagene alleine nicht carcinogen sind, ihnen aber eine mögliche co-carcinogene Aktivität zukommt. Andere Autoren, wie z. B. STERN u. MICKEY [*31*], konnten das durch Carcinogene (DMBA) induzierte Wachstum von Mammatumoren durch Enovid (Gestagen-Östrogen-Präparat zur Kontrazeption) hemmen.

Die vorsorgliche Zurücknahme des oralen Ovulationshemmers Neonovum (1969) soll hier ebenfalls erwähnt werden. Beagle-Hunde hatten in Langzeitversuchen mit 10- bis 25-fachen Hormondosen in 8,3% (5 von 60 Tieren) gutartige Fibroadenome entwickelt, für die die Gestagenkomponente verantwortlich gemacht wurde.

Das Experiment scheint in der Genese von Brustkrebs bei Mäusen zwei Fakten zu sichern: Östrogen und Erblichkeit. Die erforderliche Dosis ist meist vieltausendfach höher als die bei Therapie angewandte; eine Vermehrung von Tumoren ist meist nicht zu erzielen, lediglich ihr früheres Manifestwerden. Gestagene stimulieren oder hemmen die Wirkung von Carcinogenen, ob über zentrale Mechanismen ist offen. Wichtig erscheint, daß Rhesusaffen bisher niemals Brustkrebs entwickelten, weder spontan noch nach Hormonzufuhr.

Brustkrebs und endogenes Hormon. Nach Oophorektomie vor dem 40. Lebensjahre reduziert sich das Risiko, ein Mamma-Carcinom zu bekommen, auf weniger als ein Drittel. Frauen, deren Menopause nach dem 50. Lebensjahr auftritt, erkranken offenbar gehäuft an Brustkrebs. Die cystische Mastopathie, eine fragliche Präcancerose, scheint mit langer, endogener Hormoneinwirkung gekoppelt. Somit scheint Hyperöstrogenismus eine Rolle zu spielen. Aber wir wissen noch sehr wenig über einen präcancerösen Metabolismus der Steroidhormone, so daß Aussagen zur carcinogenen Induktion vorerst nur theoretisches Interesse zukommt. Daß ein Brustkrebs während der Schwangerschaft gewöhnlich progressiv wächst, ist nicht ein Problem der hormonellen Tumorinduktion, sondern der mechanischen Wachstums- und Metastasierungsaktivierung.

Brustkrebs und exogene Hormone. Obwohl Brustkrebs als häufigster Krebs der Frau etwa jede 20. Frau befällt, liegen nur wenige Fälle eines Zusammentreffens von Brustkrebs mit Langzeittherapie von Östrogenen vor.

WILSON [*36*] untersuchte 304 Frauen, die bis zu 27 Jahre (durchschnittlich 7,8 Jahre) wegen Osteoporose und klimakterischen Beschwerden mit Östrogenen behandelt worden waren. Die Brüste waren den Östrogenen über eine Periode von 2387 Patientenjahren exponiert. Er errechnete, daß 18 Fälle von Brust- oder Genitalkrebs zu erwarten waren. Kein einziger Fall trat auf.

Bei GORDAN's [*8*] 120 Patienten, die über 15 Jahre lang mit Östrogenen behandelt worden waren, traten ebenfalls keine Krebse von Brust und Uterus auf. Auch WALLACH u. HENNEMAN [*34*] kamen zum gleichen Ergebnis bei Langzeittherapie von Menopausepatienten mit Östrogenen.

Alle Untersucher fanden, daß eine carcinogene Wirkung der Östrogene, vor allem cyclisch verabfolgt, für die Brust der Frau nicht gesichert ist. Zu diesem Ergebnis kam auch der zweite Bericht der Food and Drug-Administration im August 1969 (HELLMAN [*10*]). Auch die offiziellen Statistiken der USA zeigen kein Anwachsen von Brust- und Corpus-Carcinom-Todesfällen, bezogen auf gleiche Altersgruppen, trotz 30 jährigem steigendem Gebrauch von Östrogenen (zur Zeit etwa 700 kg pro Jahr in den USA). Wenn man selbst bei Östrogenen die carcinogene Wirkung nicht sichern konnte, so ist eine solche von den oralen Kontrazeptiva mit ihrer antiöstrogenen Wirkung nur schwer zu erwarten.

Wo liegt das eigentliche Problem von Pille und Brustkrebs? Brustkrebs ist einer der wenigen menschlichen Krebse, bei denen eine vererbbare Bereitschaft wahrscheinlich ist: Die Tochter einer Mutter mit Brustkrebs hat ein 28mal, die Schwester einer Brustkrebskranken ein 40mal erhöhtes Risiko, ebenfalls einen Brustkrebs zu bekommen. Auch wenn der Pille keine carcinogene Wirkung zukommt, wird man diese hohe Risikogruppe aussondern, um das Milieu der Brust nicht zu beeinflussen und um die Pille nicht zu diskriminieren. Gibt man in solchen Fällen doch die Pille, so klärt man auf, achtet besonders sorgfältig auf die immer mit der Rezeptur gekoppelte ½-Jahres-Brustkontrolle und gibt der Pillenbenutzerin damit den optimalen Schutz der Früherkennung. (s. auch KISTNER [*17*].)

Endometriumkrebs

Tierversuch. Es ist praktisch nicht möglich, mit Östrogenen Gebärmutterkörperkrebs zu erzeugen (BISHOP [*1*]). Bei Kaninchen gelingt dies nur unter zusätzlicher Anwendung eines lokalen chemischen Carcinogens *in utero*. Gleichzeitige Gestagen-Medikation verhindert hier die Krebsentstehung (KISTNER [*17*]).

Endogene Hormone. Nach verbreiteter Lehrbuchmeinung sprechen für eine wachstumstimulierende Wirkung der Östrogene einmal ihre Assoziierung mit glandulärer Hyperplasie (Östrogene im Cyclus vermehrt), zum anderen das vermehrte Tumor-Auftreten bei Spätmenopause (Östrogeneinwirkung zu lange) und schließlich die offensichtlichen Beziehungen zu den Granulosazelltumoren (exzessive Überschwemmung mit Östrogenen) (DALLENBACH-HELLWEG [*4*]). Das Zusammentreffen hormonaktiver Tumoren mit Corpus-Carcinom kann Ausdruck multipler Bösartigkeit an Uterus und Ovar sein; es kann aber auch zufälliger Ausdruck einer vermehrten Einweisung in interessierte Zentren sein (zutreffend vielleicht für die bekannte Mayo-Statistik). Auch die prädisponierende Rolle der späten Menopause blieb nicht unwidersprochen: LARSON [*19*] fand bei 3045 Endometriumkrebsen als mittleres Menopausenalter 49,1 Jahre (gegenüber 48,4 Jahren bei Kontrollen).

Exogene Hormone und Endometriumkrebs. Bei 1979 langzeitig mit Östrogen behandelten Patienten entwickelten sich neben 3 Cervix- und 1 Brustkrebs nur 2 Korpus-Carcinome. Dies blieb unter der statistisch zu erwartenden Häufigkeit (BISHOP [*1*]) (Tabelle).

Tabelle. *Krebserkrankungsrate nach Östrogenbehandlung in Kollektiven (nach* BISHOP [*1*]*)*

Autoren	Beobachtungs-zeitraum	Zahl der Fälle	Cervix	Carcinom Korpus	Mamma
GEIST, WALTER u. SALOMON	1 bis 5 Jahre	206	0	0	0
GEMMELL u. JEFFCOATE	1 Jahr	43	3	0	0
A. M. A. Committee	3 Monate bis 2 Jahre	1000	0	0	0
HENNEMAN u. WALLACH	1 bis 20 Jahre	200	0	1	0
BISHOP u. MURRAY	1 bis 20 Jahre	530	0	1	1
Zusammen		1979	3	2	1

Wo liegt das eigentliche Problem von Pille und Endometriumkrebs? Die gutartige Hyperplasie des Endometriums wird durch Langzeitstimulierung mit Östrogenen verursacht. Sie ist extrem häufig bei anovulatorischem Cyclus, in Pubertät und Klimax, sie ist *der* klassische Befund bei Abrasio. Die häufige Assoziierung von glandulärer Hyperplasie mit Korpus-Carcinom scheint für eine (wenn auch nicht bewiesene) Prädisposition des hyperplastischen Endometriums für Carcinomentstehung zu sprechen.

Die sekretorische Umwandlung dieses hyperplastischen (gefährdeten) Endometriums gelingt leicht durch die Medikation von Gestagenen. So kann man in der Pille eine wirksame Prophylaxe gegen Gebärmutterkörperkrebs erblicken, indem sie die Hyperplasie beseitigt.

Daß Gestagene das Wachstum sogar des beginnenden und vorübergehend auch des invasiven Gebärmutterkörperkrebses hemmen – eine heute bewährte Therapie – wurde zuerst aus Freiburg durch den Gynäkologen THIESSEN [*32*, *33*] mitgeteilt. Unter Depostat (reines Gestagen) nimmt die Mitosefrequenz in Endometriumcarcinomen um 40–60% ab, ähnlich auch unter Östrogen-Gestagen-Kombinationen Kaiser [*15*], Kistner [*16*]).

Cervix-Carcinom

Tierversuch. Im allgemeinen gilt die Regel, daß sowohl Östrogene als auch Gestagene keine Beziehung zum Gebärmutterhalskrebs haben. Nur wenn bei Mäusen Östrogene kontinuierlich über mindestens 1 Jahr gegeben werden, können sich Cervix-Carcinome entwickeln.

Endogene Hormone und Cervix-Carcinom. Östrogene aktivieren die bis zur Pubertät ruhenden Zellen an der Epithelgrenze des äußeren Muttermundes zu krebssensiblen Epithelzellen und bestimmen die krebssensible Lebensphase. Erst in der Pubertät, d.h. unter der Wirkung der Östrogene gerät die Epithelgrenze am äußeren Muttermund in Zellbewegung. Die eindrucksvollen hormonell induzierten, metaplastischen Transformationsvorgänge in diesem Areal am äußeren Muttermund bei jungen Mädchen und in der ersten Schwangerschaft sind Vorbedingung einer Empfindlichkeit gegenüber den vielfältigen Carcinogenen (Hillemanns [*12*, *13*]. Steroidhormone als solche sind keine carcinogenen Stoffe; sie bestimmen aber das Terrain, an dem das Carcinogen angreift und der Krebs sich realisieren kann (Abb. 3).

Ein Wort zur Schwangerschaft, der eingreifendsten hormonalen Milieuänderung. Daß die Empfindlichkeit der hormonabhängigen Organe (nicht nur des Feten, sondern auch des Muttertieres) in der Schwangerschaft erhöht sein kann, zeigen jüngste Versuche von Ivankovic [*14*]. Eine einzige Dosis eines Carcinogens erzeugt Ovarialcarcinome, wenn sie an schwangere Ratten gegeben wird, während sie bei nichtschwangeren Tieren unwirksam bleibt. Versuche unter der gleichen Frage einer Empfindlichkeitssteigerung nach Vorbehandlung mit Ovulationshemmern sind im Gange. Bei der Behandlung der drohenden Frühgeburt des Menschen werden höchste Dosen von Östrogenen und Gestagenen (z. B. Gravibinon) über längere Zeit verabfolgt; es liegen bisher jedoch keine Mitteilungen über eine Krebsentwicklung bei Mutter oder Fet (im Sinne einer Empfindlichkeitssteigerung der Schwangeren gegenüber Carcinogenen) durch diese exogene Hormonzufuhr vor.

Exogene Hormone und Cervix-Carcinom. Es liegen bisher keine klaren Angaben über die Induktion von Cervixkrebs vor. Nach dem aufsehenerregenden Bericht des Hamburger Dr. Guhr (1964), der über Atypien der Cervix nach Ovulationshemmereinnahme berichtete [*9*], konzentrierte sich alle Forschung auf die Frage: Induziert die Pille Cervixkrebs?

Pincus [*26*] stellte bei 6253 Frauen, die Enovid genommen hatten, in 0,9–1,3% der Fälle verdächtige oder positive cytologische Befunde fest (bei Kontrollpersonen dagegen in 3,6% der Fälle). Unsere europäische

Statistik zeigte das gleiche (Soost u. Baier [30]). Auch in den Großraumprogrammen auf Haiti und auf Puerto Rico wurde keine carcinogene Wirkung gefunden, obwohl die Pille dort schon über ein Jahrzehnt in kontrollierter Anwendung ist.

Wie aber wirken orale Ovulationshemmer auf *manifeste Krebsvorstadien* und das *Cervix-Carcinom?*

Wir hatten in einem Forschungsprogramm in den USA die Frage zu beantworten, ob unter dem Einfluß langfristiger Östrogen-Gestagen-Medikation mit Enovid nicht bereits vorhandene, präcanceröse Veränderungen im Sinne eines schnelleren Tumorwachstums aktiviert würden

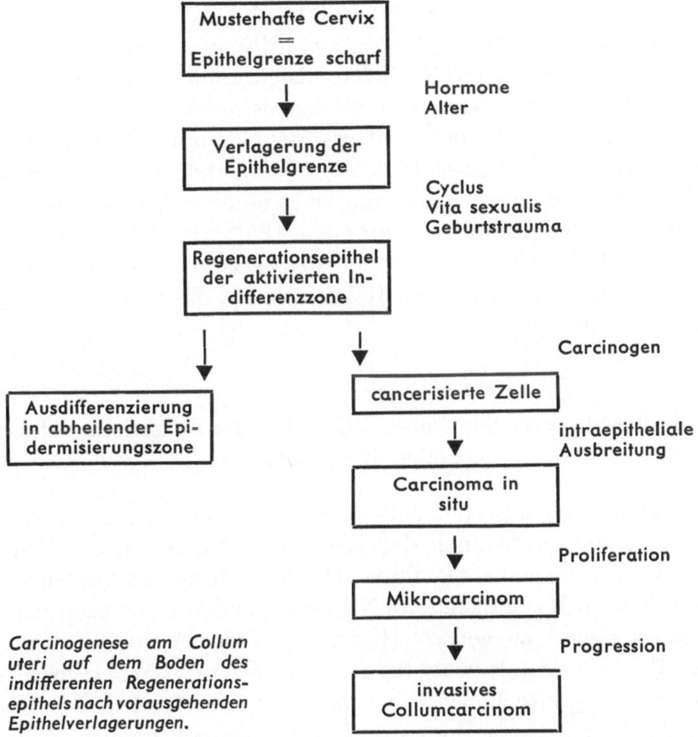

Abb. 3. Hormone disponieren das Terrain, sind aber keine Carcinogene an der Cervix uteri (Hillemanns u. Moog [13])

(Hillemanns et al. [11]). Bei 112 Patientinnen mit Dysplasie und Carcinoma *in situ* – über viele Monate und Jahre mit Enovid behandelt – fand sich die leichte Progression entsprechend dem gewohnten biologischen Verhalten von Dysplasie und Carcinoma *in situ*; kein Fall ging unter Langzeitbehandlung in ein invasives Carcinom über. Dysplasie und Carcinoma *in situ* zeigten sich hormontaub, es ergab sich kein Anhalt für eine Aktivierung durch die Östrogen-Gestagen-Kombination.

Dysplasie und Carcinoma *in situ* veränderten sich auch über Schwangerschaften, Geburten und Wochenbett nicht, dokumentierten damit die Hormontaubheit der Präcancerzellen, wie eigene Untersuchungen an 20 Fällen zeigten (Diss. GERHARD [*7*]).

Auch invasive, große Cervix-Carcinome sind hormontaub. Wir behandeln derartige Patientinnen seit 2 Jahrzehnten nach Radikaloperation und Strahlentherapie mit Östrogenen in hoher Dosierung zur Reaktivierung des Paragewebes, ohne je eine Aktivierung des Geschwulstwachstums gesehen zu haben (WIMHÖFER [37]).

Wo liegt das eigentliche Problem von Pille und Cervix-Carcinom? Erhöhte Exposition des sensiblen Zellareals gegenüber carcinogenen Reizen in der sensiblen Phase des jungen Mädchens unter dem Schutze der Pille könnte eine Steigerung von cervikalen Atypien mit sich bringen. So deuten wir die geringe, fraglich signifikante Vermehrung cervikaler Atypien bei Einnahme von Ovulationshemmern gegenüber Anwendung von Kondom oder Diaphragma (MELAMED et al. [*25*]) bzw. Nichtbenutzung der Pille (WIED [*35*]). Ob die Alteration der cervikalen Sekretion unter der Pille über lange Perioden einen Reizfaktor auf das sensible Nachbarepithel darstellt, ist ungeklärt.

F. D. A.-Bericht vom September 1969 über die möglichen Gefahren der oralen Kontrazeptiva

In diesem viel zitierten 200-Seiten-Dokument der Food and Drug Administration wurde auch das Krebsproblem untersucht. Die Kommission kam zu folgendem Schluß: „Das Verhältnis von Nutzen zu Risiko ist genügend hoch zugunsten des Nutzens, um den Kontrazeptiva die Bezeichnung ‚sicher‘ zu geben“ (Food and Drug Administration, 1969).

Die F.D.A. verlangt heute für alle Kontrazeptiva zusätzliche Tests an Affen über die ganze Lebenszeit und an Hunden für 7 Jahre. Bis heute haben die zugelassenen Präparate keine Tumoren ergeben. Nur zwei – vor allem das „Neonovum“ – führten bei 20- bis 50-facher Überdosierung zu gutartigen Mammageschwülsten bei Beagle-Hunden, die zu derartigen Tumorbildungen neigen. Brustkrebs wurde nicht beobachtet.

Einer der mit dem Problem Hormone und Krebs besonders vertrauten deutschen Pathologen, Professor DONTENWILL, hat als Gutachter diese Präparate befundet. Er kam zu der Ansicht, daß eine carcinogene Induktion bei diesen gutartigen Tumoren nicht nachweisbar war (persönliche Mitteilung).

In dem zitierten F.D.A.-Bericht wird mit Recht betont, daß die Statistik das Problem heute noch nicht lösen kann (beträgt doch die symptomlose Latenzzeit der menschlichen Tumoren etwa 10–20 Jahre). Die ersten statistisch bedeutsamen Informationen zur Frage „Pille und Krebs“ dürften erst Mitte der 70iger Jahre zu erwarten sein.

Die Prophylaxe von Brust- und Gebärmutterkrebs durch die oralen Kontrazeptiva

Schließlich ist noch eine absolut konträre, wissenschaftlich gut untermauerte Theorie auch in ihren klinischen Konsequenzen zu diskutieren. Diese Theorie besagt: Die Pille erzeugt nicht Krebs, sondern schützt vor Krebs!

Welche Argumente lassen sich für diese Theorie anführen? Zustände mit Proliferationsruhe an Uterus und Mamma stellen einen Schutzfaktor vor Krebs dar. Diese Zustände sind: Viele Schwangerschaften, lange Stillperioden (epidemiologische Ergebnisse vor allem aus Japan), auch operative Kastration und frühe Menopause. Weder in der Schwangerschaft noch während der Laktation kommt es zu mitotischem, proliferativem Wachstum. Trotz der Einwirkung hoher Östrogenkonzentrationen befindet sich der Organismus im Stadium einer Gestagen-bedingten Proliferationsruhe.

Andererseits bedeuten Hyperöstrogenismus (oft konstitutionell), Spätmenopause und generative Ovarialinsuffizienz eine Aneinanderreihung von Proliferationsphasen ohne ausreichende Unterbrechung durch Funktionsphasen. Der Mangel an Gestagenen steht im Vordergrund, wodurch über Jahre und Jahrzehnte ein erhöhter Zellumsatz sich fördernd auf eine Carcinomentstehung auswirken kann. Kommt eine genetische Disposition hinzu, so könnten diese Faktoren für die Tumorentstehung eine wichtige Rolle spielen.

So kamen R. Kaiser [*15*] in Deutschland und Robert W. Kistner [*16, 17*] in den USA zu einer gut fundierten hormonalen Prophylaxe gegen diese Krebse und zwar durch großzügige Anwendung von Gestagenen oder Ovulationshemmern zur Beseitigung kontinuierlicher Proliferationsphasen. Die proliferationsaufhebende Wirkung gerade der Ovulationshemmer stellt eine gute Begründung für ihre Anwendung als prophylaktische Maßnahme gegen Endometrium- und Mamma-Carcinome dar.

Da auch Östrogene keine Carcinogene darstellen, muß lediglich eine ungehemmte Dauereinwirkung von Östrogenen durch proliferationsbeseitigende Maßnahmen unterbrochen werden, einmal durch cyclische Gabe von Östrogenen, zum anderen durch zusätzliche Anwendung von Gestagenen bzw. von oralen Kontrazeptiva.

Zusammenfassung

Die kinetisch aktive Nucleinsäure, Angriffspunkt der Carcinogene, hat ihre größte Reaktionsbereitschaft in Phasen der stärksten funktionellen Aktivität, also in Phasen des Wachstums, der Regeneration und der östrogen-bedingten Proliferation – durchaus physiologischen Zuständen.

Die oralen Konzeptionshemmer wirken am Erfolgsorgan antiöstrogen, bedingen cyclischen Wachstumsstop und Proliferationsruhe, ja bei Daueranwendung im Genitalbereich Atrophie. Die auf den Organismus einwirkende Östrogenmenge bei hormonaler Kontrazeption liegt aufgrund der spezifischen Hemmwirkung unter der physiologischen Östrogendosis. Das aber bedeutet Resistenz gegenüber Carcinogenen im Sinne echter Prophylaxe.

Ob die Änderung des hormonalen Milieus bei entsprechender Disposition oder ob Nebenfaktoren, wie exzessive Exposition gegenüber sexuellen Reizen unter dem Schutz der Pille in sensibler Phase der Pubertät, zur vermehrten Trefferwirkung exogener Carcinogene führen, muß die Statistik zeigen.

Ein nicht zu übersehendes Faktum von größter Tragweite soll abschließend aufgezeigt werden: nichts anderes hat die Krebsvorsorge-Untersuchung und Krebsfrüherfassung, d.h. die Vermeidung invasiven Krebses, so sehr stimuliert wie die Pille!

Literatur

1. Bishop, P. M. F.: Hormones and Cancer. Clin. Obstet. Gynec. **3**, 1109 (1960).
2. Butenandt, A.: Untersuchungen über das weibliche Sexualhormon. Dtsch. med. Wschr. **55**, 2171 (1929).
3. Butenandt, A., Dannenberg, H., Friedrich-Freksa, H.: Die Mitwirkung krebserzeugender Stoffe bei der Entstehung bösartiger Geschwülste. Angew. Chemie **56**, 221 (1943).
4. Dallenbach-Hellweg, G.: Das Karzinom des Endometriums und seine Vorstufen. Verh. dtsch. Ges. Path. **48**, 81 (1964).
5. Dannenberg, H.: Steranthen, eine neue Beziehung zwischen Steroiden und krebserzeugenden Kohlenwasserstoffen. Z. Krebsforsch. **62**, 217 (1957).
6. Gardner, W. U.: The effect of estrogen on the incidence of mammary and pituitary tumors in hybrid mice. Cancer Res. **1**, 345 (1941).
7. Gerhard, Ingrid: Das Zervix-Karzinom und seine Vorstadien bei Gravidität. Diss. Freiburg 1968.
8. Gordan, G. S.: 4th Int. Congr. of Allergology, New York 1961. Abstracts of reports and communications. Int. Congr. Ser. No. 42, Amsterdam: Excerpta Med. Found. 1961.
9. Guhr, G.: Beitrag über die Wirkung von Ovulationshemmern auf das Plattenepithel der Portio uteri. Zbl. Gynäk. **88**, 815 (1966).
10. Hellman, L. M.: Report on the Oral Contraceptives. Advisory Committee on Obstetrics and Gynecology, Food and Drug Administration, August 1, 1969.
11. Hillemanns, H. G., Ayre, J. E., Le Guerrier, J. M.: Die Einwirkung von Steroiden auf Krebsvorstadien an der Cervix. Arzneimittelforsch. **14**, 784 (1964).

12. Hillemanns, H. G.: Das Cervixcarcinom. Gynäkologe **1**, 150 (1969).
13. Hillemanns, H. G., Moog, P.: Epithelgrenze und Geburtstrauma. Geburtsh. u. Frauenheilk. **26**, 519 (1966).
14. Ivankovic, S.: Erzeugung von Genitalkrebs bei trächtigen Ratten. Arzneimittelforsch. **19**, 1040 (1969).
15. Kaiser, R.: Endokrine Schutzmechanismen gegen Endometrium- und Mammakarzinome. Dtsch. med. Wschr. **94**, 2467 (1969).
16. Kistner, R. W., Griffith, C. Th., Craig, J. M.: Use of progestational agents in the management of endometrial cancer. Cancer (Philad.) **18**, 1563 (1965).
17. Kistner, R. W.: The Pill. New York: Delacorte 1969.
18. Lacassagne, A.: Apparition de cancers de la mamelle chez la souris male, soumise à des injections de folliculine. C. R. Acad. Sci. (Paris) **195**, 630 (1932).
19. Larson, J. A.: Collective review; estrogens and endometrial carcinoma. Obstet. and Gynec. **3**, 551 (1954).
20. Liebegott, G.: Mammacarcinom beim Mann nach Follikelhormonbehandlung. Klin. Wschr. **26**, 599 (1948).
21. — Mammacarcinom beim Mann nach Follikelhormonbehandlung. Klin. Wschr. **27**, 109 (1949).
22. — Follikelhormon und Mammakarzinom. Beitr. path. Anat. **112**, 235 (1952).
23. Loeb, L.: Further investigations on origin of tumors in mice. J. med. Res. **40**, 477 (1919).
24. Ludwig, H.: Hämatologische und hämostaseologische Befunde bei der Ovulationshemmung durch Östrogen-Gestagen-Kombinationen. Bibl. Gynaec. **32**, 189 (1965).
25. Melamed, M. R., Koss, L. G., Flehinger, B. J., Kelisky, R. P., Dubrow, H.: Prevalence rates of uterine cervical carcinoma in situ for women using the diaphragm or contraceptive oral steroids. Brit. med. J. **1969**, III, 195–200.
26. Pincus, G.: The Control of Fertility. New York: Acad. Press Inc. 1965.
27. Poel, W. E.: Progesterone and the prolonged progestational state: Co-carcinogenic factors in mammary tumor induction. Brit. J. Cancer **19**, 824 (1965).
28. — A differential bioassay for carcinogenic and co-carcinogenic activity of progestins. Proc. Amer. Ass. Cancer Res. **9**, 58 (1968).
29. Simmer, H. H.: Oophorectomy for breast cancer patients: Its proposal, first performance, and first explanation as an endocrine ablation. Clio Medica **4**, 227 (1969).
30. Soost, H.-J., Baier, W.: Einfluß der „Ovulationshemmer" auf das Gebärmutterhalsepithel. Dtsch. med. Wschr. **92**, 1799 (1967).
31. Stern, E., Mickey, M. R.: Effects of a cyclic steroid contraceptive regimen on mammary gland tumor induction in rats. Brit. J. Cancer **23**, 391 (1969).
32. Thiessen, P.: Die hormonrezeptorische Tumorentstehung als Ausdruck einer dienzephalhypophysären Regulationsstörung und Grundlagen einer gerichteten Hormontherapie. Z. Geburtsh. Gynäk. **137**, 138 (1952).
33. Thiessen, P.: Krebs, der neueste Stand der Forschung in Theorie und Praxis; hormonale Entstehung und Behandlung genitaler Tumoren. Medizinische **49**, 1573 (1953).
34. Wallach, S., Henneman, P. H.: Prolonged estrogen therapy in postmenopausal women. J. Amer. med. Ass. **171**, 1637 (1959).
35. Wied, G.: Pill experts perplexed by data on pap smears. Med. World News, Febr. 14, 1969.
36. Wilson, R. A.: The roles of estrogen and progesterone in breast and genital cancer. J. Amer. med. Ass. **182**, 327 (1962).
37. Wimhöfer, H.: Die hormonale und zytostatische Zusatztherapie beim Kollumkarzinom. Geburtsh. u. Frauenheilk. **28**, 609 (1968).

E.

4. Wissenschaftliche Sitzung am Freitag, den 25. 9. 1970

Vorsitz: K. E. Scheer und G. Wagner

Computer Scintigraphy

By

W. N. Tauxe

Summary

Experience of several years in data processing of scintiscan matrices by a high-speed digital computer is reported. Filters based on a system response function are used in this method. Various types of readouts are described. Using clinical examples unprocessed scans and filtered data are compared. The advantages of computer-scintigraphy in the early detection of tumors are discussed.

For further details see Tauxe, W. N.: Über die Auswertung von Radioisotop-Szintigrammdaten durch Computer. Meth. Inform. Med. 7, 96–104 (1968).

Theoretische Grundlagen zur mathematischen Bearbeitung von Szintigrammen mit digitalen Filtern

Von

H. G. Meder, W. A. Hunt, W. J. Lorenz, P. Pistor und G. Walch

Einleitung

Eine der wichtigsten Methoden für eine zuverlässige und frühzeitige Diagnose von bösartigen Geschwülsten ist die szintigraphische Lokalisation von Geschwulstgewebe. Die diagnostische Aussagekraft eines Szintigramms hängt davon ab, wie weit es gelingt, die im Szintigramm enthaltene Information dem Auge des Arztes sichtbar zu machen. Dabei muß vermieden werden, daß durch den Bearbeitungsprozeß Anomalien entstehen, denen kein klinischer Befund zugrunde liegt. In den letzten Jahren sind intensive Bemühungen gemacht worden, die szintigraphische Diagnostik zu vervollkommnen. Ein Hilfsmittel dafür ist die elektronische Datenverarbeitung [*1–6*].

Der erste Teil der folgenden Ausführungen beschreibt die Bildentstehung. Im zweiten Teil wird das Wiener-Filter vorgestellt, mit dessen Hilfe es möglich ist, einerseits die Auflösung zu erhöhen, andererseits den hochfrequenten Störpegel zu unterdrücken. Der dritte Teil zeigt auf, wo die Grenzen der Auflösungserhöhung liegen.

Mathematische Beschreibung des Szintigramms

Die Zählstatistik. Mißt man die Zahl von Gammaquanten, die von einer Strahlenquelle in kleinen Zeitintervallen im Verhältnis zur Halbwertzeit ausgesandt werden, so findet man, daß diese Zahl pro Intervall nicht immer gleich groß ist. Die statistische Gesetzmäßigkeit, die die Abweichungen der Zählraten vom Mittelwert bedingt, gehorcht einer Poisson-Verteilung. Eine wichtige Eigenschaft dieser Verteilung ist, daß ihr Mittelwert gleich der Varianz ist. Daraus folgt, daß die mittlere Zählrate pro Zeitinkrement gleichzeitig auch die Standardabweichung definiert. Bei einer mittleren Zählrate von 100 Quanten pro Zeitintervall beträgt der relative Fehler 10%, während er bei 10000 Quanten nur noch 1% ausmacht.

Was für ein Zeitintervall gilt, gilt auch für ein Flächenelement. Teilt man ein Szintigramm durch ein Raster in lauter quadratische Zellen auf, so ist die Varianz der Quantenzahl in jeder Zelle ebenfalls gleich deren Mittelwert.

Um eine Anomalie mit einem Speichereffekt oder Speicherdefekt nachzuweisen, muß die Zählrate hoch genug sein, damit der Bereich der Anomalie sich signifikant von der Umgebung abhebt.

Die Abbildungsfunktion. Das Szintigramm einer radioaktiven Punktquelle nennt man die Abbildungsfunktion des Systems. Besonders bei focussierenden Systemen ist die Abbildungsfunktion sehr stark von der Entfernung der Punktquelle von der Stirnfläche des Kollimators abhängig. Das abbildende System ist daher durch eine Schar von Abbildungsfunktionen bestimmt. Die charakteristische Größe der Abbildungsfunktion ist ihre Halbwertbreite (FWHM = Full Width at Half Maximum).

Auflösung. Befinden sich zwei radioaktive Punktquellen in genügend großem Abstand voneinander, so kann man sie im Szintigramm leicht als zwei Objekte identifizieren. Je näher diese beiden Quellen aneinanderrücken, desto schwieriger wird es, sie als Einzelobjekte wahrzunehmen. Bei einem bestimmten Abstand ist eine Unterscheidung nicht mehr möglich. Dieser Abstand wird als Maß für die Auflösung definiert. Der Betrag dieses Abstandes entspricht etwa der Halbwertbreite (FWHM) der Abbildungsfunktion.

Es gibt nun mathematische Methoden, mit denen man die Auflösung erhöhen kann, d.h. zwei Punktquellen können nach der mathematischen Bearbeitung im Szintigramm als getrennt wahrgenommen werden, während dies vorher nicht möglich war. Daraus folgt, daß die FWHM des Systems allein nicht ausreicht, um die Auflösung eines Systems zu charakterisieren. Wir werden weiter unten sehen, daß die Auflösung noch von der Anzahl der registrierten Gammaquanten abhängt.

Modulationsübertragungsfunktion. Bringt man die Abbildungsfunktion mit Hilfe der Fourier-Transformation vom Ortsbereich in den Frequenzbereich, so bezeichnet man sie dort als Modulationsübertragungsfunktion (MÜF). Sie gibt an, wie die Ortsfrequenzen des Objektes durch das abbildende System abgeschwächt werden. Mathematisch leicht beschreibbare Verhältnisse ergeben sich, wenn man die Abbildungsfunktion durch eine Gauß-Kurve approximiert, da die Fouriertransformierte einer Gauß-Kurve wieder eine Gauß-Kurve ist.

Autokorrelation, Kreuzkorrelation und Wiener-Spektrum. Die Autokorrelationsfunktion einer diskreten Zahlenfolge u_i ist im eindimensionalen Fall definiert durch

$$\varphi_j = \sum_i u_i \cdot u_{i+j}\,;\, j = 0, 1, 2, \ldots \tag{1}$$

Die Fouriertransformierte der Autokorrelationsfunktion nennt man das Wiener-Spektrum. Diese Bezeichnung geht auf den Mathematiker NORBERT WIENER *[10]* zurück, der die Anwendung der Fourier-Transformation auf Zufallsprozesse untersuchte. Autokorrelationsfunktion und Wiener-Spektrum sind die wesentlichen Bestandteile im Wiener-Filter, das im nächsten Abschnitt genauer betrachtet wird.

Die Kreuzkorrelation zweier Zahlenfolgen u_i und v_i ist definiert durch

$$\mathrm{Sj} = \sum_i u_i \cdot v_{i+j}\,;\, j = 0, 1, 2, \ldots \qquad (1\,\mathrm{a})$$

Für $v_i = u_i$ geht (1 a) in (1) über.

Faltung und Entfaltung. Es seien in einer Ebene parallel zur Stirnfläche des Kollimators eines szintigraphischen Systems mehrere radioaktive Punktquellen lokalisiert. Das Szintigramm dieser Objektverteilung kann man sich durch Superposition entstanden denken, was bedeutet, daß man jedes Objekt für sich mißt und die Einzelszintigramme addiert. Man spricht daher von Bildentstehung durch Superposition.

Wenn die Abbildungsfunktion von der Lage der Punktquelle unabhängig ist, läßt sich die Superposition durch einen speziellen Algorithmus, die Faltung (Convolution), ersetzen. Einer der Vorteile der Convolution liegt darin, daß es spezielle Zusätze für Computer gibt, mit deren Hilfe die Convolution sehr schnell ausgeführt werden kann (Array processor). Ein anderer Vorteil ist die Umkehrbarkeit der Faltung, die sog. Entfaltung.

Die Faltung zweier Zahlenfolgen c_i und d_i ist definiert durch

$$b_j = \sum_i c_i \cdot d_{j-i}. \qquad (2)$$

Dabei sei c die Objektfunktion und d die Abbildungsfunktion. Das Ergebnis der Faltung ist das Szintigramm b im eindimensionalen Fall. Zur Abkürzung verwendet man die Schreibweise

$$b = d * c = c * d. \qquad (3)$$

Es gilt jetzt festzustellen, unter welchen Umständen, in welchem Umfang und mit welchen Methoden es möglich est, den Abbildungsvorgang umzukehren und die Objektfunktion c aus dem Szintigramm b unter Zuhilfenahme der Abbildungsfunktion d zu bestimmen. Gesucht ist ein Operator f, der – gefaltet mit dem Szintigramm b – die Objektverteilung c liefert. Die Bedingung für f ergibt sich durch

$$f * b = f * d * c = \delta * c = c \qquad (4)$$

oder

$$f * d = \delta. \qquad (5)$$

Dabei ist δ die Kroneckersche Deltafunktion: $\delta = 1$ für $x = 0$ und $\delta = 0$ für $x \neq 0$.

Eine einfache Lösung ergibt sich, wenn man (5) in den Frequenzbereich transformiert. Die Faltung wird dort zur Multiplikation und die Fouriertransformierte der δ-Funktion ist gleich der Zahl 1.
Damit ist

$$F \cdot D = 1 \tag{6}$$

und daher

$$F = \frac{1}{D}. \tag{7}$$

F und D sind die Fouriertransformierten von f und d.

Den Filteroperator f im Ortsbereich kann man aus F durch inverse Fouriertransformation gewinnen.

Wie man aus (5) und (7) erkennt, hängt der inverse Filteroperator nur von der Abbildungsfunktion d bzw. der MÜF D ab. Da D im Nenner auftritt, ist die Gefahr der Instabilität vorhanden, wenn Werte von D in die Nähe von Null kommen. Die Form der Abbildungsfunktion spielt daher eine wesentliche Rolle bei der Rückgewinnung der Objektverteilung aus dem Szintigramm.

Das Wiener-Filter

Die Anwendung des inversen Filters verbietet sich aus folgenden Gründen: Das Szintigramm darf nicht gestört und der Filteroperator muß unendlich lang sein. Beide Forderungen sind in der Praxis nicht erfüllbar. Aus diesem Grund verzichtet man auf die exakte Lösung und wählt eine Methode, die Störungen mitberücksichtigt und einen Filteroperator endlicher Länge benutzt.

Das Wiener-Kriterium. Verzichtet man auf die exakte Berechnung der Objektfunktion c aus dem Szintigramm b, so muß man jetzt noch eine Bedingung angeben, der das Lösungssystem genügen soll. Diese Bedingung kann ein Maß für die Qualität der Approximation zwischen der durch den Filteroperator errechneten Objektverteilung $\hat{c}$ und der tatsächlichen Objektverteilung c sein. NORBERT WIENER wählte dafür die Summe der Quadrate der Abweichungen zwischen $\hat{c}$ und c und verlangte, daß diese Summe zu einem Minimum werden soll.

$$I = \sum_i \sum_j (\hat{c}_{i,j} - c_{i,j})^2 = \text{Minimum}. \tag{8}$$

Diesen Ausdruck nennt man das Wiener-Kriterium.

Das Wiener-Filter für störungsfreie Szintigramme. Die Bildentstehung ist in diesem Fall gegeben durch $b = c * d$ und das mit dem endlich langen

Operator f gefilterte Szintigramm folglich durch $\hat{c} = b * f = c * d * f = c * w$. Verlangt man nicht die Rückrechnung von b auf die exakte Objektverteilung c, sondern auf die mit dem Operator z, der „neuen Abbildungsfunktion“, geglättete Objektverteilung c, so ist $\bar{c} = \bar{c} * z$.
Das Wiener-Kriterium lautet dann

$$I = \sum_i \sum_j (w_{i,j} - z_{i,j})^2 = \text{Minimum}. \tag{9}$$

Die gesuchten Koeffizienten f_{ij} des Wiener-Filters erhält man in bekannter Weise durch partielle Ableitung von I nach den f_{ij} und durch Nullsetzen dieser Ableitungen. Das dadurch entstehende Gleichungssystem lautet

$$\sum_m \sum_n f_{m,n} \cdot r_{i-m,\, j-n} = g_{i,j} \;, \tag{10}$$

wobei r die Autokorrelationsfunktion der Abbildungsfunktion d, und g die Kreuzkorrelationsfunktion zwischen d und der neuen Abbildungsfunktion z sind.

Das Wiener-Filter für Szintigramme mit „weißem“ Störpegel. Die durch begrenzte Quantenzahlen verursachte statistische Fluktuation im Szintigramm ist zufallsverteilt und ihre Autokorrelation daher eine δ-Funktion. Das bedeutet, daß im Wiener-Spektrum des Störpegels alle Frequenzen gleich stark vertreten sind, weshalb man auch von einem weißen Störpegel spricht. Bezeichnet man diese durch Quantenrauschen verursachte Störung mit n, so wird das Szintigramm jetzt dargestellt durch

$$b = c * d + n\,. \tag{11}$$

Führt man diesen Ausdruck in $\hat{c}$ ein, so ist $\hat{c} = f * b = c * d * f + n * f$.
Das Wiener-Kriterium lautet dann

$$I = \sum_i \sum_j (\hat{c}_{i,j} - c_{i,j})^2 = \text{Minimum} \tag{12}$$

mit

$$\hat{c}_{ij} = \sum_i \sum_j f_{m,n} \cdot b_{i-m,\, j-m} \;,$$

wobei hier als Ergebnis des Filterns die exakte Objektverteilung c gewünscht wird. Im Gegensatz zum störungsfreien Szintigramm ist jetzt das Gleichungssystem zur Bestimmung der Filterkoeffizienten außer von der Autokorrelation r und der Kreuzkorrelation g noch von der Objektverteilung c abhängig.

Durch partielle Ableitung von I nach den Filterkoeffizienten f_{ij} erhält man wieder ein lineares Gleichungssystem

$$\sum_m \sum_n f_{m,n}\left(r_{i-m,\, j-n} + \frac{\sigma_N^2}{\sigma_c^2}\,\delta_{i-m,\, j-n}\right) = d_{-i,-j} \;, \tag{13}$$

aus dem die Filterkoeffizienten bestimmt werden können. Dabei sind σ_N^2 und σ_c^2 die Autokorrelationskoeffizienten des Störpegels und der Objektverteilung.

Interessant sind in diesem Zusammenhang zwei Spezialfälle:

1. $\sigma_N^2 = 0$, d. h. der Fall des störungsfreien Szintigrammes Gl. (13) geht in Gl. (10) über, jedoch ist die Kreuzkorrelation g zu ersetzen durch $d * \delta = d$, die Abbildungsfunktion selbst. Dasselbe Ergebnis erhält man, wenn man in (9) an Stelle von z die δ-Funktion als gewünschte Form der „neuen Abbildungsfunktion" wählt.

2. $\sigma_N^2 \gg \sigma_c^2$. In diesem Fall kann man die Autokorrelation r gegenüber dem Störglied vernachlässigen, und man erhält

$$f_{ij} = \alpha\, d_{-i,\,-j}\ ,$$

d. h., bei starkem Rauschen ist das Wiener-Filter identisch mit der Abbildungsfunktion, jedoch mit negativen Indices. Man nennt dieses Filter auch das „systemangepaßte Filter" oder „matched filter". In der Szintigraphie wird dieses Filter von TAUXE [*8, 9*] schon seit einigen Jahren mit Erfolg auf Szintigramme mit niedriger Zählstatistik angewendet.

Die Grenzen der Auflösungserhöhung durch inverse Filter

Ähnlich wie man eine Photographie nur begrenzt vergrößern kann und auf die Schärfe des Originals und die Feinkörnigkeit des Films Rücksicht nehmen muß, kann man auch in Szintigrammen die Auflösung nicht beliebig erhöhen. Die Frage, die hier beantwortet werden soll, lautet, wie weit bei vertretbarem Aufwand mit Hilfe von digitalen Filtern die Auflösung erhöht werden kann.

Nimmt man als Abbildungsfunktion d eine Gauß-Kurve der Form

$$d = \frac{N}{s\sqrt{2\pi}}\, e^{-\frac{x^2}{2s^2}} \tag{14}$$

an, wobei s die Standardabweichung und N die Anzahl der von einem Objekt ausgesandten und im Szintigramm registrierten Gammaquanten darstellt, so ist die Fouriertransformierte D von d gegeben durch

$$D = N\, e^{-2\pi^2 s^2 \nu^2} \tag{15}$$

mit ν als Ortsfrequenz.

Das Wiener-Spektrum der MÜF D ist

$$R = D^2 = N^2 e^{-4\pi^2 s^2 \nu^2}\,. \tag{16}$$

Diese Beziehungen gelten für die ungestörte Abbildungsfunktion einer Punktquelle. Dadurch, daß nur eine begrenzte Anzahl von Gammaquanten registriert werden kann, ist aber immer ein Störpegel vorhanden. Da er rein zufälliger Natur ist, besitzt er ein „weißes" Spektrum, was bedeutet, daß sein Wiener-Spektrum alle (Orts-) Frequenzen in gleicher Stärke enthält.

Es läßt sich theoretisch und durch Messung nachweisen, daß der Betrag der Autokorrelation des Störpegels gleich der Anzahl der Quanten N ist, die von der Punktquelle ausgesandt und vom Detektorsystem registriert werden,

$$R_N = N. \tag{17}$$

Das Wiener-Spektrum R der Abbildungsfunktion hat die Form einer Gauß-Kurve mit dem Wert N^2 für $\nu = 0$, während das Wiener-Spektrum des Rauschens R_N eine im Abstand N zur Abszisse ν parallele Gerade ist.

Die Frequenz ν_N, bei der der Störpegel R_N und das Signal R gleich groß sind, ergibt sich aus (16) und (17) zu

$$\nu_N = \frac{1}{2\pi s} \sqrt{\ln N}. \tag{18}$$

Je höher die Zahl der vom interessierenden Objekt empfangenen Gammaquanten ist, desto höher sind die Ortsfrequenzen, die über dem Störpegel liegen, und desto besser ist folglich die zu erzielende Auflösung.

Ein auflösungerhöhendes Filter, gleich welcher Art, wirkt dadurch, daß es die Frequenzen des Signals in allen Bereichen möglichst gleich groß, d. h. zu einem weißen Spektrum macht. Da das Spektrum außer dem Signal aber auch Störungen enthält, wird bei Verwendung auflösungserhöhender Filter der Störpegel mit angehoben. Aus diesem Grunde kann die „Kontrastverstärkung" nicht beliebig weit getrieben werden.

Eine Abschätzung der zu erzielenden Auflösungserhöhung ergibt sich aus den in (18) bestimmten Frequenzen ν_N wie folgt:

Angenommen, es wäre möglich, durch ein Filter alle Frequenzen ν, $0 \leq \nu \leq \nu_N$, der MÜF R auf den Betrag 1 zu verstärken und alle Frequenzen $\nu > \nu_N$ auf Null zu bringen.

Dieser Rechteckfunktion im Frequenzbereich entspricht im Ortsbereich die Funktion

$$y = \frac{\sin(2\pi \cdot x \cdot \nu_N)}{\pi \cdot x}. \tag{19}$$

Aus dieser ergibt sich als Maß für die Auflösung die Halbwertbreite $\overline{\text{FWHM}}$ zu

$$\overline{\text{FWHM}} \approx \text{FWHM} \cdot \frac{1}{\sqrt{\log_{10} N}}. \tag{20}$$

FWHM ist die im ersten Abschnitt definierte Halbwertbreite der Abbildungsfunktion d. Definiert man die Auflösungsverbesserung durch den Quotienten $k = \mathrm{FWHM}/\overline{\mathrm{FWHM}}$, so ist

$$k \approx \sqrt{\log_{10} N}. \tag{21}$$

Diese Auflösungsverbesserung stellt eine obere Grenze dar, die von dem hier besprochenen Wiener-Filter annähernd erreicht wird.

Man erkennt, daß bei einer Zählrate $N = 10$ die Auflösung nicht verändert wird. Bei $N = 10000$ ergibt sich eine Erhöhung der Auflösung um den Faktor 2. Wollte man eine Auflösungsverbesserung um den Faktor 3 erzielen, so wären dafür 10^9 Gammaquanten von dem betreffenden Objekt zu registrieren.

Legt man die Leistung der heutigen Meßgeräte zugrunde, dann läßt sich aufgrund von (21) feststellen, daß digitale Filterung eine Auflösungserhöhung um den Faktor 2 ermöglicht.

Literatur

1. Gregg, E. C.: Modulation transfer function, information capacity and performance criteria of scintiscans. J. nucl. Med. **9**, 116 (1968).
2. Hunt, W. A., Lorenz, W. J., Luig, H., Meder, H. G., Pistor, P., Schmidlin, P., Walch, G., Schmitt, H. G.: Digital Processing of Scintigraphic Images. IBM Scientific Center Technical Report No. 70.03.001, Wiss. Zentrum Heidelberg 1970.
3. Hunt, W. A., Lorenz, W. J., Luig, H., Meder, H. G., Pistor, P., Schmidlin, P., Walch, G., Schmitt, H. G.: Optimum Sample Size in Digital Radioscintigraphy. IBM Scientific Center Technical Report No. 70.08.004, Wiss. Zentrum Heidelberg 1970.
4. Meder, H. G.: Digitale Filter und ihre Anwendungen. IBM-Nachrichten **19**, 843 (1969). IBM Form 78.300.2.70.
5. Pistor, P.: Digital Processing of Scintigraphic Images by Two-Dimensional Recursive Wiener-Filters. IBM Scientific Center Technical Report No. 70.12.006, Wiss. Zentrum Heidelberg 1970.
6. Robinson, E. A.: Multichannel Time Series Analysis with Digital Computer Programs. New York: Holden-Day 1967.
7. Röhler, R.: Informationstheorie in der Optik. Stuttgart: Wiss. Verlagsanstalt 1967.
8. Tauxe, W. N., Chaapel, D. W., Sprau, A. C.: Contrast enhancement of scanning procedures by high-speed digital computer. J. nucl. Med. **7**, 647 (1966).
9. Tauxe, W. N.: Über die Auswertung von Radioisotop-Szintigrammdaten durch Computer. Meth. Inform. Med. **7**, 96 (1968).
10. Wiener, N.: Extrapolation, Interpolation and Smoothing of Stationary Time Series. Cambridge/Mass.: The M. I. T. Press 1949.

Anwendung von digitalen Filtern auf Szintigramme

Von

W. J. Lorenz, P. Georgi, H. Luig, H. G. Meder und P. Schmidlin

Einleitung

Der Einsatz von digitalen Rechenanlagen und die Anwendung von mathematischen Methoden zur Bearbeitung von Szintigrammen hat zu einer wesentlichen Verbesserung der Aussagekraft der nuclearmedizinischen Lokalisationsdiagnostik geführt [1–6]. Ein wichtiges Anwendungsgebiet dieser Untersuchungsmethode ist der Nachweis und die Lokalisation von Tumoren und Metastasen. Bei der Untersuchung werden den Patienten radioaktiv markierte Verbindungen verabreicht, die sich entweder im Tumorgewebe anreichern und szintigraphisch als sog. „heiße Knoten" erkennbar sind oder sich im umgebenden gesunden Gewebe anreichern und dadurch Tumoren oder Metastasen als sog. „kalte Knoten" darstellen. Die Aktivitätsdifferenzen zwischen Tumorgewebe und gesundem Gewebe werden mit szintigraphischen Systemen, wie bewegten Detektoren (Scannern) oder stehenden Detektoren (Gammakameras), von außen gemessen.

Für eine rechtzeitige und damit erfolgversprechende Behandlung einer Tumorerkrankung ist der möglichst frühzeitige Nachweis von vorhandenem neoplastischen Gewebe von größter Wichtigkeit. Eine vordringliche Aufgabe der nuclearmedizinischen Forschung ist daher die Verbesserung und Weiterentwicklung der nuclearmedizinischen Lokalisationsdiagnostik. Dabei wird das Ziel verfolgt, bösartige Tumoren möglichst im Frühstadium zu erkennen, d. h. möglichst kleine neoplastische Zellansammlungen zu diagnostizieren. Aufgrund dieser Aufgabenstellung werden z. Z. in der nuclearmedizinischen Lokalisationsdiagnostik drei Hauptforschungsrichtungen verfolgt:

1. Die Entwicklung von Radiopharmaka, die sich möglichst selektiv im Tumorgewebe anreichern.

2. Die Entwicklung und der Bau von szintigraphischen Detektorsystemen mit hoher Auflösung und Nachweisempfindlichkeit.

3. Die Entwicklung von mathematischen Verfahren zur Bearbeitung von Szintigrammen, um den Informationsgehalt der szintigraphischen

Messung möglichst vollständig für die diagnostische Beurteilung des Szintigramms nutzbar zu machen.

In der vorliegenden Arbeit wird über Ergebnisse berichtet, die durch mathematische Bearbeitung von Szintigrammen der Anger-Kamera mit Wiener-Filtern erzielt wurden. Die theoretischen Grundlagen dieses Filterverfahrens werden in der vorangehenden Arbeit behandelt [7].

Ergebnisse

Zur Erläuterung des Filterverfahrens möge Abb. 1 dienen. Im oberen Teil der Abbildung ist in Analogie zur Radioaktivitätsverteilung in einem Untersuchungsobjekt das Modell eines Autos mit Fahrer durch schwarze und weiße Rasterfelder dargestellt. Dieses Modell wurde mit Hilfe eines Computers simuliert. Der mittlere Teil der Abbildung entspricht einem Bild des fahrenden Autos, das mit zu langer Belichtungszeit aufgenommen wurde. Dieses Bild wurde aus dem Original durch Faltung mit einer trapezförmigen Funktion errechnet. Das ist analog zu der Messung einer Radioaktivitätsverteilung in einem Untersuchungsobjekt mit einem szintigraphischen System, dessen Abbildungsfunktion keine nadelförmige Funktion ist und deshalb unscharfe Bilder ergibt. Aus der Kenntnis der Abbildungsfunktion kann ein mathematischer Filter berechnet werden, der auf die unscharfe Aufnahme angewandt. wieder das Original ergibt. Das untere Bild in Abb. 1 ist die gefilterte Aufnahme, die mit dem Original identisch ist. Diese idealen Verhältnisse sind allerdings nur bei Objekten gegeben, deren Aufnahme ohne Rauschen, d. h. ohne statistisch bedingte Zählratenschwankungen erhalten wurde. Bei szintigraphischen Aufnahmen gibt es keine rauschfreien Aufnahmen, so daß durch Anwendung von mathematischen Filterverfahren auf das Szintigramm nur eine Annäherung an eine ideale Abbildung des radioaktiven Verteilungsmusters im Untersuchungsobjekt erreicht werden kann.

Abb. 2. zeigt auf der linken Seite zwei Aufnahmen des IAEA-Leberphantoms mit einer Szintillationskamera nach Anger. Das Leberphantom ist mit radioaktiver Lösung gefüllt und enthält acht kalte Knoten mit Durchmessern zwischen 4,0 und 0,8 cm. Die Kameraszintigramme wurden digital gespeichert und mit einem Computer IBM 360/50 ausgedruckt. Das Szintigramm links oben ist im Bereich von 20–80% der maximalen Zählrate in 10 Graustufen dargestellt. Das Szintigramm links unten zeigt die Darstellung für den Bereich von 20–50% der maximalen Zählrate. Die kleinen kalten Knoten sind in beiden Szintigrammen nicht zu erkennen.

Die rechte Seite der Abbildung zeigt die gleichen Szintigramme nach Korrektur von Inhomogenitäten des Detektors und nach Anwendung eines Wiener-Filters mit einem Filterfaktor von $F = 3{,}0$. Bei der Dar-

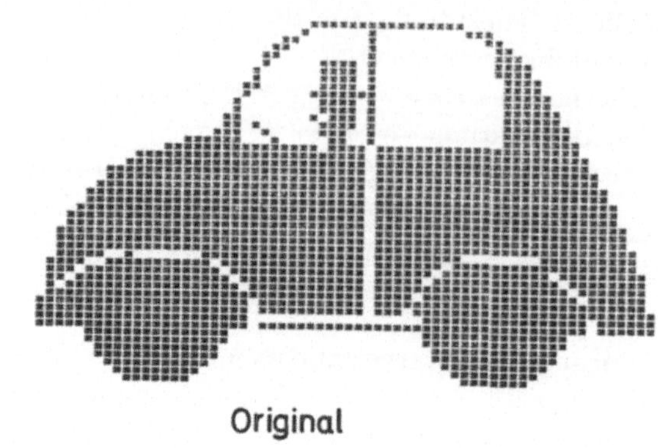

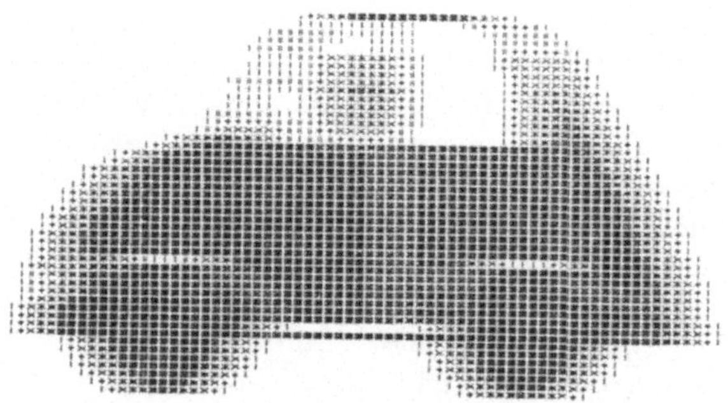

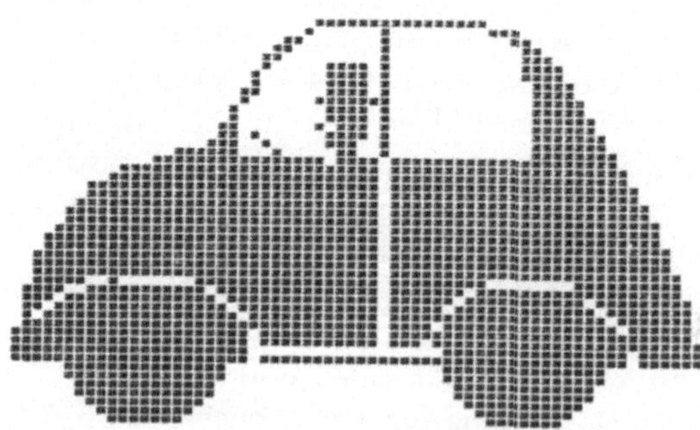

Abb. 1. Computersimuliertes Modell einer Radioaktivitätsverteilung: Original, unscharfe Aufnahme nach Anwendung einer trapezförmigen Abbildungsfunktion auf das Original und gefilterte Aufnahme nach Anwendung eines mathematischen Filters auf die unscharfe Aufnahme

stellung im Bereich 20–80% der maximalen Zählrate ist das Szintigramm noch recht unruhig. Bei der Darstellung im Intervall von 20–50% entspricht das Szintigramm sehr gut der Radioaktivitätsverteilung im Phantom. Auch die kleinen Knoten mit 1,0 bzw. 0,8 cm Durchmesser sind jetzt deutlich zu erkennen. Dieses Beispiel zeigt, daß neben der Entwicklung und

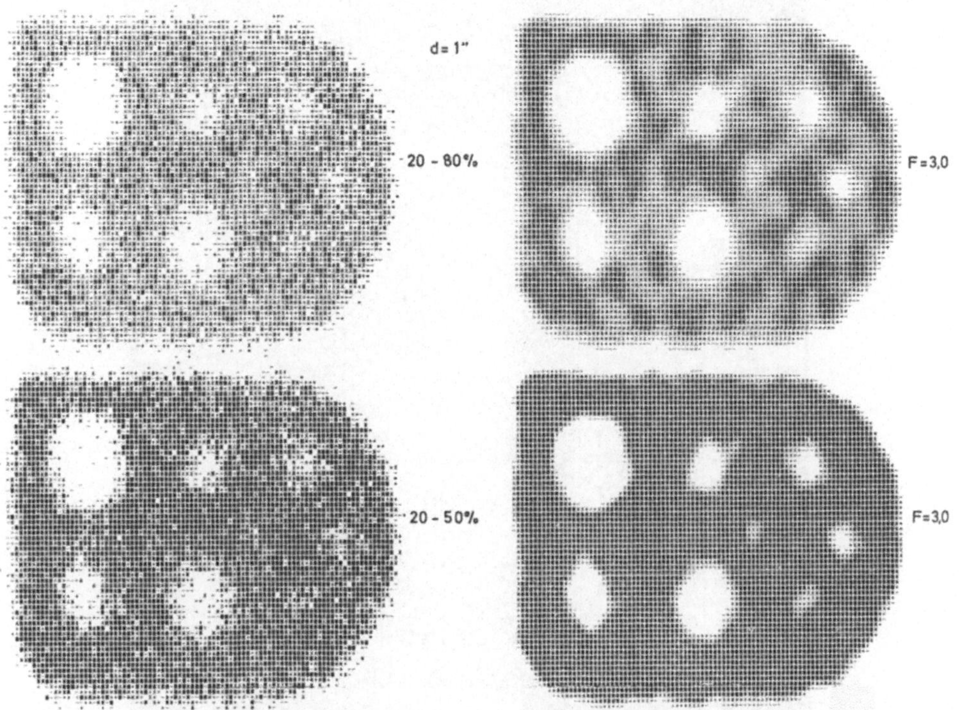

Abb. 2. Szintigraphische Aufnahmen des IAEA-Leberphantoms mit einer Anger-Kamera (linke Spalte) und gefilterte Szintigramme der Original-Kameraaufnahmen (rechte Spalte). Darstellung in 10 Schwärzungsstufen. Dargestellter Bereich: 20–80% bzw. 20–50% der maximalen Zählrate. Abstand zwischen Kollimator und Phantom 1". Filterfaktor $F = 3,0$

Anwendung von geeigneten mathematischen Bearbeitungsverfahren auch die Art der Darstellung die Aussagekraft des Szintigramms und damit den diagnostischen Aussagewert der szintigraphischen Messung wesentlich beeinflußt.

Abb. 3 zeigt Szintiphotos des Schädels einer Patientin (10137) mit einem links temporal gelegenen Hirntumor. Die Frontalaufnahme oben links und die Lateralaufnahme oben rechts wurden nach Gabe von ^{18}F-

Hexafluoroaluminat, die Frontalaufnahme unten links und die Lateralaufnahme unten rechts wurden nach Gabe von $^{99}Tc^{m}$-Pertechnetat gewonnen. Eine umschriebene pathologische Aktivitätsanreicherung im Gehirn ist in beiden Lateralaufnahmen zu erkennen.

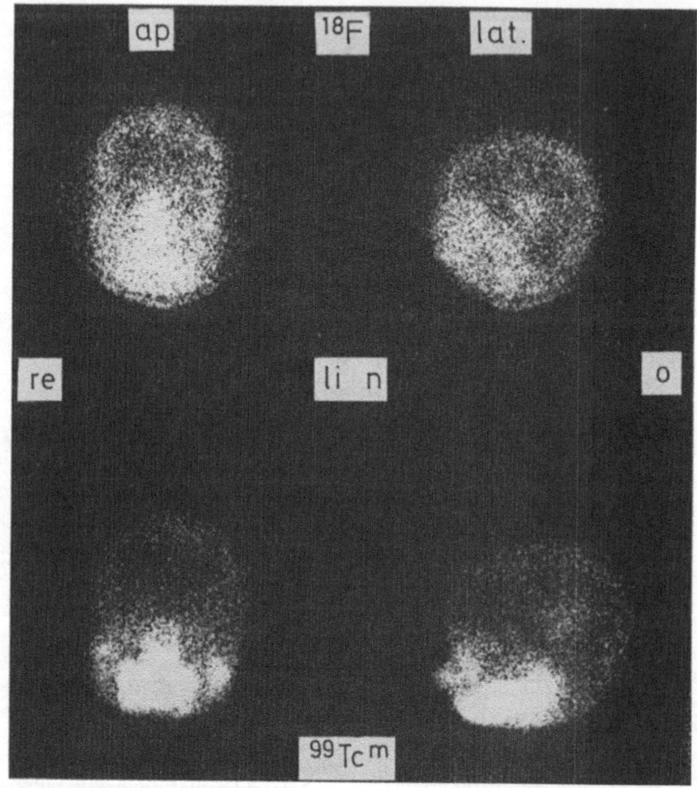

Abb. 3. Szintiphotos des Schädels einer Patientin (10137) mit einem links temporal gelegenen Hirntumor. Die Kameraaufnahmen wurden nach Gabe von ^{18}F-Hexafluoroaluminat (oben) und $^{99}Tc^{m}$-Pertechnetat (unten) gemacht. In beiden Fällen ist bei den lateralen Aufnahmen der Speicherherd gut zu erkennen

Abb. 4 zeigt die Computerszintigramme (10137) der lateralen $^{99}Tc^{m}$-Aufnahmen. Sowohl im ungefilterten als auch im gefilterten Bild ist der Tumor deutlich zu erkennen. Im gefilterten Szintigramm können darüberhinaus Einzelheiten des radioaktiven Verteilungsmusters im Bereich des Tumors festgestellt werden.

Abb. 5 zeigt die Computerszintigramme (10137) in lateraler Aufnahme nach Gabe des ^{18}F-Komplexes. Der Tumor ist im ungefilterten und im

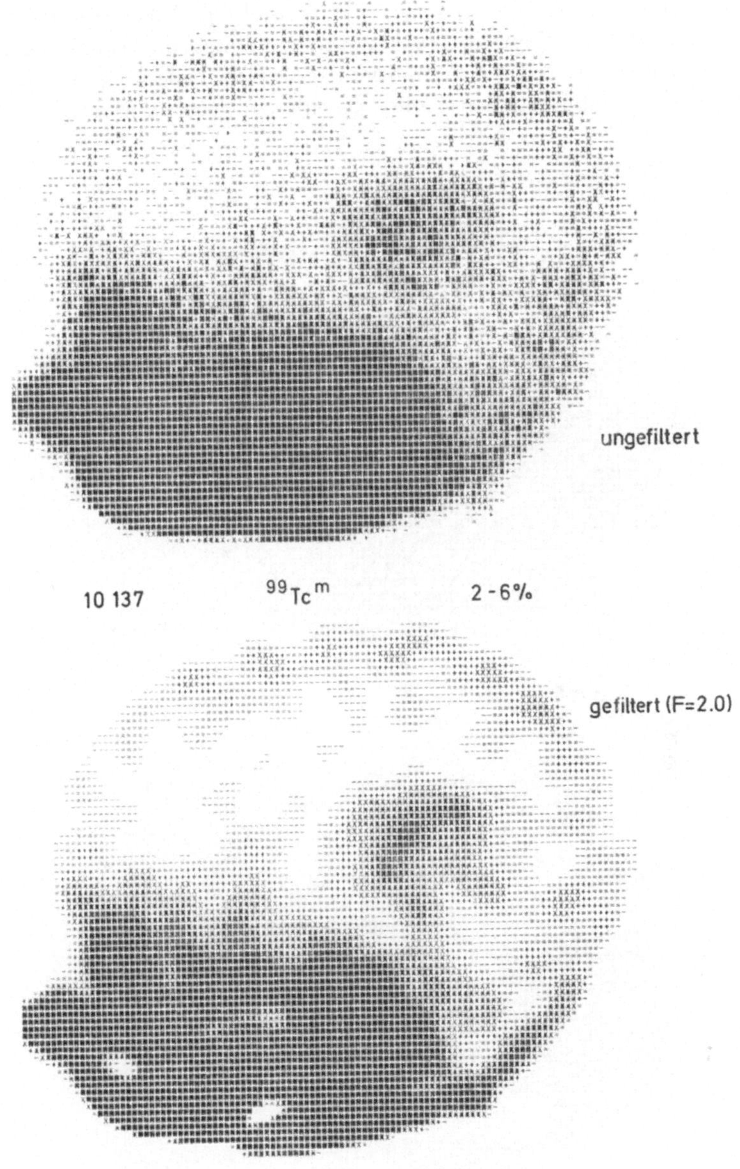

Abb. 4. Kameraszintigramm der Patientin 10137 (oben) und gefiltertes Kameraszintigramm der gleichen Patientin (unten) nach Gabe von $^{99}Tc^{m}$-Pertechnetat. Deutliche Darstellung des Tumors in beiden Aufnahmen. Einzelheiten der Aktivitätsverteilung im Tumorbereich sind im gefilterten Szintigramm sichtbar

gefilterten Szintigramm gut dargestellt. Außerdem kommen Bereiche des knöchernen Schädels deutlich zur Abbildung. Das gefilterte Szintigramm zeigt Einzelheiten der Aktivitätsverteilung im Tumor, aus denen entweder auf eine Nekrotisierung von zentralen Teilen des Tumors oder auf einen metastasierenden Tumor geschlossen werden kann.

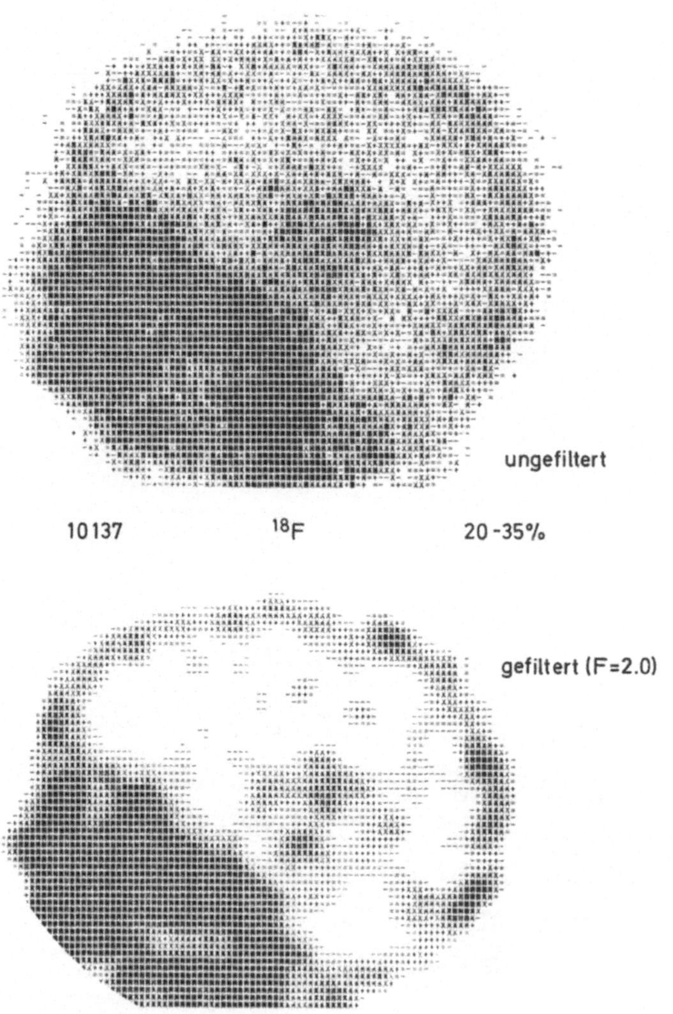

Abb. 5. Kameraszintigramm der Patientin 10137 (oben) und gefiltertes Kameraszintigramm der gleichen Patientin (unten) nach Gabe von ^{18}F-Hexafluoroaluminat. In beiden Szintigrammen ist der Tumorbereich gut abgebildet. Das gefilterte Szintigramm zeigt Einzelheiten der Aktivitätsverteilung im Tumor

Schlußbemerkung

Aufgrund von eingehenden theoretischen Überlegungen und aufgrund der bisher vorliegenden praktischen Erfahrungen erscheint der Wiener-Filter ein geeignetes mathematisches Hilfsmittel zur Bearbeitung von Szintigrammen zu sein. Durch Anwendung dieses Filters auf digitale Szintigramme wird nahezu der gesamte Informationsgehalt der szintigraphischen Messung zur diagnostischen Beurteilung der Radioaktivitätsverteilung im Untersuchungsobjekt verfügbar gemacht. Voraussetzung für die Anwendbarkeit dieses mathematischen Analyseverfahrens ist allerdings die Verfügbarkeit eines relativ großen Digitalrechners. Wir konnten daher unsere bisherigen Analysen nur mit dem Rechner IBM 360/50 des Wissenschaftlichen Zentrums Heidelberg der IBM Deutschland durchführen, da der Computer IBM 360/30 des DKFZ sowohl hinsichtlich Speicherkapazität als auch Rechengeschwindigkeit für die Anwendung von Filterverfahren in der Szintigraphie nicht ausreichend dimensioniert ist.

Um den Wert des Filterverfahrens für die Frühdiagnostik von Tumorerkrankungen beurteilen zu können, ist es notwendig, eine größere Zahl von Patienten zu untersuchen. Diese Untersuchungen werden zur Zeit in Zusammenarbeit mit mehreren Heidelberger Kliniken durchgeführt.

Literatur

1. Lorenz, W. J., Adam, W. E.: Digitale und analoge Auswertung von Aufnahmen mit der Szintillationskamera. Nucl. Med. **6**, 367 (1967).
2. Lorenz, W. J., Luig, H., Meder, H. G., Pistor, P., Schmidlin, P., Walch, G.: Mathematische Methoden zur Verbesserung der Aussagekraft von Szintigrammen. (7. Symposium der Sektion Nuklearmedizin der Gesellschaft für Radiologie der DDR, Reinhardsbrunn/Thüringen, 6.–8. 4. 1970) (Im Druck).
3. Lorenz, W. J., Ammann, W., Krauss, O., Ostertag, H., Pistor, P., Schmidlin, P., Walch, G.: Ergebnisse der Anwendung von digitalen Wiener-Filtern auf Szintigramme der Anger-Kamera. (8. Jahrestagung der Gesellschaft für Nuclearmedizin, Hannover, 16.–19. 9. 1970) (Im Druck).
4. Lorenz, W. J., Luig, H., Meder, H. G., Pistor, P., Schmidlin, P., Walch, G.: Kontrastverstärkung in Szintigrammen mit Hilfe von digitalen Filtern. Z. Krebsforsch. **74**, 344 (1970).
5. Meder, H. G.: Digitale Filter und ihre Anwendungen. IBM-Nachrichten **19**, 843 (1969).
6. Meder, H. G., Lorenz, W. J., Luig, H., Pistor, P., Schmidlin, P., Schmitt, H. G.: Digitale Filter in der Computerszintigraphie. (7. Jahrestagung der Gesellschaft für Nuklearmedizin, Zürich, 25.–27. 9. 1969) (Im Druck).
7. Meder, H. G., Hunt, W. A., Lorenz, W. J., Pistor, P., Walch, G.: Theoretische Grundlagen zur mathematischen Bearbeitung von Szintigrammen mit digitalen Filtern. In H. Lettré, u. G. Wagner (Hrsg.): Aktuelle Probleme aus dem Gebiet der Cancerologie III, S. 174. Berlin-Heidelberg-New York: Springer 1971.

Möglichkeiten einer positiven Tumorszintigraphie

Von

P. Georgi, P. Schenck und H. Sinn

Tumorspezifische Radiopharmaka für den szintigraphischen Nachweis eines malignen Wachstums stehen der medizinischen Diagnostik auch heute noch nicht zur Verfügung. Maligne Tumoren zeichnen sich dadurch aus, daß sie keine oder eine weitgehend eingeschränkte spezifische Funktion der Ausgangsorgane erkennen lassen. In vielen Fällen wird daher ein sogenannter „negativer Nachweis" eines Tumors möglich; während das Organparenchym eine selektive Speicherung des Radionuklids zeigt, findet im Tumorgewebe keine Ablagerung statt.

Der Nachweis dieser sogenannten „kalten Bezirke" stellt besonders hohe technische Anforderungen und ist nur möglich, wenn die Impulsrate über dem Tumor um 10–15% niedriger als über dem umgebenden Gewebe ist. Größe und Lage des Tumors sind ebenfalls von Bedeutung. Je höher die radionuklidspeichernde Gewebsschicht über dem nichtspeichernden Tumor ist, um so schwieriger gelingt der Nachweis. Der Mindestdurchmesser eines kalten Bezirks, der mit einem konventionellen Szintigraphen nachgewiesen werden kann, beträgt im günstigsten Fall 1 bis 1,5 cm.

Der positive szintigraphische Tumornachweis ist aus meßtechnischen Gründen einfacher zu führen. Mit modernen Szintigraphen ist es möglich, weitgehend unabhängig von den Abmessungen 1 μCi eines Radionuklids mit einer mittleren Gamma-Energie nachzuweisen, wenn das umgebene Gewebe keine Radionuklidspeicherung aufweist. Diese sog. „positive Tumordiagnostik" hat ihre Leistungsfähigkeit beim Nachweis von radiojodspeichernden Schilddrüsenmetastasen, sowie Knochen- und Hirntumoren bewiesen. Bei keinem der Fälle handelt es sich jedoch um einen spezifischen Nachweis des neoplastischen Wachstums.

Voraussetzung für den szintigraphischen Tumornachweis ist die Photonenemission eines Radiopharmakons. Es wurden daher Versuche mit geeigneten Gamma-Strahlern durchgeführt. Von den wesentlichen Elementen des Gewebes: Kohlenstoff, Sauerstoff, Wasserstoff, Stickstoff, Schwefel und Phosphor stehen jedoch keine geeigneten γ-Strahler außer ^{11}C zur Verfügung.

BENDER u. BLAU [1] konnten 1964 nachweisen, daß die schwefelhaltige Aminosäure Methionin auch dann in viele Körperproteine eingebaut wird, wenn der Schwefel durch das Selenisotop ^{75}Se ersetzt wurde. Gewebe mit erhöhter Proteinsynthese zeigt eine hohe initiale Selenmethioninanreicherung. Es gelingt daher, mit ^{75}Se-Methionin Adenome der Nebenschilddrüsen nachzuweisen (Abb. 1). In den letzten Jahren wurde auch die Verwendung von Selenmethionin für den Nachweis einer malignen Reticulose beschrieben [2].

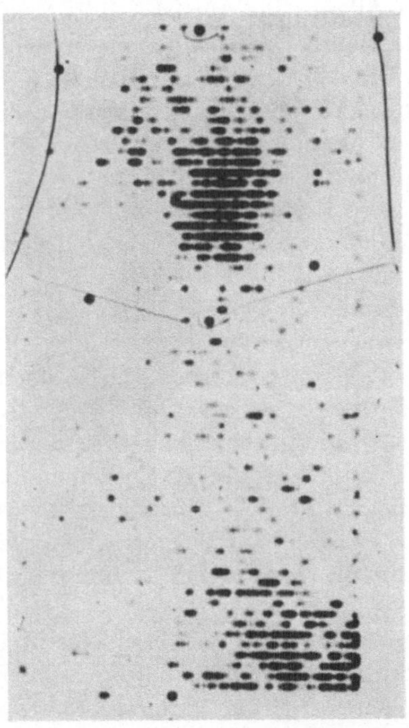

Abb. 1. Photoszintigramm eines Adenoms der Nebenschilddrüse 1 Std nach i.v Applikation von 250 μCi ^{75}Se-Methionin

Eine bessere Möglichkeit, den erhöhten Stoffwechsel im Tumor szintigraphisch zu erfassen, verspricht das Kohlenstoffisotop ^{11}C. Seine Halbwertzeit beträgt 20,3 min. Da ^{11}C nur im Cyklotron hergestellt werden kann und ein längerer Transport wegen der kurzen Halbwertzeit nicht möglich ist, liegen bisher noch keine ausreichenden Untersuchungsergebnisse vor. Eine weitere Schwierigkeit ist in der notwendigen, sehr schnellen Präparation der erforderlichen Precursor zu sehen, die schnell in den Tumorstoffwechsel eingebaut werden.

Von verschiedenen Tumoren ist bekannt, daß sie Serumproteine extravasal speichern. Eine besonders hohe Albuminanreicherung zeigen im Tierexperiment transplantierte Tumoren. Da Humanserumalbumin mit ^{131}J relativ leicht zu markieren ist, lag es nahe, radiojodmarkiertes Humanserumalbumin bei der Tumordiagnostik zu verwenden. Hiermit konnte eine positive Tumordarstellung bei Patienten mit Bronchial-Ca, Larynx-Ca und Reticulumzellsarkomen im Szintigramm erhalten werden [*6*]. Eine vermehrte Nuklidkonzentration gegenüber gesundem Gewebe wurde bei Tumoren des Magendarmkanals nach intraarterieller Injektion von ^{131}J markierten Albuminmakropartikeln beobachtet [*8*]. Das hitzedenaturierte Serumalbumin wird im neoplastischen Gewebe langsamer als in der gesunden Umgebung abgebaut, so daß 3–4 Tage nach der Injektion Anreicherungsfaktoren gefunden werden, die zwischen 4,5 und 22 liegen. Mit dieser Methodik konnten über 90% der untersuchten Neoplasmen nachgewiesen werden.

Neben Albumin wird in verschiedenen Tumoren auch eine hohe Fibrinanreicherung gefunden [*9*]. 1967 gelang es der italienischen Arbeitsgruppe um Monasterio mit ^{131}J markiertem Fibrinogen Tumoren beim Menschen szintigraphisch darzustellen [*11*].

Es war naheliegend, auch Fibrinogenantikörper zu markieren. Von Marrak et al. [*10*] wurden Antikörper des Kaninchens gegen Humanfibrinogen bei 137 Patienten getestet. 80% der untersuchten Tumoren konnten von ihnen szintigraphisch nachgewiesen werden. Hierbei ließen sich Sarkome und Melanome besser als Carcinome darstellen. Der Speicherungsmechanismus ist für ^{131}J-Fibrinogen und markierte Fibrinogenantikörper gleich; er hängt von der intra- und peritumoralen Fibrinanreicherung ab und stellt somit ebenfalls keine spezifische Tumoranreicherung dar.

Als weitere Möglichkeit eines positiven Nachweises eines malignen Geschehens haben wir die szintigraphische Darstellung der pathologischen Gefäßversorgung des Tumors gewählt. Bereits 1826 gelang es Schroeder van der Kolk durch Injektionsstudien *in vitro* normales und neoplastisches Gewebe visuell zu differenzieren. Fast im gesamten folgenden Jahrhundert dominierten mikroskopische *In-vitro*-Untersuchungen über die Tumorzirkulation. In den beiden letzten Jahrzehnten ermöglichte dann die Röntgenangiographie den *In-vivo*-Nachweis einer pathologischen Gefäßversorgung des Tumors.

Bereits vor etwa 2 Jahren haben wir eine einfache szintigraphische Methode der positiven Tumorgefäßdarstellung mit der Szintillationskamera nach Anger angegeben und uns auf die einfache bolusartige intravenöse Applikation eines möglichst vorher leicht zu präparierenden Radiopharmakons beschränkt. Wir geben heute kurzlebigen, hochspezifischen Aktivitäten wie dem ^{99}Tc^{m}-Pertechnetat und dem ^{113}In^{m}-Serumalbumin

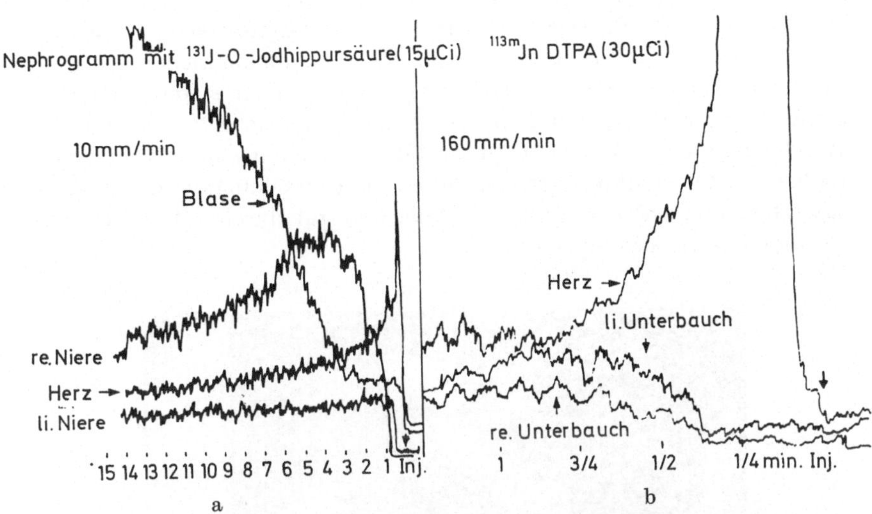

Abb. 2a u. b. Schleimbildendes Adenocarcinom des linken Beckens. a) Das Isotopennephrogramm mit 16 μCi ^{131}J-o-Jodhippursäure zeigt eine funktionslose Niere links; b) Das Isotopennephrogramm mit 30 μCi ^{113}In ^{m}-DTPA zeigt eine vermehrte Tumordurchblutung im Gebiet der linken Niere

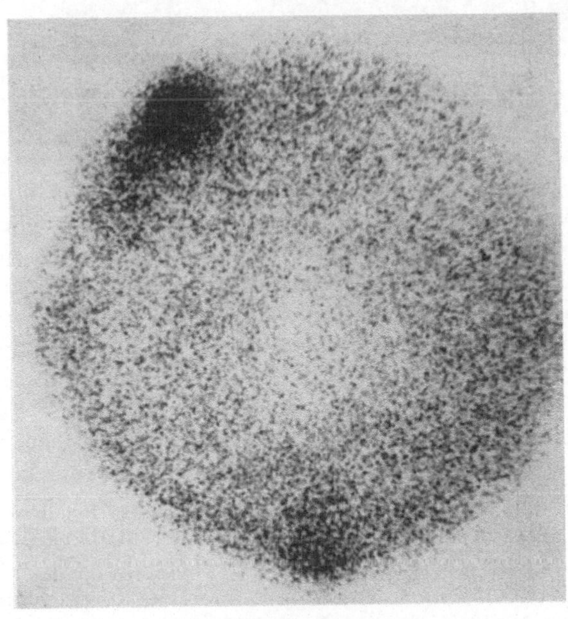

Abb. 3. Szintifoto des in Abb. 2 dargestellten Adenocarcinoms des linken Beckens (2 mCi ^{113}In ^{m}-DTPA)

den Vorzug. Als günstigster Termin zum szintigraphischen Nachweis einer Tumordurchblutung – insbesondere von abdominellen malignen Geschehen – hat sich eine Expositionszeit der Szintiphotos von 0–20 sec p. i. bewährt; ein Zeitraum, in dem noch keine wesentliche Radioaktivitätsausscheidung in die Blase erfolgt ist. Zu subtrahieren sind hierbei der mit Radioaktivität gefüllte Herzinnenraum, die Darstellung der diagnostisch zusätzlich verwertbaren großen Gefäße und gut durchbluteten Organe, insbesondere Leber und Nieren.

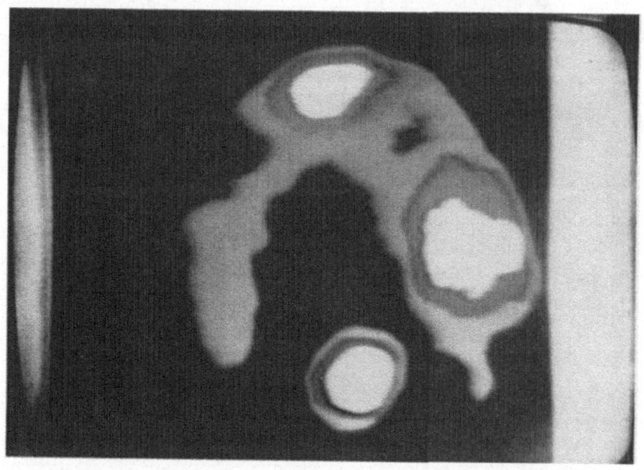

Abb. 4. Kontrastanhebung der Abb. 3. (Chromoscan II. Fa. Nuclear Chicago.)

In Abb. 2 erkennt man im Isotopennephrogramm eine durch ein schleimbildendes Adeno-Carcinom des linken Unterbauches induzierte funktionslose Niere links. Auf der rechten Bildhälfte ist der Nachweis einer vermehrten Tumordurchblutung im linken Unterbauch durch 2 ventral über beiden Beckenhälften angelegte Kollimatoren möglich. Das Szintiphoto, das bei der gleichen Patientin ebenfalls nach der Injektion von $^{113}In^{m}$-DTPA angefertigt wurde, zeigt in der oberen Bildhälfte das untere Polgebiet der funktionstüchtigen rechten Niere. Die Blase und der vermehrt durchblutete Tumor sind jedoch nicht sicher voneinander abzugrenzen (Abb. 3). Erst durch eine Kontrastanhebung kommt der Tumor deutlich zur Abbildung (Abb. 4).

Welche falschen Interpretationsmöglichkeiten diese doch sehr einfache Tumorsuchmethode beinhalten kann, zeigt das nächste Szintiphoto. Es handelt sich um einen Patienten mit einem Hypernephrom rechts. 0–30 sec nach der Injektion von 2 mCi $^{113}In^{m}$-Serumalbumin stellt sich neben dem Herzinnenraum eine gleichmäßig von $^{113}In^{m}$-Serumalbumin perfundierte Leber dar (Abb. 5). Zunächst hatten wir eine isolierte vermehrte Metastasendurchblutung erwartet, nachdem das kurz vorher angefertigte konventionelle Szintigramm nach Gabe von ^{198}Au-Kolloid einen deutlichen Speicherdefekt im cranialen Polgebiet des rechten Leberlappens erkennen ließ (Abb. 6).

Schon vor 40 Jahren wiesen HEVESY u. KAHN [7] auf die besondere Tumoraffinität von Schwermetallen hin. Für die Lokalisationsdiagnostik maligner Geschwülste wurden daher ^{64}Cu, ^{74}As, ^{86}Rb, ^{131}Cs, ^{203}Hg und

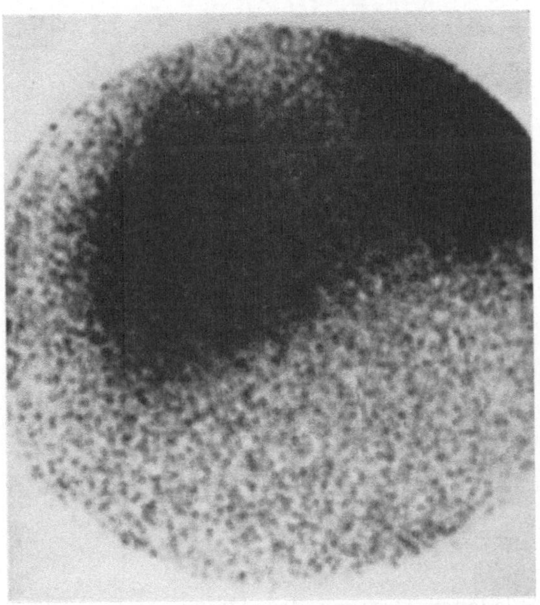

Abb. 5. Szintifoto der Leber eines Patienten mit einem Hypernephrom rechts (Aufnahme 0–30 sec nach Injektion von 2 mCi ^{113}In^{m}-Humanserumalbumin)

^{206}Bi eingesetzt. Obwohl ^{206}Bi von allen bisher untersuchten Radionukliden die höchsten Speicherraten zeigt, wurde es aufgrund seiner ungünstigen physikalischen Eigenschaften in der Diagnostik nicht oder nur selten verwendet. Eine Tumorspezifität wird jedoch trotz der hohen Anreicherungsraten sowohl von Wismut als auch von Kupfer von GERHARD u. MUNDINGER abgelehnt [5].

Nachdem von WOLF u. FISCHER [12] 1965 beobachtet worden war, daß Quecksilberchlorid nicht nur in Hirntumoren, sondern auch in Geschwülsten anderer Organe des Körpers eingelagert wird, wurde in den letzten Monaten und Wochen von verschiedenen Autoren die Beobachtung der ^{67}Ga-Citrat-Speicherung im neoplastischen Gewebe bestätigt

[3, 4]. Auf Grund seiner physikalischen Eigenschaften ist ^{67}Ga für szintigraphische Untersuchungen gut geeignet. Es handelt sich hierbei um ein Cyclotronprodukt mit einer Halbwertzeit von 78 Std und einer γ-Strahlung von 184 und 296 keV, das trägerfrei gewonnen werden kann. Nachteilig ist sowohl für ^{203}Hg als auch für ^{67}Ga die physiologische Anreiche-

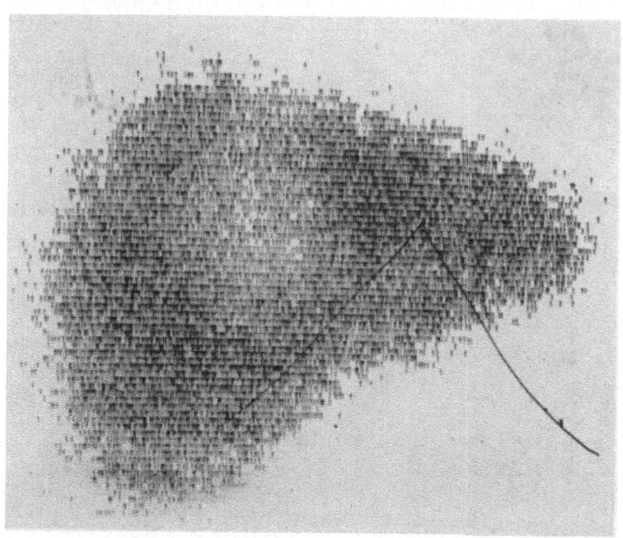

Abb. 6. Szintigramm der in Abb. 5 dargestellten Leber 1 Std nach i.v. Applikation von 120 μCi ^{198}Au-Kolloid

rung in verschiedenen Organen des Abdomens bzw. die Ausscheidung über den Darm. Über den Mechanismus der Anreicherung im neoplastischen Gewebe liegen bisher keine Angaben vor; Hayes et al. [4] berichteten lediglich, daß ^{67}Ga im Cytoplasma der neoplastischen Zellen abgelagert wird, wobei nach Ultrazentrifugation des Homogenats 80% der Aktivität im Niederschlag gefunden wurde.

Erste szintigraphische Untersuchungen bei Patienten zeigten, daß mit ^{67}Ga-Citrat Carcinome der Schilddrüse und des Respirationstraktes sowie Systemerkrankungen bevorzugt dargestellt werden können. Ein Zusammenhang zwischen der Morphologie eines Tumors und seiner Fähigkeit, ^{67}Ga anzureichern, konnte jedoch bisher nicht nachgewiesen werden, ebenso konnte kein Tumortyp gefunden werden, der in jedem Fall ein positives Szintigramm ergab. Für ^{67}Ga kann daher ebenso wie für die oben genannten Schwermetallisotope keine echte Tumorspezifität angenommen werden.

Zusammenfassend kann also gesagt werden, daß schon heute mit verschiedenen Methoden in der nuclearmedizinischen Diagnostik eine positive Darstellung von Tumoren möglich ist, die sich auch in einer Vielzahl der Fälle klinisch bewährt hat, daß aber der Beweis eines neoplastischen Wachstums mit Radiopharmaka noch immer aussteht.

Literatur

1. Bender, M. A., Blau, M.: Pancreas-scanning with ^{75}Se-1-selenomethionine. Scintillation scanning in clinical medicine. Philadelphia: Saunders 1964.
2. Britton, K. E., Keeling, D.: The use of ^{75}Se-selenomethionine in the detection of malignant reticuloses. In McCready, V. R., Taylor, D. M., Trott, N. G., et al. (Eds.): Radioactive Isotopes in the Localization of Tumours. London: Heinemann 1969.
3. Edwards, C. L., Hayes, R. L.: Tumor scanning with ^{67}Ga-citrate. J. nucl. Med. **10**, 103 (1969).
4. Edwards, C. L., Hayes, R. L.: Gallium-67 for tumor scanning. XII. Internat. Congress of Radiology, Tokyo 1969, Abstracts, p. 92.
5. Gerhard, H., Mundinger, F.: Biochemische Untersuchungen über Tumorspeicherung der zur Hirntumordiagnostik verwendeten Radioisotope. Acta radiol. Ther. Phys. Biol. **5**, 118 (1966).
6. Hisada, K., Hiraki, T., Ohba, S.: Positive delineation of human tumors with ^{131}I-human-serum-albumin. J. nucl. Med. **7**, 41 (1966).
7. Kahn, H.: Die Ablagerung von aktivem Wismut in malignen Tumoren. Strahlentherapie **37**, 751 (1930).
8. Kaneko, M., Sasaki, T., Kido, C.: Positive scintigraphy of tumor by means of intra-arterial injection of radioiodinated macroaggregated albumin (MAA). Amer. J. Roentgenol. **102**, 81 (1968).
9. Magnenat, G., Isliker, H.: Transport d'agents cytostatiques par les proteins plasmatiques. Europ. J. Cancer **5**, 25 (1969).
10. Marrack, D., Dewey, W. C., Corry, P., Spar, J. L., Bale, W. F.: ^{131}J-antihuman fibrinogen as an agent for the localisation of tumors in man – a comparison with other agents. In McCready, V. R., Taylor, D. M., Trott, N. G., et al. (Eds.): Radioactive Isotopes in the Localization of Tumors. London: Heinemann 1969.
11. Monasterio, G., Beccini, M. F., Riccioni, N.: Detection of tumours in man by means of 131-J-fibrinogen. Progr. Radiol. Vol. II, p. 1270. Amsterdam: Exerpta Medica Foundation 1967.
12. Wolf, R., Fischer, J.: Tumorszintigraphie mit radioaktiven Quecksilberverbindungen ($^{197}HgCl_2$ und ^{197}Hg-Neohydrin). In G. Hoffmann (Hrsg.): Radionuklide in der klinischen und experimentellen Onkologie, S. 223–228. Stuttgart: Schattauer 1965.

Probleme der Versuchsplanung in der Krebsforschung

Von

H. Immich

Zusammenfassung

Versuche in der Krebsforschung sind dadurch ausgezeichnet, daß im allgemeinen Summationseffekte betrachtet werden. Diese sind nicht unabhängig von der Zeit. Infolgedessen erhalten wir stets vermengte Effekte. Diese Tatsachen schließen die Anwendung bestimmter statistischer Verfahren deswegen aus, weil die Voraussetzung der Unabhängigkeit in den meisten Fällen nicht gewährleistet ist. Für die Berechnung relativer Häufigkeiten ist es unvorteilhaft, daß der Nenner eines Bruchs durch die Zahl der Tiere beeinflußt wird, welche vorzeitig absterben. Aus allen diesen Gründen empfiehlt sich die Einführung einer neuen Variablen, die nur auf das Versuchstier bezogen und daher unabhängig ist. Diese Variable ist die Zeitdauer zwischen Beginn der Behandlung und dem ersten Auftreten des Effekts, beispielsweise des Tumors oder des Todes. An einem Beispiel wird die Zweckmäßigkeit dieser Variablen gezeigt.

Erschienen in Med. Welt **22**, 1127–1129 (1971).

From Literature Documentation to Medical Documentation

By

M. Wolff-Terroine

Als mich Professor Wagner vor einigen Monaten bat, auf diesem Symposium über die Grundlinien des SABIR-Systems vorzutragen, habe ich sofort und ohne Vorbehalte zugesagt. Angesichts dieses Auditoriums sehe ich mich jedoch vor gewisse Probleme gestellt, nämlich

1. ein Problem des Inhalts: was soll ich Ihnen von unserer Arbeit auf dem Gebiet der nichtnumerischen Datenverarbeitung vortragen? Sie sind ja Cancerologen und keine Informationswissenschaftler!

2. ein Problem der Form: in welcher Sprache soll ich vortragen: französisch, deutsch oder englisch? Natürlich spreche ich am besten französisch, aber ich bin nicht sicher, ob mich dann alle Anwesenden gut verstehen würden. Mein Deutsch ist, wie Sie ja selbst hören, nicht so ganz glänzend. Daher möchte ich – wenn Sie erlauben – englisch sprechen.

Information retrieval constitutes at the present time a complex problem which the individual research worker is often incapable of solving because the number of conventional media of information (journals, books, congress proceedings etc.) is constantly increasing. You all know this tremendous growth in the number of scientific journals (Fig. 1) and also of secondary journals (Fig. 2).

This problem, difficult enough to cope with in other fields of science, is even more complicated in cancerology, since cancerology in both its clinical and experimental aspects is essentially a multidisciplinary subject. Recent progress in experimental cancerology has been due principally to the links that have been forged between it and a large number of basic sciences. Research workers in cancerology are, therefore, obliged to consult a vast number of articles and indexes in many fields of science and are never sure that they did not miss anything, because the information they are seeking might be available in a paper relating to a completely different branch of study.

Being aware of these difficulties, French cancerologists decided to create a Department of Scientific Documentation at the Institut Gustave-Roussy. After a modest beginning in the sixties with conventional equipment this center went through a phase of rapid expansion thanks, in particular, to the installation of a relatively powerful computer (UNIVAC 1107, with a central memory of 65,536 words of 36 bits).

One of the aims of the department was to use the recent information processing methods for facilitating the dissemination of scientific information. During many years the department has given special attention to these aspects of the problem of scientific communication and has tried to perfect the instruments required to achieve this aim.

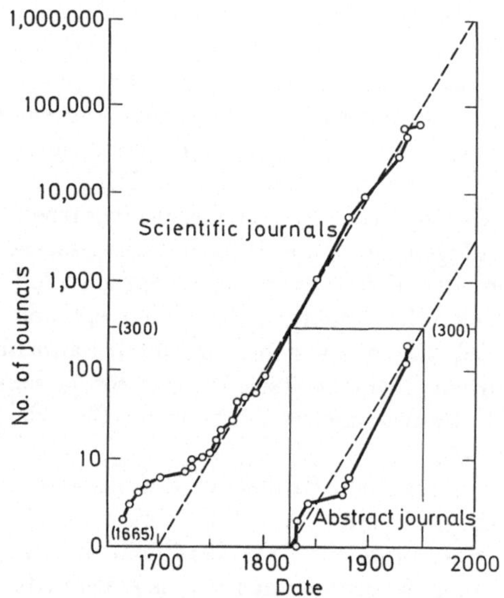

Fig. 1. Growth of the scientific journals. (from Cahn, R. S.: Survey of chemical publications, London, 1965)

It has been important to plan an organisation

- covering the entire clinical and experimental carcinology;
- analysing the literature at a very high level of specificity;
- giving a quick and selective diffusion of information and also retrospective searches;
- registering once and only once the information with all its criteria, whatever future use may be made of this information.

The SABIR-System ("*S*ystème *A*utomatique de *B*ibliographie, d'*I*nformation et de *R*echerche en Carcinologie"), a system for the analysis and automatic retrieval of data in the field of cancerology, has been elaborated to serve this fourfold purpose.

I should like to add that, when I speak about cancerology, I use this word in its widest sense; it covers all aspects of the subject, i.e. clinical, experimental, public health etc. (Fig. 3).

This system could not have been devised without close collaboration between a large number of doctors and research workers at the Gustave-Roussy Institute and the Scientific Documentation Service responsible for designing the system. The staff of the Information Department includes people with a high level background: M. Ds, Ph. Ds, engineers etc.

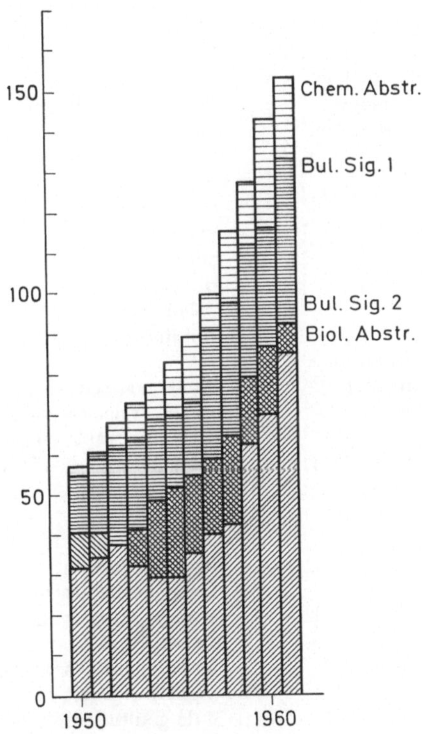

Fig. 2. Growth of the abstracts journals. (from Cahn, R. S.: Survey of chemical publications, London, 1965)

Without entering into the technicological problems and difficulties of non-numeric data processing, I should like to stress some important points relating to this processing:

1. One of the basic principles of the system is in fact that the literature must be analysed by specialists in the various subjects concerned and not by general practitioners or students. Thus articles on virology are

read by a virologist, those on paediatrics by a paediatrician etc. Only specialists working in a clinical or research department are capable of extracting important and original ideas from articles concerned with their own sphere of interest. Thanks to the work of these specialists,

I	II
	II – Clinical Medicine
	Statistics, geographical pathology
	Fight against cancer, ethics, psychology
	Etiopathogeny, theory, natural history
	of cancer, multiple tumors . . .
	Child
I – Experimentation and Research	Human pathology (cytological diagnosis..)
Biochemistry, molecular biology	Clinical diagnosis
Exp. cytology, exp. histology,	Para-clinical diagnosis (endoscopy,
ultrastructure, cell proliferation,	serological, hematological diagnosis . . .)
caryotype	Radiological diagnosis
Tissue culture	Radiationtherapy
Transplantation	Chemotherapy
	Surgery
	Hormonotherapy
	Other treatments: myelotherapy,
	immunotherapy, dietetics . . .
Spontaneous tumours in animals	
Carcinogenesis (mechanisms),	Head and neck, respiratory and alimentary
chemical carcinogenesis	upper tract, salivary glands . .
Viral carcinogenesis, virology	Digestive tract: esophagus, bowel, anus ...
Radiocancer (exp.), radiobiology,	Adnexial glands of the digestive tract:
radiophysics (ionizing rays, laser,	liver, bile ducts, pancreas, . . .
ultrasounds . . .)	
	Urinary tract: kidney, ureter, urinary
	bladder, urethra.
	Chest, bronchus, pleura, heart, media-
	stinum, chest wall, . . .
	Breast
Tumour physiology (hormonal	Female genital tract: ovary, vulva,
factors . . .)	vagina, uterus, . . .
Immunology	Male genital tract: prostate, testicle,
	penis, . . .
	Endocrine glands: hypophysis, thyroid,
	adrenal gland, . . .
	Nervous system: central N. S., sympa-
	thetic N. S., meninges, eye, . . .
	Skin
Therapeutic experimentation	Bone and articulations
	Soft tissues
	Malignant hemopathias
	Miscellaneous

Fig. 3. Fields covered by the SABIR system

the Scientific Documentation Service is able to cover more than 1000 journals and to abstract about 20,000 articles a year.

2. The analysis of the literature is carried out in a normalized documentary language. The cooperation of many members of the Gustave-Roussy Institute proved indispensable in the preparation of this basic instrument without which no automatic data-processing system can function efficiently. This normalized language is the *thesaurus*. A thesaurus is a sort of dictionary which is fed into the computer and used by the abstractor; it includes all concepts that are of importance in cancerology and indicates all possible relationships between these concepts.

```
CHONDRODYSPLASIE DEFORMANTE HEREDITAIRE
   EMPL MALADIE EXOSTOSANTE

CHONDROMATOSE
   TL CHONDROME
   TR OLLIER (MAL.DE)
   ALL CHONDROMATOSE
   ANG CHONDROMATOSIS

CHONDROME
   EP ECCHONDROME
   EP ENCHONDROME
   TE CHONDROMATOSE
   TE OLLIER (MAL.DE)
   ALL CHONDROM
   ANG CHONDROMA
```

Fig. 4. Thesaurus ordered alphabetically

Thus, when planning a search of the literature, it is possible with the aid of the thesaurus to envisage every conceivable aspect of a problem and thus to reduce the number of "silences" (i.e. relevant documents which the computer fails to produce in reply to a question). If, for example, one wants to search the literature for data on Ewing's tumour, the thesaurus will indicate that, since the proper designation of this tumour has for a long time been a matter of considerable controversy, it might be useful to look for papers on "bone reticulosarcoma" as well, especially in cases where the question of differential diagnosis is involved. The thesaurus also classifies terms under various headings; it shows for instance that the Friend, Moloney, Gross and Rauscher viruses belong to the larger group of "mouse leukaemia viruses" which, in turn, may by either "RNA viruses" or "leukaemia viruses" (Fig. 4 and 5).

Such a thesaurus is a mirror, a new means of expressing the actual state of knowledge in a given field. To compile a thesaurus of this type, the aim of which is to reveal the links between various concepts, is a difficult task which calls for the assistance of a large number of experts.

Moreover, a thesaurus can never be regarded to be complete, since the science with which it is dealing is constantly developing. It, therefore, has to be revised at regular intervals and these revisions may affect some of the data previously stored in the computer. Consequently, the work of adding adjustments and corrections has to be carefully programmed.

Immunology I. Immunity

Antibody	R. T. gammaglobulin
	R. T. immunoglobulin
	R. T. immune serum
	R. T. macroglobulin
Cellular immunity	R. T. delayed hypersensitivity
Humoral immunity	
Natural immunity	R. T. isoimmunity
Acquired immunity	R. T. immunotherapy
	R. T. immunoprotection
N. T. active immunity	R. T. sensitization
	R. T. immune serum
	R. T. vaccination
	R. T. immunological adjuvant
N. T. passive immunity	
N. T. adoptive immunity	R. T. marrow graft
	R. T. splenic graft
	R. T. immunological competent cell
Autoimmunity	R. T. collagenosis
	N. T. dermatomyositis
	N. T. Wegener's granuloma
	N. T. Heerfordt's syndrome
	N. T. Lupus erythematosus
	N. T. rhumatism
	N. T. dermatosclerosis
	N. T Sjögren's syndrome
	....
	R. T. Hashimoto's thyroiditis
Isoimmunity	R. T. rhesus factor
	R. T.
....	

Fig. 5. Thesaurus ordered by semantic fields (extract)

Special attention has been paid to the problem of synonyms and to the different ways of spelling a given term. When we requested doctors and research workers to abstract the literature, we could not, of course, force them to adopt an unduly rigid terminology. Hence, *Polycythaemia vera/Vaquez (maladie de)/Vaquez (Mal. de)/Maladie de Vaquez/Poly-*

cythémie vraie/*Polycythémie essentielle*/*Polyglobulie vraie*/and *Polyglobulie essentielle* are all accepted by the computer. As a result, of course, the preparation of the material to be fed into the computer takes a considerable amount of time.

What are the products delivered by SABIR? The system makes it possible to

1. obtain answers to specific bibliographical questions;
2. obtain a monthly information service on new literature, taking into consideration the user's profile of interest;
3. print out a current awareness bulletin listing the most recent articles under 40 different headings.

The selective dissemination of information is built up on a documentary profile. This profile can be modified according to the user's wishes. We have here a feed-back allowing an optimization of the system.

I believe that you as users of the system will be interested to know what kind of questions you will be able to put to the system. SABIR can answer either a broad question or a very precise one. It has been conceived to be as flexible as possible. If the subjects of this symposion were regarded as questions to the system, SABIR could process and answer all of them with the exception of some technical problems such as "Reliefautoradiographie in der Mäusehaut".

To ensure that this automatic data-processing system can be used on a wider scale, we decided to translate the thesaurus into English and German. Some years ago we got in contact with Professor WAGNER who planned to create a similar information system on cancer literature at Heidelberg. As it seemed unnecessary to duplicate such efforts in two nearby countries at a time when data transmission systems are in a state of development, we decided to cooperate in the development of the SABIR system. This was the first mesh in an international network.

Now the SABIR system has become operational and can

- process data analysed either in French or in English or in German;
- answer questions formulated either in French or in English or in German;
- give answers with bibliographic citation and description of the article in French, English or German (Fig. 6).

By this time the system is cooperating not only with Germany but also with other European countries.

What are the other possible fields of application of the SABIR system?

We use SABIR for medical records, autopsies, biopsies, X-ray-diagnosis. On account of its normalized terminology a number of mistakes can be avoided.

For one year we have been working on an extension to SABIR, namely the creation of a special file devoted to chemical compounds.

```
***************************************************
* 011644                                          *
* 48/3/1/69                                       *
* DE VITA V.T.,EMMER M.                           *
* MED.BRANCH,NAT.CANCER INST.,BETHESDA,MD.,USA    *
* THE SUCCESSFUL TREATMENT OF PNEUMOCYSTIS        *
*   CARINII PNEUMONITIS IN AN ADULT WITH          *
*   LYMPHOSARCOMA.A COMMENT ON PENTAMIDINE        *
*   ISETHIONATE NEPHROTOXICITY.                   *
* REUSSITE D'UN TRAITEMENT DE LA PNEUMONIE A      *
*   PNEUMOCYSTIS CARINII CHEZ UN ADULTE           *
*   ATTEINT DE LYMPHOSARCOME.DISCUSSION SUR LA    *
*   NEPHROTOXICITE DE L'ISETHIONATE DE            *
*   PENTAMIDINE.                                  *
* REV.FRANC.ETUD.CLIN.BIOL.,14,55-56,1969         *
* LYMPHOSARCOME,LEUCEMIE AIGUE LYMPHOBLASTIQUE,   *
*   CHIMIOTHERAPIE,PNEUMONIE,THERAPEUTIQUES       *
*   (COMPLICATIONS),REIN,TOXICITE,                *
***************************************************
```

```
***************************************************
* 011644                                          *
* 48/3/1/69                                       *
* DE VITA V.T.,EMMER M.                           *
* MED.BRANCH,NAT.CANCER INST.,BETHESDA,MD.,USA    *
* THE SUCCESSFUL TREATMENT OF PNEUMOCYSTIS        *
*   CARINII PNEUMONITIS IN AN ADULT WITH          *
*   LYMPHOSARCOMA.A COMMENT ON PENTAMIDINE        *
*   ISETHIONATE NEPHROTOXICITY.                   *
* REUSSITE D'UN TRAITEMENT DE LA PNEUMONIE A      *
*   PNEUMOCYSTIS CARINII CHEZ UN ADULTE           *
*   ATTEINT DE LYMPHOSARCOME.DISCUSSION SUR LA    *
*   NEPHROTOXICITE DE L'ISETHIONATE DE            *
*   PENTAMIDINE.                                  *
* REV.FRANC.ETUD.CLIN.BIOL.,14,55-56,1969         *
* LYMPHOSARCOMA,LEUKEMIA'ACUTE LYMPHOBLASTIC,     *
*   CHEMOTHERAPY,PNEUMONIA,THERAPEUTIC SIDE-      *
*   EFFECTS,KIDNEY,TOXICITY,                      *
***************************************************
```

```
***************************************************
* 011644                                          *
* 48/3/1/69                                       *
* DE VITA V.T.,EMMER M.                           *
* MED.BRANCH,NAT.CANCER INST.,BETHESDA,MD.,USA    *
* THE SUCCESSFUL TREATMENT OF PNEUMOCYSTIS        *
*   CARINII PNEUMONITIS IN AN ADULT WITH          *
*   LYMPHOSARCOMA.A COMMENT ON PENTAMIDINE        *
*   ISETHIONATE NEPHROTOXICITY.                   *
* REUSSITE D'UN TRAITEMENT DE LA PNEUMONIE A      *
*   PNEUMOCYSTIS CARINII CHEZ UN ADULTE           *
*   ATTEINT DE LYMPHOSARCOME.DISCUSSION SUR LA    *
*   NEPHROTOXICITE DE L'ISETHIONATE DE            *
*   PENTAMIDINE.                                  *
* REV.FRANC.ETUD.CLIN.BIOL.,14,55-56,1969         *
* LYMPHOSARKOM,LEUKAEMIE'AKUTE LYMPHOBLASTISCH,   *
*   CHEMOTHERAPIE,PNEUMONIE,THERAPEUTISCHE        *
*   NEBENWIRKUNG,NIERE,GIFTIGKEIT,                *
***************************************************
```

Fig. 6. A trilingual answer of a bibliographical citation

It is known that neither the fragmentation-notation nor the line-notation yield good results when one is not looking for a complete structure but for a substructure. We should like to find a way out of the difficulties presented by the existing chemical compounds systems. However, it will take a long time to achieve this end, the work being especially difficult as far as the machine is concerned, and I do not believe that the extension to the system will become operational before 1973.

In conclusion I should like to emphasize the following points:

1. The progress now achieved in information processing is opening up new ways and means for the communication of scientific information. However, we are not yet accustomed to make full use of them.

2. International cooperation, which for a long time seemed utopian, becomes a reality in the field of scientific information processing. This German-French cooperation offers an example.

Erste Erfahrungen mit dem SABIR-System in Heidelberg

I. Datenerfassung und Datenverarbeitung

Von

L. SANDOR

Eine wesentliche Aufgabe des Instituts für Dokumentation, Information und Statistik am Deutschen Krebsforschungszentrum ist es, ein computergesteuertes System zur Erfassung der Krebsliteratur aufzubauen, das in der Lage ist, allen interessierten Wissenschaftlern schnelle und gezielte Auskünfte über spezielle Fragen und den neuesten Stand der Kenntnisse auf dem Gebiet der Krebsforschung zu geben.

Gemeinsam mit dem französischen Krebsforschungszentrum in Villejuif hat das Institut in den letzten Jahren ein Information-Retrieval-System auf elektronischer Basis entwickelt, das den Namen SABIR (*S*ystème *A*utomatique de *B*ibliographie, d'*I*nformation et de *R*echerche) erhalten hat. Dieses System befindet sich zur Zeit in Paris in Operation und in Heidelberg in der Testphase.

Zu den Voraussetzungen dieser französisch-deutschen Zusammenarbeit gehörte es, einen Thesaurus der zu benutzenden Deskriptoren und ein französisch-deutsches Übersetzungslexikon aufzubauen.

Abb. 1 zeigt als Beispiel aus diesem Wörterbuch einige Deskriptoren zum Leukämieproblem in französischer und deutscher Sprache. Es ging bei der Übersetzung weniger um eine wörtliche als vielmehr um eine konzeptionsgerechte Übersetzung der rund 4000 französischen Deskriptoren, wobei insbesondere die spezifischen Eigenheiten der beiden Sprachen und der verschiedenen medizinischen Schulmeinungen zu berücksichtigen waren.

Unsere externen Mitarbeiter aus allen Fachgebieten der experimentellen und klinischen Krebsforschung arbeiten mit einem offenen, das heißt erweiterungsfähigen Synonymenlexikon (Abb. 2).

In diesem stehen links die Hauptbegriffe (sog. preferred terms) alphabetisch geordnet untereinander; die Synonyme sind drei Spalten nach rechts eingerückt. Rechts hinter ihnen stehen die zugehörigen Hauptbegriffe. Das Synonymenlexikon stellt ein Schlagwörterverzeichnis dar, in dem alle Deskriptoren erfaßt sind, die für die Analyse einer Arbeit benützt werden dürfen. Der Indexer kann auch die Synonyme verwenden; aus Gründen des maschineninternen Verarbeitungsprogramms werden aber vom Computer nur preferred terms ausgedruckt.

```
0000702  1 LEUCEMIE                              2 LEUKAEMIE
0003563  1 LEUCEMIE A BASOPHILES                 2 LEUKAEMIE BASOPHIL
0000706  1 LEUCEMIE A CELL.SOUCHES               2 LEUKAEMIE'STAMMZELL-
0000707  1 LEUCEMIE A EOSINOPHILES               2 LEUKAEMIE EOSINOPHIL
0003565  1 LEUCEMIE A MASTOCYTES                 2 LEUKAEMIE'MASTOZYTEN-
0000710  1 LEUCEMIE A MEGACARYOCYTES             2 LEUKAEMIE'MEGAKARYOZYTEN-
0000709  1 LEUCEMIE A MONOCYTES                  2 LEUKAEMIE'MONOZYTEN-
0000711  1 LEUCEMIE A PLASMCCYTES                2 LEUKAEMIE'PLASMAZELL-
0006538  1 LEUCEMIE A VIRUS                      2 LEUKAEMIE'VIRUS-
0000703  1 LEUCEMIE AIGUE                        2 LEUKAEMIE AKUT
0000705  1 LEUCEMIE AIGUE LYMPHOBLASTIQUE        2 LEUKAEMIE AKUT LYMPHOBLASTISCH
0004214  1 LEUCEMIE AIGUE MONOBLASTIQUE          2 LEUKAEMIE AKUT MONOBLASTISCH
0000704  1 LEUCEMIE AIGUE MYELOBLASTIQUE         2 LEUKAEMIE AKUT MYELOBLASTISCH
0002294  1 LEUCEMIE AIGUE PROMYELOCYTAIRE        2 LEUKAEMIE AKUT PROMYELOZYTAER
0000708  1 LEUCEMIE ALEUCEMIQUE                  2 LEUKAEMIE ALEUKAEMISCH
0000713  1 LEUCEMIE AVIAIRE                      2 LEUKAEMIE'HUEHNER-
```

Abb. 1. Ausschnitt aus dem französisch-deutschen Übersetzungslexikon

```
0000702  LEUKAEMIE
0000703  LEUKAEMIE AKUT
0000705  LEUKAEMIE AKUT LYMPHOBLASTISCH
0004214  LEUKAEMIE AKUT MONOBLASTISCH
0000704  LEUKAEMIE AKUT MYELOBLASTISCH
0002294  LEUKAEMIE AKUT PROMYELOZYTAER
0000708  LEUKAEMIE ALEUKAEMISCH
0003563  LEUKAEMIE BASOPHIL
0000714  LEUKAEMIE CHRONISCH
0000718  LEUKAEMIE CHRONISCH LYMPHATISCH
0000719  LEUKAEMIE CHRONISCH MYELOISCH
0000707  LEUKAEMIE EOSINOPHIL
0000715  LEUKAEMIE EXP.
0000715     LEUKAEMIE EXPERIMENTELL                    LEUKAEMIE EXP.
0008729  LEUKAEMIE L1210
0002296  LEUKAEMIE NAEGELI
0000720  LEUKAEMIE STRAHLENINDUZIERT
0002296     LEUKAEMIE TYP NAEGELI                      LEUKAEMIE NAEGELI
0008212  LEUKAEMIE'FRIEND-
```

Abb. 2. Ausschnitt aus dem deutschen Synonymenlexikon

Das SABIR-System ist als ein internationales Informations-Netzwerk konzipiert, in das jedes beteiligte Land die nationale Literatur einbringen soll, wobei es gleichzeitig in den Genuß des insgesamt eingespeicherten Materials kommt. Die beiden ersten Kristallisationspunkte des Systems sind Paris und Heidelberg. Der deutsche Anteil an dem System besteht zur Zeit darin, die neu erscheinenden deutschsprachigen Publikationen aus dem Bereich der experimentellen und klinischen Krebsforschung nach bestimmten Regeln zu indexen, auf Band zu nehmen, zu kontrollieren und schließlich nach Paris zur Eingliederung in das Gesamtsystem zu schicken.

In der Phase des Aufbaus einer Heidelberger Indexer-Gruppe wurden zunächst 80 deutschsprachige Zeitschriften ausgewählt, aus denen alle Artikel über experimentelle und/oder klinische Krebsforschung registriert und geindext werden.

Deutsches Krebsforschungszentrum
Institut für Dokumentation, Information und Statistik

ANALYSENBOGEN KREBSLITERATUR

1 Dokument-Nr.: — Indexer: Dr. Sandor

2 Verarbeitungsmerkmale: 4 3 | 2 | 7 0 (Klassifikation, Proz.-Code, Erf.-Stelle, Erfass-jahr)

3 Autoren: Bokelmann D., Doerr D., Linder F., Oellers B., Roeher H. D., Rudolph H., Trumm F. A.

4 Herkunft der Arbeit: Chir. Univ. Klin., Heidelberg, Deutschland

5 Originaltitel: Zur Pathologie und Therapie der Struma maligna

6 Übersetzter Titel: A propos de la pathologie et du traitement du goitre malin

7 Bibliograph. Zitat: Dtsch. Med. Wschr., 95:666-671, 1970

8 Deskriptoren: THYREOIDEA (T), HISTOPATHOLOGIE, KLASSIFIKATION TNM, DIAGNOSTIK RADIOLOGISCH, SZINTIGRAPHIE, JOD 131, BEHANDLUNG,CHIRURGIE' RADIKAL-, RADIOTHERAPIE' HOCHENERGIE, THERAPIE KOMBINIERT, HORMONTHERAPIE, UEBERLEBENSZEIT (MEHR ALS FUENF JAHRE), PROGNOSE,

9 Zusätzliche Suchmerkmale:

D M W O	Coden	0	Übersichts-arbeit?
G E	Sprache	1	Beobachtungs-reihe?
1	Publikationstyp	0	Experiment Arbeit?
0	Zusammenfassung (D, E, F,)	0	Arbeit aus IGR bzw. DKFZ?
1	Graphiken u. Tabellen	1	TNM-Klassif?
1	Abbildungen, Fotos	1 2	Zahl Deskript.?
1	Bibliographie?	0 2 2	Lit.-Angaben?
1	Wert des Artikels	2	Orig vorhanden?
			Reserve

Bemerkungen:

F 5/69

Abb. 3. Analysenbogen für Krebsliteratur

Auf einem speziellen Analysenbogen (Abb. 3) werden von jeder Arbeit die wichtigsten bibliographischen Angaben, wie Namen der Autoren, Herkunft der Arbeit, Originaltitel der Arbeit, übersetzter Titel, bibliographisches Zitat und einige zusätzliche Suchmerkmale erfaßt. Gemeinsam mit dem Analysenbogen wird die Arbeit dann dem sie bearbeitenden Fachwissenschaftler übersandt. Dieser analysiert ihren Inhalt unter Benutzung der im Synonymenlexikon festgelegten Deskriptoren und vermerkt die jeweils in Frage kommenden Schlagwörter in Rubrik 8 des Analysenbogens.

Der Indexer muß sich also mit dem Inhalt des Artikels vertraut machen und ihn mittels der Deskriptoren – sozusagen im Telegrammstil – wiedergeben. Eine Arbeit sollte im Durchschnitt durch 10–15 Deskriptoren so charakterisiert werden, daß die wichtigsten in ihr enthaltenen Informationen damit erfaßt sind.

Die Angaben auf dem Analysenbogen werden dann auf Lochstreifen übertragen, wobei zugleich eine Klartext-Kopie geschrieben wird. Eventuell im Klartext gefundene Fehler werden sofort auf dem Lochstreifen korrigiert. Der Inhalt des Lochstreifens wird anschließend auf Magnetband übertragen. Dabei werden die Deskriptoren und ihre Schreibweise maschinenintern mit dem Synonymenlexikon verglichen. Auf diese Weise können formale Fehler entdeckt und korrigiert werden. Erst nach dieser maschineninternen Kontrolle werden die Neuzugänge endgültig auf Magnetband gespeichert. Abb. (4) zeigt die Zahl der in verschiedenen Bereichen der experimentellen und klinischen Krebsforschung in Heidelberg in den letzten 6 Monaten 1970 geindexten Arbeiten.

Zum Wiederauffinden der gespeicherten Informationen sind die Suchfragen in eine maschinenadäquate Form (Boole'sche Algebra) umzusetzen. Bei der Formulierung einer Anfrage muß nach allen dabei zu berücksichtigenden Deskriptoren und ihren Relationen abgefragt werden. Für eine Computer-Recherche über beispielsweise „Sarkome der Weichteile" (Abb. 5) benötigt man als Deskriptoren nicht nur die Oberbegriffe – wie „Weichteilgewebe-Tumor", „Sarkom" oder „Muskel-Tumor" – sondern auch die im Schlagwörterverzeichnis vorkommenden spezifischen Begriffe, wie etwa Chondrosarkom, Fibrosarkom, Myxosarkom usw.

Das Retrieval wird mit speziellen Suchprogrammen durchgeführt, über die im nächsten Vortrag berichtet wird; die Recherche-Ergebnisse werden dann vom Computer ausgedruckt.

Vorerst sollen die wissenschaftlichen Interessensprofile der am System teilnehmenden Wissenschaftler ermittelt und diesen dann in monatlichen Abständen Computer-Ausdrucke der sie voraussichtlich interessierenden neuen Publikationen zugänglich gemacht werden. Außerdem soll das System gezielte individuelle Anfragen unter Berücksichtigung der gesamten eingespeicherten Informationen beantworten.

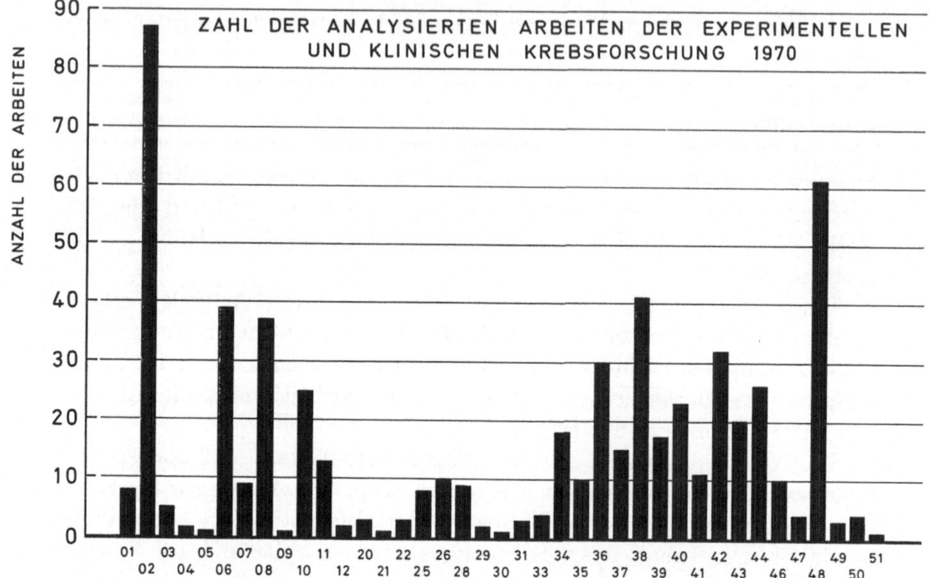

01 (8) Exp. Zytologie
02 (87) Biochemie
03 (5) Gewebekultur
04 (2) Transplantation
05 (1) Spontane Tiertumoren
06 (39) Chemische exp. Carcinogenese
07 (9) Genetik
08 (37) Tumor-Virologie
09 (1) Tumorphysiologie
10 (25) Exp. Therapie
11 (13) Immunologie
12 (2) Radiobiologie
20 (3) Ätio-pathogenese
21 (1) Klinische Diagnostik
22 (3) Paraklinische Diagnostik
25 (8) Röntgendiagnostik
26 (10) Strahlentherapie
28 (9) Chemotherapie
29 (2) Andere Therapieformen
30 (1) Humanhistologie
31 (3) Humanzytologie
33 (4) Kinderheilkunde
34 (18) Haut
35 (10) Kopf und Hals
36 (30) Verdauungssystem
37 (15) Leber
38 (41) Thorax
39 (17) Uropoetisches System
40 (23) Brustdrüse
41 (11) Genitalsystem, männlich
42 (32) Genitalsystem, weiblich
43 (20) Endokrine Drüsen
44 (26) Nervensystem
46 (10) Knochen und Gelenke
47 (4) Weichteilgewebe
48 (61) Hämoblastosen
49 (3) Statistik, geograph. pathol.
50 (4) Krebsbekämpfung
51 (1) Varia

Abb. 4. Anzahl und Fachgebiete der von Juli bis Dezember 1970 in Heidelberg geindexten Publikationen.

Frage Nr. 701: SARKOME DER WEICHTEILE

GEWEBE'WEICHTEIL (T)-
UND
SARKOM

ODER

MUSKEL (T)
UND
SARKOM

ODER

CHONDROSARKOM
ODER
FIBROSARKOM
ODER
FIBROMYOSARKOM
ODER
FIBROMYXOSARKOM
ODER
HAEMANGIOENDOTHELIOM MALIGNE
ODER
SARKOM HISTIOZYTAER
ODER
LIPOSARKOM
ODER
MYXOSARKOM
ODER
MYXOLIPOSARKOM
ODER
SARKOM ALVEOLAER
ODER
SARKOM BOTRYOID

Abb. 5. Beispiel der Formulierung einer Anfrage nach „Sarkomen der Weichteile“

Das System kann auf die Dauer nur dann optimal funktionieren, wenn wir auf die Mitarbeit der Fachwissenschaftler des Deutschen Krebsforschungszentrums und die Kooperation von sonstigen interessierten Wissenschaftlern bezüglich der Aufschließung der neuen deutschsprachigen Literatur – das heißt: das ständige „Füttern“ des Computers mit neuen einschlägigen Informationen – rechnen können.

Erste Erfahrungen mit dem SABIR-System in Heidelberg

II. Programmtechnische Aspekte

Von

C. Köhler und G. Wagner

Der Aufbau des SABIR-Systems in Heidelberg wurde in den letzten Jahren nicht nur durch personelle Engpässe, sondern auch durch zahlreiche, meist nicht voraussehbare technische Schwierigkeiten behindert, die offenbar bei internationalen Projekten unvermeidlich sind. So gingen beispielsweise in der ersten Projektphase die Institute in Paris und Heidelberg von der Annahme aus, daß der Systemaufbau an beiden Stellen identisch und mit austauschbaren Programmen gestaltet werden könnte. Leider erwies sich diese Hoffnung als trügerisch; in Paris wurde eine elektronische Datenverarbeitungsanlage angeschafft, die mit der in Heidelberg vorhandenen nicht kompatibel ist. Das hatte zur Folge, daß die bis dato in Heidelberg geleisteten Vorarbeiten nicht mehr verwendbar waren und eine ganz neue Systemkonfiguration mit allen zugehörigen Programmen entwickelt werden mußte. Im Verlaufe des Systemaufbaus in Paris sich ergebende Änderungen machten mehrfach wiederum Änderungen in den Heidelberger Programmen erforderlich; als lästig und zeitraubend erwiesen sich auch die notwendigen Umcodierungsarbeiten.

Die größten Schwierigkeiten beim Aufbau des Systems ergaben sich jedoch aus der Tatsache, daß der in Heidelberg vorhandene Computer (IBM 360/30) für ein so umfangreiches Projekt der Literaturdokumentation stark unterdimensioniert ist. Wegen des zu kleinen Kernspeichers mußten praktisch alle Programme gestückelt werden. Das wiederum führt in der Verarbeitung zu unerwünscht langen Maschinenzeiten, insbesondere bei der Übersetzung der Schlagwörter und beim Recherchieren. Hierauf wird weiter unten noch näher eingegangen.

Programme zur Literaturerfassung

Die für die Erfassung, Speicherung und Verarbeitung der Literatur notwendigen Arbeitsschritte sollen im folgenden durch einige Ablaufdiagramme erläutert werden. Abb. 1 zeigt die Erfassung der in Heidelberg geindexten Literatur. Die von den Indexern abgelieferten und von

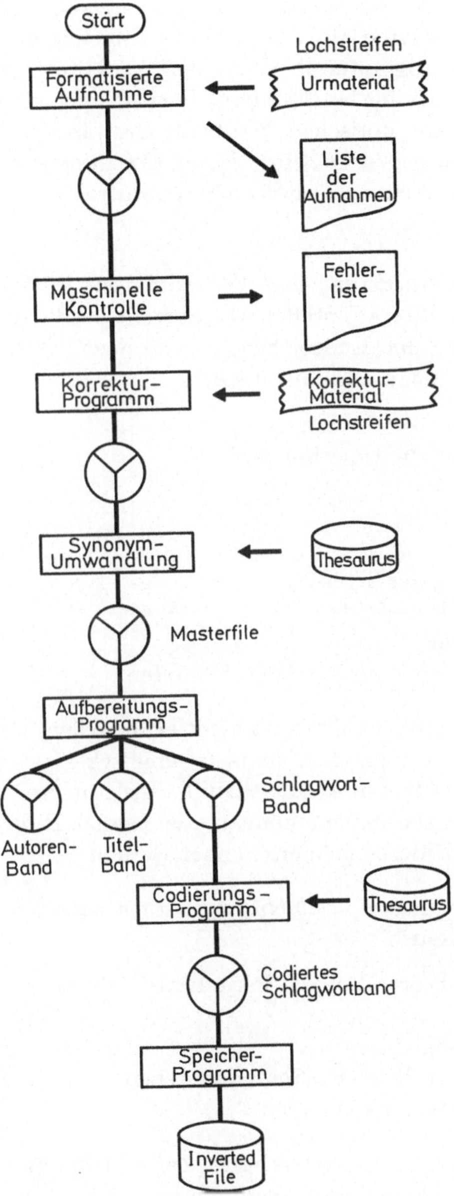

Abb. 1. Ablaufdiagramm über die Erfassung und Kontrolle der in Heidelberg geindexten Krebsliteratur

der Literatur-Dokumentationsgruppe des Instituts durchgesehenen und ergänzten Analysenbogen werden zunächst mittels eines programmierbaren Schreibautomaten auf Lochstreifen aufgenommen. In einem speziellen Aufnahmeprogramm überträgt der Computer in mehreren Schritten das Urmaterial in bestimmtem Format auf Magnetband, wobei gleichzeitig eine zur optischen Kontrolle des Bandsatzes Verwendung findende Liste ausgedruckt wird. Parallel zu der menschlichen Sichtkontrolle läuft im Computer ein formales Kontrollprogramm ab. Hierbei werden geprüft:

1. *die richtige Gliederung und Vollständigkeit jedes logischen Records* (jeder geindexten Literaturstelle). Dabei stellt der Computer fest, ob die speziellen Anfangs- und Endzeichen für jede einzelne Arbeit und folgende näheren Angaben dazu vorhanden sind:

a) laufende Nr. der Arbeit,
b) sog. Verarbeitungsmerkmale,
c) Autor(en),
d) Herkunftsstelle,
e) Originaltitel,
f) Übersetzung des Titels,
g) bibliographisches Zitat,
h) Schlagwörter,
i) zusätzliche Suchmerkmale (z. B. Coden).

Eine Übersetzung des Titels ist nicht erforderlich, wenn die Arbeit in einer der drei Arbeitssprachen deutsch – englisch – französisch publiziert wurde; die Herkunft der Arbeit (Klinik, Institut etc.) ist nicht immer angegeben. In diesen Fällen können die beiden Rubriken d) bzw. f) durch jeweils drei Sterne gekennzeichnet werden.

2. *die korrekte Angabe des bibliographischen Zitats.*
Diese muß enthalten:

a) den nach „World Medical Periodicals" abgekürzten Zeitschriftentitel,
b) die Bandzahl,
c) die erste und die letzte Seite der Arbeit,
d) das Erscheinungsjahr.

Die Maschine erkennt fehlerhafte Zeitschriftenkurztitel und prüft z. B. nach, ob die letzte Seite einen höheren Zahlenwert hat als die erste Seite (Kontrolle von Schreibfehlern). Nach einer gewissen Anlaufzeit sollen als Erscheinungsjahr neu ins System kommender Literatur nur noch das jeweils laufende und das Vorjahr als richtig akzeptiert werden.

3. *die richtige Schreibweise der benutzten Schlagwörter.* Die Maschine erkennt aufgrund eines Vergleichs mit dem maschinenintern gespeicherten Thesaurus nur die dort in gleicher Schreibweise aufgeführten Schlagwörter als „richtig" an. Eine abweichende Schreibweise vorhandener oder die Verwendung von im Thesaurus (noch) nicht enthaltener Deskriptoren werden als „Fehler" registriert.

Das automatische Prüfprogramm schreibt eine Liste mit genauer Lokalisation jedes gefundenen Fehlers. Die Korrekturen dieser maschinell und visuell gefundenen Fehler werden wiederum auf Lochstreifen aufgenommen. Mittels eines Korrekturprogramms werden dann die fehlerhaften Angaben durch die berichtigten ersetzt, wobei ein bereinigter Bandsatz erstellt wird.

Ein weiteres Programm wandelt schließlich alle verwendeten Synonyme in die festgelegten Hauptbegriffe um. Ein Doppel des endgültigen Bandes wird nach Paris geschickt.

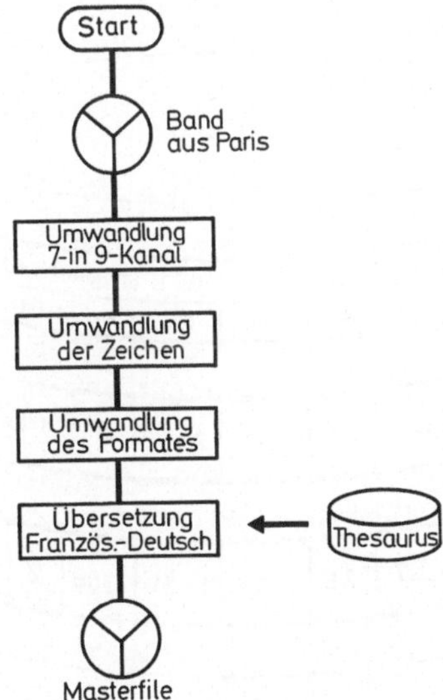

Abb. 2. Die erforderlichen Aufarbeitungsschritte für die aus Paris gelieferte Literatur

Abb. 2 zeigt die nötigen Verarbeitungsschritte für das aus Paris kommende Material. Hierbei sind vier Programme zu durchlaufen:

1. Umwandlung des 7-Kanal- in 9-Kanal-Code,
2. Umwandlung der Zeichenvercodung,
3. Umwandlung des Satzformates,
4. Übersetzung der französischen Schlagwörter.

Der aus diesen Verarbeitungsschritten resultierende Neuzugang wird in den vorhandenen Bestand (Masterfile) übernommen. (Neben diesen monatlich durchzuführenden Routineprozeduren muß der maschinenintern gespeicherte Thesaurus in bestimmten Intervallen auf den neuesten Stand gebracht werden.)

Aus dem Masterfile werden drei weitere Bestandsbänder erstellt:

1. Das Autorenband (für die Suche nach Autoren),
2. Das Titelband (für die Suche nach Titeln),
3. Das Schlagwortband (für die Suche nach Schlagwörtern).

Die Suche nach Schlagwörtern ist die bei weitem häufigste, aber auch aufwendigste Art der Literaturrecherche. Sie wird aus Gründen der Zeitersparnis nicht seriell, sondern im sog. „inverted file" durchgeführt, in dem jedes Schlagwort durch einen Code (Schlagwort-Nr.) repräsentiert ist, hinter dem die laufenden Nummern aller Arbeiten erscheinen, die dieses Schlagwort enthalten.

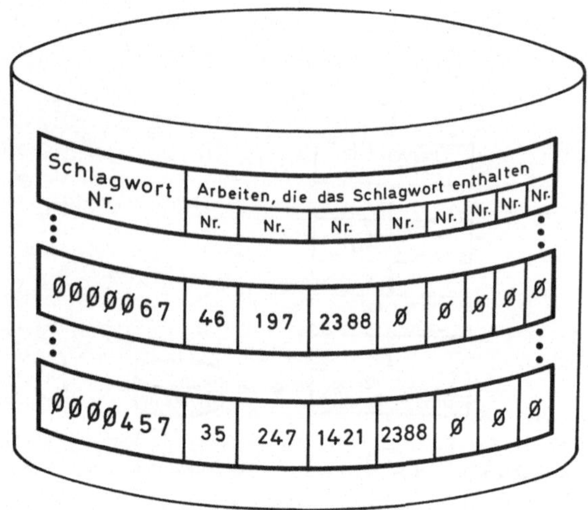

Abb. 3. Der Aufbau des „Inverted File" im Heidelberger System

Abb. 3 zeigt schematisch den Aufbau des auf zwei Magnetplatten mit Direktzugriff lokalisierten „inverted file". Dieser Bestand besteht nur noch aus Zahlen, die ein schnelleres Suchen und Vergleichen ermöglichen, als es mit alphabetischen Zeichen möglich wäre. Hinter jeder Schlagwort-Nummer ist Platz für die Nummern aller Arbeiten, in denen das entsprechende Schlagwort vermerkt ist. Diese Art der Speicherung gestattet ein ökonomischeres Retrieval als der rein serielle Betrieb.

Das Prinzip der Literatursuche

Jedes elektronische „Information Retrieval" gehorcht den Gesetzmäßigkeiten der von dem Engländer George Boole Mitte des vorigen Jahrhunderts entwickelten symbolischen oder Schalt-Algebra mit ihren zwei Hauptverknüpfungen, dem logischen „Und" (&) und dem logischen „Oder" (|). Abgesehen von einigen Besonderheiten lassen sich aus den beiden Grundformen A | B und A & B nach den Regeln der Boole'schen Algebra alle nur denkbaren logischen Verknüpfungen zwischen bestimmten Suchbegriffen bilden, z. B.

(A | B) & (C | D) – (sprich: A oder B und C oder D)
(A & B) | (C & D)
[A & (B | C | D)] | [E & (F | G | H)] | I | J | K
[(A | B) & (C | D)] | [(E & F) | G | H]
{(A & B) | [C & (D | E | F) & G]} & (H | I | J).

Die „Oder"-Verknüpfung von zwei (oder mehr) Suchbegriffen besagt, daß eine Arbeit dann als relevant gilt und ausgedruckt werden soll, wenn entweder der eine oder der andere (oder einer von mehreren) Suchbegriffen als Schlagwort vorliegt; bei der „Und"-Verknüpfung gilt eine Arbeit nur dann als „Treffer", wenn sie sämtliche so verbundenen Suchbegriffe als Schlagwörter enthält. Im Beispiel der Abb. 3 würde die Suchanfrage „67 ODER 457" die 6 Arbeiten Nr. 35, 46, 197, 247, 1421 und 2388 als Ergebnis liefern, die Anfrage „67 UND 457" dagegen nur die Arbeit Nr. 2388.

Leider sind auch die Suchprogramme in unserer kleinen Anlage nur mit Schwierigkeiten unterzubringen, wobei der ungenügende Kernspeicherplatz einen erhöhten Zeitbedarf bei der Recherche bedingt. Generell wird die benötigte Suchzeit in erster Linie durch die Anzahl der Arbeiten bestimmt, die hinter einem entsprechenden Schlagwort gespeichert sind; die Komplexität der Anfrage und die Anzahl der abzufragenden Schlagwörter sind bezüglich des Zeitbedarfs für die Recherche weniger bedeutsam. Zwei Beispiele aus der Praxis sollen dies verdeutlichen:

1. Suchanfrage: (A | B | C | D | E) & (F | G)
Anzahl der Schlagwörter = 7
Anzahl der dabei insgesamt gespeicherten Arbeiten = 2506
Anzahl der relevanten Arbeiten = 21
Zeitaufwand für die Recherche: $1^1/_2$ Std.

2. Suchanfrage: [A & (B | C)] | [D & (E | F)] | G | H | I | J
Anzahl der Schlagwörter = 10
Anzahl der dabei insgesamt gespeicherten Arbeiten = 224
Anzahl der relevanten Arbeiten = 62
Zeitaufwand für die Recherche: 15 min.

Bei der Recherche im „inverted file“ werden zunächst nur die Nummern der zutreffenden Arbeiten ermittelt und auf einer Magnetplatte zwischengespeichert. In einem zweiten Arbeitsgang werden dann aufgrund dieser Nummern für beliebig viele Anfragen gleichzeitig die vollständigen Zitate aus dem Masterfile herausgesucht und über den Drucker ausgegeben. Der Zeitaufwand hierfür beträgt bei unseren recht langsamen Bandeinheitena. ca. 8–10 min pro 1000 im Masterfile vorhandener Arbeiten.

Sachverzeichnis

„f.“ bedeutet, daß das betr. Wort auch noch auf der folgenden Seite auftritt. „ff.“ bedeutet, daß das betr. Wort mindestens auf den beiden folgenden Seiten auftritt.